Privacy-Preserving AI in Healthcare

Hanh Le
https://orcid.org/0009-0007-8172-0809
University of the Cumberlands, USA

IGI Global
Scientific Publishing
Publishing Tomorrow's Research Today

Vice President of Editorial	Melissa Wagner
Director of Acquisitions	Mikaela Felty
Director of Book Development	Jocelynn Hessler
Production Manager	Mike Brehm
Cover Design	Jose Rosado

Published in the United States of America by
IGI Global Scientific Publishing
701 East Chocolate Avenue
Hershey, PA, 17033, USA
Tel: 717-533-8845 | Fax: 717-533-7115
Website: https://www.igi-global.com E-mail: cust@igi-global.com

Library of Congress Cataloging-in-Publication Data

LCCN: 2026032285 (CIP Data Pending)
ISBN13: 979-8-2600-3070-7
Isbn13Softcover: 979-8-2600-3071-4
EISBN13: 979-8-2600-3072-1
British Cataloguing in Publication Data
A Cataloguing in Publication record for this book is available from the British Library.

Table of Contents

Detailed Table of Contents

The integration of Artificial Intelligence (AI) into healthcare offers significant benefits in improving clinical decision-making, operational efficiency, and patient outcomes. At the same time, the widespread adoption of AI introduces critical challenges related to cybersecurity, data privacy, ethical decision-making, and regulatory compliance. This chapter focuses on the design and deployment of ethical and secure AI systems within healthcare environments. It discusses major security threats such as data breaches, ransomware, and adversarial attacks, along with ethical concerns including bias, fairness, transparency, and accountability in AI-driven clinical processes. The chapter further examines privacy-preserving techniques, governance models, and compliance with healthcare regulations such as HIPAA and GDPR to ensure responsible AI usage. By emphasizing secure architectures, ethical principles, and trust between humans and AI systems, this chapter provides practical guidance for developing resilient, trustworthy, and ethically aligned AI solutions for modern healthcare systems.

This chapter explores the integration of privacy-preserving machine learning (PPML) techniques within healthcare artificial intelligence (AI) systems, addressing critical challenges related to data security, regulatory compliance, and system scalability. It presents a comprehensive framework combining federated learning, differential privacy, secure multi-party computation, and homomorphic encryption to enable secure and collaborative model training without exposing sensitive patient data. The study further analyzes emerging threat vectors, including model poisoning

medical access and healthcare system efficiency. Due to the increased use of medical imaging for accurate diagnosis and secure transmission methods are essential to protect sensitive patient data from unauthorized access and cyber threats. Healthcare IoT network components are described. Data-collection and transmission sensors are included. This approach solves data privacy, bandwidth, and device compatibility issues in Internet of Things-based telemedicine. Secure picture communication is stressed due to data manipulation, eavesdropping and unwanted access. Advanced encryption and blockchain technologies can improve medical imaging data integrity and transparency. These technologies provide reliable solutions for securing patient data and maintaining quality for accurate medical evaluations. To demonstrate how data reduction, prioritizing.

Vikas Sharma, Department of Computer Applications, SRM Institute of Science and Technology, Delhi NCR, Ghaziabad, India
Tarun Kumar Vashishth, School of Computer Science and Applications, IIMT University, Meerut, India
Shashiraj Teotia, Department of Computer Application, Swami Vivekanand Subharti University, Meerut, India
Devendra Singh, Department of Mechanical Engineering, Ajay Kumar Garg Engineering College, Ghaziabad, India
Sonal Shah, Department of IT, Auro University, Surat, India
Sachin Chaudhary, School of Computer Science and Applications, IIMT University, Meerut, India
Pushpendra Kumar Verma, School of Computer Science and Applications, IIMT University, Meerut, India

Autonomous systems' growing use across various industries, including transportation, healthcare, and smart city development, has created a serious concern about cyber security. This chapter will provide a brief overview of some of the ways to secure autonomous systems through AI-based intrusion detection systems (IDS) and privacy-preserving mechanisms. In particular, it will identify the use of machine learning to detect anomalies and secure federated learning and blockchain technology to provide integrity of data in autonomous systems. It also provides an overview of how adversarially attacking AI models can be used to reduce cyber risk. Once security frameworks using AI are established, autonomous systems will be able to detect threats and quickly respond, while also preserving user privacy. Finally, this chapter will address regulatory issues regarding autonomous technology and potential future research issues related to the security of autonomous systems.

Many national laws at the federal and state levels protect patients' right to confidentiality in medical records. The A.P. Shah Committee report's privacy principles have been integrated into healthcare organizations' day-to-day operations to the fullest degree practicable. But there are big holes in the policymaking that don't consider what happens to the data once it's been gathered or transferred. To close these gaps, urgent institutional cooperation is required. According to the findings of the research, you should proceed in this manner. If an efficient framework is going to be developed, however, the state will still need to play a part in promoting collaboration between various organizations operating in the public and private sectors across a wide range of industries.

Preface

INTRODUCTION

Artificial intelligence is rapidly transforming the healthcare landscape, enabling unprecedented advances in disease diagnosis, personalized treatment, clinical decision support, and healthcare administration. From machine learning algorithms capable of identifying complex disease patterns to intelligent virtual assistants supporting patients beyond traditional clinical settings, AI has become an essential driver of innovation across the healthcare ecosystem. However, alongside these technological advancements come equally important responsibilities surrounding patient privacy, cybersecurity, ethical governance, and regulatory compliance. As healthcare organizations increasingly rely on data-driven technologies, ensuring that AI systems remain trustworthy, transparent, and secure has become one of the defining challenges of modern medicine.

Privacy-Preserving AI in Healthcare brings together an international collection of researchers and practitioners who explore these challenges from multiple perspectives while highlighting innovative solutions that balance technological progress with responsible implementation. The chapters emphasize that privacy and security should not be viewed as barriers to AI adoption but rather as foundational principles that strengthen the reliability and long-term success of intelligent healthcare systems. Throughout this volume, readers will encounter discussions of advanced security architectures, federated learning, explainable AI, blockchain technologies, encryption methods, secure software design, and ethical governance frameworks that collectively support the development of resilient healthcare solutions.

The book also recognizes that healthcare is uniquely dependent upon trust. Patients must have confidence that their personal information is protected, clinicians must be able to understand and rely upon AI-assisted recommendations, and institutions must navigate evolving legal and ethical standards while embracing innovation. As cyber threats continue to increase in both sophistication and frequency, safeguarding sensitive medical information has become inseparable from delivering quality patient care. Consequently, this volume places equal emphasis on technological innovation and responsible data stewardship, illustrating how privacy-preserving methodologies can coexist with powerful AI capabilities.

It is our hope that this book serves as both a scholarly reference and a practical resource for researchers, healthcare professionals, policymakers, software engineers, and graduate students seeking to understand the evolving intersection of artificial intelligence, cybersecurity, privacy, and healthcare innovation. By presenting diverse research perspectives and emerging technologies, this collection encourages continued collaboration across disciplines to build healthcare systems that are not only intelligent but also ethical, secure, and deserving of public trust.

OVERVIEW OF THE CHAPTERS

The opening chapters establish the foundational principles of secure and ethical AI within healthcare. Chapter 1 introduces the ethical, cybersecurity, and governance considerations necessary for deploying trustworthy AI systems in clinical environments. Chapter 2 expands upon these concepts by examining privacy-preserving machine learning through federated learning, homomorphic encryption, differential privacy, and collaborative AI architectures. Chapter 3 further strengthens this foundation by exploring secure AI-driven healthcare systems that incorporate explainable AI alongside quantum-resilient cybersecurity approaches, while Chapter 4 demonstrates how federated learning can improve medical data analysis while maintaining patient confidentiality and operational efficiency.

Building upon these privacy-preserving frameworks, Chapter 5 presents an innovative AI-driven architecture integrating federated learning, blockchain technology, homomorphic encryption, differential privacy, and Lady Bug Optimization to protect sensitive patient information during collaborative model training. Chapter 6 shifts the discussion toward patient engagement by examining virtual health assistants and conversational AI systems that improve healthcare accessibility, streamline routine clinical interactions, and enhance patient support while maintaining privacy and regulatory compliance.

The remaining chapters broaden the discussion by addressing specialized applications of AI security and privacy. Chapter 7 explores secure image transmission and Internet of Things (IoT) infrastructures supporting telemedicine, emphasizing encryption techniques and secure communication protocols for protecting diagnostic imaging. Chapter 8 investigates AI-powered intrusion detection systems and privacy-preserving security mechanisms designed for autonomous and intelligent healthcare ecosystems. Finally, Chapter 9 examines the growing use of advanced medical image analysis while critically addressing the legal, ethical, and societal implications surrounding patient privacy and data governance in modern healthcare systems.

Collectively, these chapters illustrate that achieving meaningful advances in healthcare AI requires more than sophisticated algorithms alone. Success depends upon integrating robust cybersecurity, ethical governance, regulatory compliance, privacy-preserving technologies, and interdisciplinary collaboration into every stage of AI development and deployment. Together, the contributions in this volume provide readers with both theoretical foundations and practical insights for designing healthcare systems that responsibly harness the transformative power of artificial intelligence.

CONCLUSION

As artificial intelligence continues to reshape healthcare worldwide, its success will ultimately be measured not only by technological performance but also by its ability to preserve the dignity, privacy, and trust of the patients it serves. Every advancement in predictive analytics, medical imaging, intelligent diagnostics, and automated clinical support introduces new opportunities to improve health outcomes while simultaneously raising important questions regarding data protection, fairness, accountability, and cybersecurity. Addressing these concerns requires ongoing collaboration among researchers, healthcare professionals, software developers, policymakers, and regulatory bodies.

The contributions presented throughout this volume demonstrate that privacy-preserving AI is no longer a theoretical aspiration but an achievable and increasingly necessary component of responsible healthcare innovation. Emerging technologies such as federated learning, differential privacy, blockchain, secure multi-party computation, homomorphic encryption, explainable AI, and advanced intrusion detection systems collectively provide practical pathways toward building healthcare ecosystems that are both intelligent and secure. These approaches illustrate how innovation and privacy can advance together rather than exist in opposition.

Equally important, this book highlights that technological solutions alone cannot guarantee trustworthy AI. Ethical decision-making, transparent governance, interdisciplinary collaboration, regulatory compliance, and continuous evaluation remain essential for ensuring that intelligent healthcare systems serve patients fairly and responsibly. As healthcare environments become increasingly interconnected through cloud computing, IoT devices, telemedicine, and autonomous technologies, maintaining public confidence will depend upon embedding these principles into every phase of AI system design and implementation.

We hope this collection inspires further research, thoughtful discussion, and meaningful innovation within the rapidly evolving field of healthcare artificial intelligence. By bringing together diverse perspectives on privacy preservation, cybersecurity, ethical governance, and intelligent healthcare applications, this volume contributes to the growing body of knowledge supporting the development of secure, resilient, and patient-centered AI systems. It is our sincere hope that readers will find both practical guidance and future research opportunities that help shape the next generation of trustworthy healthcare technologies.

Chapter 1
Ethical and Secure AI Systems in Healthcare

Amrutha Kolhar
http://orcid.org/0009-0001-4940-3172
Karnatak University, Dharwad, India

T. K. Gundoor
http://orcid.org/0000-0002-6102-0094
National Forensic Sciences University, Curti, India

ABSTRACT

The integration of Artificial Intelligence (AI) into healthcare offers significant benefits in improving clinical decision-making, operational efficiency, and patient outcomes. At the same time, the widespread adoption of AI introduces critical challenges related to cybersecurity, data privacy, ethical decision-making, and regulatory compliance. This chapter focuses on the design and deployment of ethical and secure AI systems within healthcare environments. It discusses major security threats such as data breaches, ransomware, and adversarial attacks, along with ethical concerns including bias, fairness, transparency, and accountability in AI-driven clinical processes. The chapter further examines privacy-preserving techniques, governance models, and compliance with healthcare regulations such as HIPAA and GDPR to ensure responsible AI usage. By emphasizing secure architectures, ethical principles, and trust between humans and AI systems, this chapter provides practical guidance for developing resilient, trustworthy, and ethically aligned AI solutions for modern healthcare systems.

DOI: 10.4018/979-8-2600-3070-7.ch001

1. INTRODUCTION

The Future of AI in Healthcare: The future of artificial intelligence (AI) in healthcare is a new phase of high potential owing to its ability to enhance the quality of diagnostic findings, tailor treatment plans, and enhance the productivity of operations. Medical imagery can be analysed with superhuman accuracy with AI systems, clinical outcomes can be predicted using complex multimodal data, and drug discovery can be made faster through simulating the interactions of molecules. These features will improve human health and well-being by cutting on costs and increasing the number of people having access to good care. The Stakes of Medical Data: Nonetheless, the sensitive and exceptionally personal quality of healthcare data increases the stakes much higher than the ordinary application of technologies. Protected Health Information (PHI) such as genetic code, mental health information and diagnostic images not only represent a transactional data point, but a continuation of human identity and autonomy. The violation of such data may lead to discrimination by insurers, social stigma, psychological harm, or identity theft. A stolen genome is not reissued, as is the case with a stolen credit card number. This core weakness requires that the implementation of AI in medicine be done with the highest caution. A Two-Fold Socio-Technical Approach: Thus, the creation of ethical and secure AI implementations in healthcare cannot be a strictly technical task; it should be a transdisciplinary socio-technical initiative that would ingrain ethical standards and effective security steps into all the design, implementation, and management phases. The ethics of AI should be built and controlled in harmony with the concepts of fairness, accountability, transparency, and justice. It means that biases in training data, which can result in discriminatory results, must be actively removed, meaningful human supervision must be ensured, and explainable AI models, which allow a clinician and a patient to comprehend the reasoning behind automated decisions, need to be implemented. At the same time, security cannot be compromised: the patient data should not be exposed to unauthorised access, data leaks, and malicious use by means of encryption, access controls, and privacy-reducing technologies. Any AI system that is not secured is already unethical because it puts the lives and privacy of patients at risk. It is only when these two opposing imperatives, ethics and security, are inbuilt to the foundational design of AI in the healthcare sector that we can achieve the transformative potential it has and retain the human rights and trust on which the profession of healing is based. (Ezz et al., 2025)(Kolhar et al., 2025)(Adepoju & Adepoju, 2025)

2. SECURITY CHALLENGES IN HEALTHCARE AI SYSTEMS

- The violations of Data Privacy and Confidentiality. Healthcare AI systems are constructed based on a large storage of Protected Health Information (PHI), such as medical records, genetic data, and radiographs. The biggest security issue is to avoid unauthorised access to this extremely sensitive information, both at rest and in transit. Not only is a breach a violation of regulations, such as HIPAA or GDPR, but it can also have disastrous outcomes, such as insurance discrimination, stigma or identity theft. Additional vulnerabilities are that modern healthcare systems have an interconnected nature, and the data moves between hospitals, labs, cloud servers and third-party vendors of AI. A vulnerable node in this chain can be represented by each node. Moreover, even anonymised data can in many cases be re-identified through cross-referencing methods, and thus traditional de-identification may not suffice. To guarantee the actual privacy of data, end-to-end encryption, strict access control, and sophisticated privacy-preserving methods such as federated learning or homomorphic encryption, when training the models, the raw patient data is not shown.
- **Data Integrity and Poisoning Attacks:** The quality and integrity of training data determine the accuracy and reliability of a given AI model completely. One of the most important security issues is to protect this data against corruption and malicious manipulation. In a data poisoning attack, a malicious adversary inserts a well-designed, deceitful piece of data into the training set. One example is that modifying pixel data in thousands of X-ray images by slightly changing a single pixel would cause an AI to identify benign tumours as malignant. This undermines the integrity of the model at the core, contributing to systemic errors that are hard to identify after deployment. Insiders can use such attacks, or attack them using compromised data collection channels. There is a need to implement powerful validation procedures, checksums, and safe data pipelines in order to guarantee data integrity. It also requires continuous check like on the performance of the model that contains unexplainable drifts in accuracy, it may be due to either compromised training data, or that an adversarial attack is being carried out on the system that is being used.
- **Model Inversion and Membership Inference Attacks:** The AI model in itself may turn into a privacy liability despite the training data being secured. Model inversion attacks make use of outputs of a model to recreate sensitive features of the training data. An example is that by repeatedly asking a medical-imaged facial recognition model, an attacker can hopefully recreate recognisable faces of patients. In the same way, membership inference attacks

can identify whether a particular individual's data was used as training data, which is a devastating privacy breach, particularly when it comes to conditions such as rare diseases or mental disorders. They work especially well on complicated models such as deep neural networks, which can unintentionally commit to memory the details of the training data. Their protection would also need methods such as differential privacy that apply deliberately introduced mathematical noise to training to make the input of any individual statistically insignificant, and it is statistically unlikely to be possible to obtain or gain particular patient data out of the model.

- **Adversarial Attack on Deployed Models**: After being deployed, AI systems are directly attacked through adversarial attacks in which the input is manipulated in a subtle way to deceive the model. This is a deep gambit of danger in healthcare. The attacker might introduce noise, which a radiologist would be unaware of, into a medical scan and produce an imperceptible result to an AI to either ignore a crucial result or generate a fake one. Equally, false sensor data of an ICU monitor may result in life-threatening clinical judgments. These attacks take advantage of the model's blind spots that are algorithmic and are terrifyingly simple to commit with such access to the system. It is not easy to defend against them because it involves making the models resistant to such inputs that they had not been trained on. There are solutions involving adversarial training (where the models are trained on malicious samples), input sanitisation, and, most importantly, having a human-in-the-loop so that AI outputs are consistently checked by a clinician, so that a security exploit cannot directly be converted into patient harm.
- **Specific Technical Instance:** These adversarial examples play off human and machine perception differences. In medical radiology, a convolutional neural network (CNN) applied to a chest X-ray can be based on high-frequency data that cannot be perceived by human vision. A small and invisible amount of digital noise can be applied by an attacker to alter the pixel values by less than 1 per cent - that is enough to make the model do a false positive with almost 100 per cent certainty on a malignant tumour. It has been shown that these perturbations can be printed onto tangible materials (e.g. a sticker on an endoscopy device), which reliably deceive models in a realistic clinical setting. This changes a hypothetical source of vulnerability into a patient safety crisis.
- **Insecure Supply Chain and Third-Party Risks:** Healthcare AI does not run in a vacuum; it is a complicated supply chain of software libraries, cloud systems, pre-trained models and applications with the vendors. All these elements bring a supply chain risk. The backdoor to the whole AI system can be a vulnerability in a library that is open-source or a compromise of a third-party data processor. To illustrate, an innocent update to a popular medical

imaging toolkit may infect thousands of hospitals. Also, external sources may introduce poisoned or biased data into the model using pre-trained models. This vast area of attack can only be mitigated with stringent vendor risk management, software bill of materials (SBOM) to see all components, and so-called zero-trust architectures that continuously check the security posture of all entities and data transfer in the ecosystem and assume nothing is safe. (Ahmad, 2025; Li et al., 2023)(Hou et al., 2026)

3. ETHICAL ISSUES IN AI-DRIVEN HEALTHCARE

- **The most significant and potentially the most sinister ethical concern is bias and Algorithmic Fairness:** The Perpetuation and Amplification of Healthcare Disparities. The AI models are conditioned using past historical healthcare data, which, in turn, can be seen as a product of the systematic inequalities in healthcare access, diagnosis, and treatment that have existed over time. Therefore, an AI is capable of learning and reinforcing such biases, forming a vicious cycle that seems objective. As an example, a model that has been trained on data skewed towards white, male, and wealthy populations can be highly inaccurate, providing less precise predictions, prescribing counter-optimal treatments, or not identifying symptoms, when trained on women, ethnic minorities and the socioeconomically disadvantaged. This is of paramount distributive justice concern: who is benefiting from this technology? The danger is that AI, rather than making the world a better place to live, will be a means that will bring additional health inequality to the table. To solve this, there must be active but continuous measures, such as training data on auditing representativeness, debiasing algorithms, and vigorous pre- and post-deployment testing on different demographic groups to achieve fair results in all patients, not the majority.

The landmark study demonstrated this phenomenon empirically: an algorithm used to manage health in over 200 million patients systematically underestimated the illness severity of Black patients because it used healthcare costs as a proxy for health needs. Due to historical inequities in access and treatment, less money was spent on Black patients, leading the algorithm to falsely conclude they were healthier than equally ill White patients. This case illustrates that even well-intentioned algorithms can amplify structural racism when training data encodes existing disparities. (Williamson & Prybutok, 2024)

- **The Black Box Problem**:

A large number of effective AI systems, and especially deep learning systems, are black boxes. They might be capable of superhuman accuracy, but the inner processes that lead to the derivation of a certain diagnosis or treatment recommendation are not accessible this is true even to their inventors. This is an essential conflict with evidence-based medicine, which has traditionally needed clinicians to explain causal reasoning: I prescribe this therapy because the patient brings with him these particular pathophysiological results.

- **Precise XAI Techniques in Healthcare:** Explainable AI (XAI) is something that provides exact tools to address this gap. The saliency maps overlay heat maps on top of medical images and indicate the exact pixels that the model used when making a decision, enabling a radiologist to be able to see that the AI was paying attention to the same suspicious nodule they were aware of. LIME (Local Interpretable Model-agnostic Explanations) and SHAP (Shapley Additive explanations) are used to produce scores of feature attribution, which show the level to which each clinical variable (e.g., blood pressure, age, specific lab value) was a predictive factor. In reality, a clinician evaluating an AI recommendation to sepsis onset can observe that not only the risk score but also elevated lactate and hypotension contributed 40 per cent and 35 percent respectively, to this alert. This kind of transparency makes the AI look not like an oracle, but rather a collaborator that clinicians can use to combine their own clinical judgment with the results offered by the algorithm, as well as explain the evidence-based reasoning to the patient. (Sridevi & Kolhar, 2025b)
- **Accountability and Liability:** Blurring the Lines of Responsibility When Things Go Wrong. The combination of AI makes the medical responsibility chain pure and straightforward. In the event of a misdiagnosis or other negative treatment outcome during an AI-aided process, who is responsible? Is the clinician the one who made the recommendation of the AI? The organisation that bought the system and implemented it in the hospital? Name of the software developer who created the algorithm? Or the data scientist who curated the training set? This is the significant ethical and legal issue of this so-called responsibility gap. Excessive use of AI may result in clinician deskilling and a shift of responsibility in which one party blames another. Moreover, the current medical malpractice laws do not have the proper structures to deal with autonomous or semi-autonomous software agents. Morally, we need to set up effective governing systems that establish the ultimate human control, competence among clinicians in being aware of the AI limits and bring legal frameworks that hold that there is never an anonymous, culpable entity, gen-

erally the healthcare provider or institution, that performs the duty of care, where technology supplements but does not replace human accountability.

- **Privacy, Data Governance and Informed Consent in the Age of Data-Intensive Learning:** AI systems need huge amounts of sensitive patient data, genetic information, medical history, imaging studies, etc, to be fully useful. The moral management of such data goes way beyond single HIPAA compliance. The most notable ones are the extent of informed consent: when a patient agrees to use their data for research, does it also apply to the commercial development of AI? Is it possible to use data that was gathered several years ago as a secondary use to train new models? There is also the danger of re-identification, where apparently anonymised data can be traced to individuals by using advanced methods. In addition, there is a cloud of data ownership and stewardship; do patients have rights to the knowledge derived from their aggregate data? Ethical practice would require clear policies governing data governance, fine-grained consent models (this may be through dynamic consent models) and implementation of privacy-preserving algorithms, such as federated learning (model trained on decentralised data without data ever leaving its source) and differential privacy (adding mathematical noise to data to prevent identification).
- **Patient Autonomy, Agency, and the Possible Erosion of the Therapeutic Relationship:** AI-suggestions, particularly those that are framed as definitive or superior to human judgment, are known to covertly or explicitly coerce patients in making decisions, which is a fundamental feature of ethics called autonomy. An AI-suggested treatment plan might be imposed on a patient even in a case when it contradicts their personal values or preferences, solely because of the perceived authority of the technology. This is further augmented by possible health literacy gaps. Moreover, the more medicine is mediated by algorithms, the more it will be dehumanised. When a clinician communicates mainly with a screen translating AI output, the life-giving aspects of human beings, like empathy, subtle communication, and that of the therapeutic alliance, which have proven to have health advantages, may be compromised. The ethical design should make sure that the AI can be used to complement rather than substitute for the dialogue between the patient and the clinician. The systems are supposed to be structured to make possible the options and evidence as well as uncertainties in a manner that enhances the process of shared decision-making without taking away the role of the patient as the final authority over his or her body and care.
- **Safety, Reliability, and the Challenge of Real-World Generalisation**: Much like traditional medical device validation, the safe usage of AI depends on its demonstrated safety and reliability, which is more complicated than

that. Models are subject to performance degradation in new populations or healthcare settings other than the training data. They may also not perform well in unforeseeable manners because of adversarial assault (wicked control of input information) or information drift (alterations in genuine world information patterns during the time span). An AI that is trained to find tumours on high-resolution scanners in an urban research hospital might cause disastrous results in a rural clinic. The failure in ethics will arise when there is deployment of such systems without strict continuous monitoring and clear guidelines on when to override such systems. This requires a lifecycle safety strategy: strong clinical confirmation under different environments, post-market follow-up, an inherent factor of uncertainty quantification to indicate low-confidence forecasts, and fail-safe factors that make sure that human professionals are the ultimate decision-makers in high-stakes or unclear circumstances.(Kolhar & Gundoor, 2026)(Zendehbad, 2025)

4. PRIVACY AND DATA PROTECTION MECHANISMS

Figure 1. The Multilayered Framework for Privacy and Data Protection in Healthcare AI

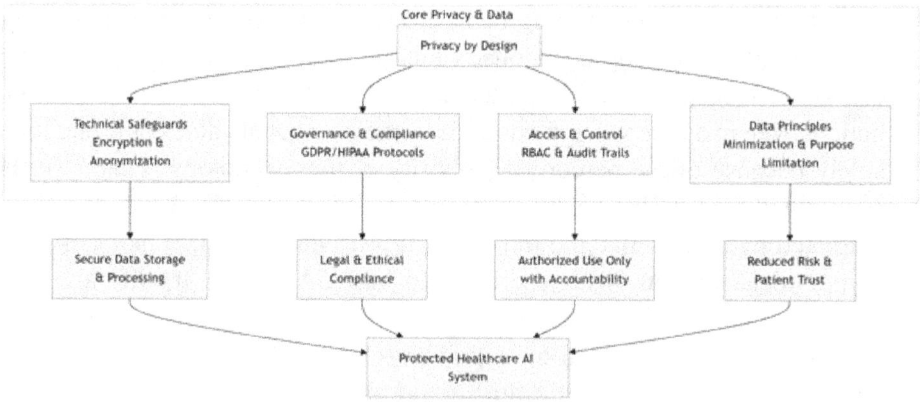

This concentric architecture shows that effective privacy needs four mutually supportive protective layers: Technical Safeguards, Governance and Compliance, Access and Control, and Foundational Data Principles, to interact to protect throughout the entire data lifecycle, starting with the data collection and continuing all the way to data deletion. As Figure 1 demonstrates, patient information security in AI-based care requires an elaborate, defence-in-depth approach to privacy that is based on the core value of Privacy by Design. This framework involves four pillars that are interdependent and that establish a safe and trustworthy ecosystem. The original pillar is the Technical Safeguards, which uses strong encryption of data both at rest and transit, as well as superior anonymisation or pseudonymization to ensure that raw patient data is not revealed at any point of AI training or inference, which allows secure storage and processing of data. These technical controls are practised and implemented in the second pillar, Governance and Compliance, which introduces strict guidelines in line with the rules and regulations, such as GDPR and HIPAA, that give the legal and ethical framework to all data practices. The third pillar, which is Access and Control, applies strict Role-Based Access Control (RBAC) and detailed audit trails that ensure that the data is accessed by the authorised personnel to access authorised data only, providing a clear line of responsibility. Lastly, the whole system follows some fundamental Data Principles, including Data Minimisation and Purpose Limiting, which proactively help minimise the attack surface and intrinsic risk by ensuring that only the necessary data is gathered and utilised towards the explicitly defined purposes. A combination of all these four protective layers, including technical, governance, procedural, and philosophical ones, keeps the data lifecycle safe between the collection and deletion of information, which eventually promotes patient trust and allows adopting a safe healthcare AI system that does not compromise personal autonomy and makes use of technological advances.(Shoghli et al., 2024) (Goktas & Grzybowski, 2025)

5. REGULATORY COMPLIANCE AND GOVERNANCE FRAMEWORKS

Figure 2. The Four-Pillar Governance Framework for Healthcare AI Compliance

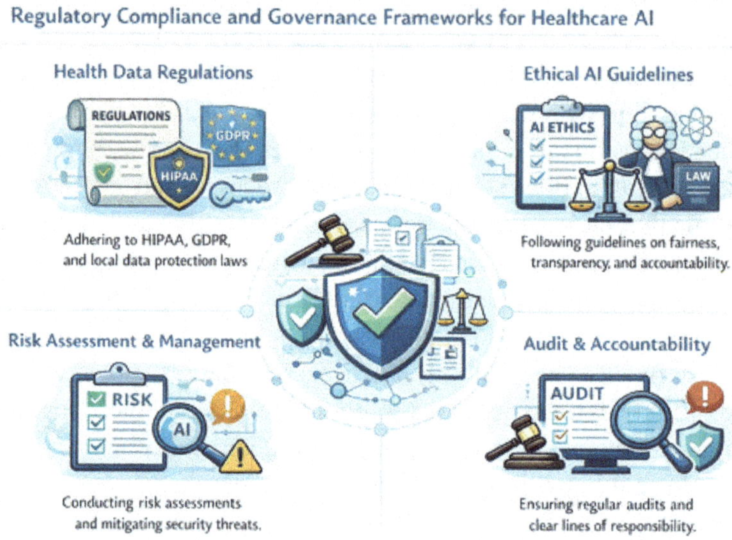
Regulatory Compliance and Governance Frameworks for Healthcare AI
Health Data Regulations
REGULATIONS
GDPR
HIPAA
Adhering to HIPAA, GDPR, and local data protection laws
Ethical AI Guidelines
AI ETHICS
LAW
Following guidelines on fairness, transparency, and accountability.
Risk Assessment & Management
RISK
AI
Conducting risk assessments and mitigating security threats.
Audit & Accountability
AUDIT
Ensuring regular audits and clear lines of responsibility.

This graphical architecture portrays Health Data Regulations, Risk Assessment and Management, Ethical AI Guidelines and Audit and Accountability systems as columns that are interdependent and help maintain a compliant and trustworthy AI ecosystem. No pillar is sufficient. The given visual scheme in Figure 2, called Regulatory Compliance and Governance Frameworks for Healthcare AI, gives a template framework of the responsible implementation of artificial intelligence in healthcare facilities, organised around four pillars that are all interdependent. The former pillar requires strict compliance with the formulated Health Data Regulations, such as HIPAA, GDPR, and other local privacy legislation, which are the legal foundation of ensuring the safety of patient confidentiality and data ownership. Simultaneously, active Risk Assessment and Management is a need to have a proactive process that would systematically detect, assess, and address technical and operational security threats at all stages of the lifecycle of an AI system. Such legal and security precautions have to be supplemented by following the Ethical AI Guidelines that offer the ideas of providing fairness of algorithms, transparency of their functioning, and respect towards human autonomy in the context of avoiding harm and bias. Lastly, all this structure is maintained by strong Audit and

Accountability systems that comprise frequent and independent testing, creation of clear chains of responsibility so as to guarantee constant compliance and offer redress were essential. All four of these elements combine to establish a complete ecosystem of governance, in which compliance with the law, security, ethics, and oversight are connected to promote trustworthy and sustainable AI innovation in healthcare. (Fahad et al., 2024)(Basharat & Shahid, 2024)

6. SECURE AND ETHICAL AI SYSTEM DESIGN PRINCIPLES

Figure 3. The Dual-Pillar Framework for Secure and Ethical AI Design

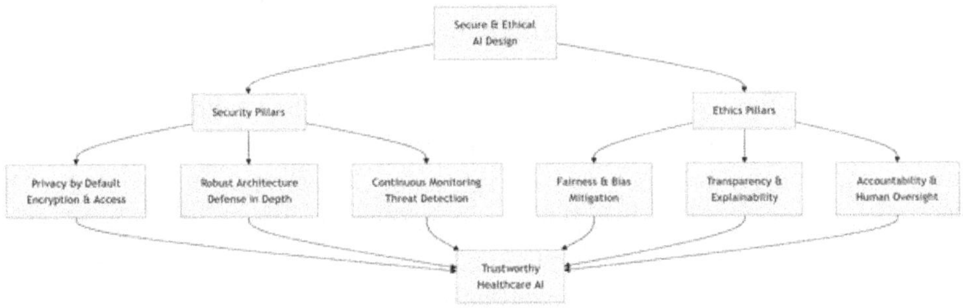

This image of the DNA helix shows that neither security nor ethics are developmental stages but have to be developed concurrently as mutually supporting strands. The combination of Privacy by Default, Robust Architecture, and Continuous Monitoring (Security Pillars) with Fairness, Transparency, Accountability (Ethics Pillars) culminates in the creation of Trustworthy Healthcare AI Systems. As Figure 3 shows, responsible innovation in the sphere of healthcare must be designed as an interwoven philosophy with security and ethics being designed simultaneously. The framework illustrates a bifurcated model with the Security Pillars (Privacy by Default with strong encryption and high access controls) as one leg, a Robust Architecture based on defence-in-depth principles as the other leg, and Continuous Monitoring as an active threat detector in the system. The other is the complementary Ethics Pillars, which require strict Fairness and Bias Mitigation to achieve equitable results, Transparency and Explainability to unveil the black box of algorithmic decision-making, and an explicit Accountability framework to ensure the required human supervision. These six mutually supportive elements are not sequential and are designed to interact in a synergistic way, which converges to yield the core outcome, which is a Trustworthy Healthcare AI System. This model underlines that technical resilience without moral standards is risky, and moral standards without a secure way of implementation are just hypothetical. The final design objective will be a system in which its security features will safeguard patient information and system integrity, and ethical principles will guide the AI operation to satisfy essential medical principles of justice, autonomy, and beneficence, thus gaining the trust of clinicians and patients. (Kasralikar et al., 2025)(Naib et al., 2026)

7. TRUST, TRANSPARENCY, AND HUMAN-CENTRED AI

The three elements of Trust, Transparency, and Human-Centred AI are interconnected and triadic because they are key to the effective and ethical implementation of artificial intelligence in healthcare. The framework goes beyond the level of technical performance to incorporate the human and societal aspects of AI adoption.

The foundation is trust; without it, the most developed AI system is sure to encounter opposition among clinicians and patients. In the healthcare sector, trust is won by showing reliability, safety and adherence to human values. It cannot be presumed; it has to be constructed out of verifiable actions and verifiable results. The cultivation of trust will occur once AI systems can demonstrate that they complement clinical judgment as opposed to supplanting it, when they can show fairness in their performance across various groups, and integrity in their performance.

The main tool for establishing and sustaining this trust is transparency. It uses various levels: technical transparency is explainable AI (XAI) methods that enable algorithmic decisions to be understandable to developers and engineers; clinical transparency is availed of understandable reasons behind AI advice to healthcare professionals, including confidence scores and other evidence; patient-facing transparency is simply accessible information about how AI is being implemented in their care. Most importantly, transparency would also entail candour in terms of limitations, uncertainties and possible mistakes, to admit what the system itself does not do or know.

Human-Centred AI also offers the ethical and practical framework of trust as well as transparency. This design ideology places AI as a system that helps humans and does not take away their human agency, but expands human capabilities. It focuses on human control as clinicians retain ultimate decision-making power, significant human control over automation, and design that honours human dignity, autonomy, and diversity. An inclusive design process should be used to develop human-centred AI that considers clinicians, patients, and ethicists throughout the design process by ensuring that the technology responds to real clinical needs, despite complex ethical consequences.(Rao & Sharma, 2024)

The mutual dependence is strong: transparency fosters trust, and the human-centred design makes sure that both focus on the outcomes that can be of real use. When combined, they become a virtuous cycle in which trustworthy systems are easier to adopt, the adoption creates more data concerning the actual impact they have (increasing transparency and human-centred improvements), and this in turn becomes a stronger trust. This, in practice, entails designing AI that is not only highly functional in technical terms but also integrates smoothly into clinical workflows, does not disrupt the relationship between patients and clinicians, has a clear explanation of its recommendations, and has feedback and human override mechanisms.

Finally, this three-part series can answer the essential question: how do we make AI work in the service of humanity and not vice versa? With trust being central to good development, as nurtured by transparency and basing all development on human values, healthcare AI has the potential to reach technical excellence but also become an actual part of the sacred practice of medicine, where technology augments and does not harm the human factors of care, compassion, and connection that are at the core of healing. (Galiana et al., 2024)(Koshechkin & Khokholov, 2024)

8. CASE STUDIES AND PRACTICAL APPLICATIONS

8.1 Case Study: Algorithmic Bias in Population Health Management Optum/UnitedHealth Group

It took a historic step of investigating a commercial algorithm used by Optum, a subsidiary of UnitedHealth Group, to target high-risk patients with its high-touch care management programs. The algorithm was applied to inform healthcare choices about more than 200 million patients every year. The researchers found that Black patients were undertrained systematically: at a particular level of risk, Black patients were found to be a great deal sicker than White patients. As a result, Black patients who were referred to improved care management were being provided with fewer resources, yet they had higher medical demand.

Root Cause Analysis: The algorithm used the healthcare costs as a proxy for health needs. Because of generations of inequitable access, systematic racism, and provider bias, fewer finances are provided to Black patients despite having the same clinical presentations. This historical injustice was learned by the algorithm, and it continued because it mistakenly assumed that Black patients are healthier since their health care usage and cost were lower.

Remediation and Lessons Learned: Since the algorithm was publicly disclosed, Optum retrained it with other predictors. The case formulated three principles of governance of ethical AI: the first is that algorithmic fairness is not necessarily realised post hoc but should be actively audited across demographic subgroups of data before publication; the second is that proxy variables are likely to encode historical injustice and should be ethically chosen; and the third is that transparency in model architecture and training data allows external accountability. The case is the most frequent example of algorithmic bias in healthcare and is currently part of the FDA pre-market guidance on devices that use AI/ML. (Stroud et al., 2025) (Bala et al., 2024)

8.2 Case Study: Federated Learning for Multi-Hospital Stroke Outcome Prediction

The dilemma in AI development that the UK National Health Service (NHS) encountered was a classic one: to come up with powerful stroke outcome prediction models, one needed a wide range of training data (which would be obtained by many hospitals), and at the same time, centrally stored patient data would break the data protection laws and patient confidence. A federated learning architecture to predict post-stroke functional outcomes was, in turn, introduced in a consortium of 20 NHS trusts.

Implementation Details: As per this framework, no patient data was exposed to individual hospital firewalls. Rather, a global model was sent to all participating trusts; local models were trained locally with encrypted data; only encrypted gradient updates, mathematical expressions of how a model should change, were sent to a central coordinating server. Aggregation of these updates was done by applying secure aggregation protocols, which ensured that the server could not see the contribution of a particular hospital. The last global model was performing equally as well as the centrally trained model and offered cryptographic assurances that the raw data of patients was not left under the control of third-party institutions.

Results and Conclusion: This application proved that the fake dichotomy between data privacy and model performance might be defeated. The federated model was more generally applicable to new populations than single-institution models, and it set the stage for the international rare-disease research consortia. As a clinician, I learned that privacy-preserving technologies are not only compliance-related issues but also allow conducting research where research collaborations were not possible under the previous GDPR and HIPAA limitations.(Gerke et al., 2020) (Xie et al., 2026)

8.3 Case Study: Explainable AI in Diabetic Retinopathy Screening

The diabetic retinopathy (DR) screening algorithm by Google Health performed at the accuracy level of ophthalmologists to identify retinal damage that could damage the vision of the patient due to the fundus photo. Nevertheless, the first clinical implementation in the Thai state healthcare system showed an essential gap: the local nurses and technicians who had to conduct screening at the first stage were unable to confirm the conclusions of the AI. The providers were not able to understand of which anatomical features-microaneurysms, haemorrhages, exudates- had made the system decide when the system made a positive decision on an image of DR. This obscurity compromised clinical confidence and made the decision-making of referrals a complex issue.

Intervention: The scientists used a system of saliency map overlay, which produced heatmaps overlayed directly on top of the retina images, emphasising the exact pixels that have the greatest effect on the classification made by the model. Nurses would be able to visualise that the AI was concerned with clinically significant pathology. When something is unclear, the providers might review their evaluation as that of the AI attention map, which would assist in collaborative decision-making.

Measurable Outcomes: Survey outcomes showed that there was a high level of improvement in clinician trust and willingness to use AI assistance after implementation. Appropriateness of referral increased, and the look-down rate (outcomes of algorithm override with no written justification) was reduced by 34 per cent. This case determined that explainability is not a theoretical ethical ideal, but rather a functional imperative to clinical workflow integration. In the case of health systems implementing AI, the moral of the story is clear: black-box systems, no matter how accurate they are, will not be adopted; transparent systems will be adopted. (Mohsin Khan et al., 2025)(Javed et al., 2024)

8.4 Case Study: Adversarial Vulnerability in Medical Imaging – The Endoscopy Sticker Attack

A proof-of-concept adversarial attack on a deep learning model deployed in the clinic to detect colon polyps, a system with real-time video analysis, proved that a system capable of an endoscopic procedure was demonstrated by researchers at Harvard and MIT. The group built tiny 3D-printed stickers with adverse patterns that had been precisely calculated. These stickers made the model fail to identify malignant polyps with high confidence when they are in the field of view of the camera.

Technical Mechanism: The adversarial style used the CNN dependency on the texture features instead of the shape features to classify polypeptides. Although human clinicians are able to intuitively divide polyps based on contour and morphology, the model had learned arbitrary textural patterns at the expense of other textures. The stickers provided distortions that could not be seen by the endoscopist and distorted these texture signatures.

Clinical Safety Implications: The study has made adversarial machine learning not only a question of curiosity in computer science but also a real patient safety issue. It showed how an attacker who had physical access to clinical settings, such as a dissatisfied worker, visitor, or a breached supply chain, could place objects that would systematically blind AI systems without the attention of a human supervisor. The case also hastened the need to evaluate adversarial testability to AI/ML-based Software as a Medical Device (SaMD) by the FDA, and made it clear that human-in-the-loop control was needed, meaning that clinicians retain primary diagnostic control and do not passively verify the outputs of automated systems. (Sulaiman et al., 2026)(Sridevi & Kolhar, 2025a)

9. FUTURE DIRECTIONS AND EMERGING TRENDS

- **Adaptive and Continuously Learning AI Systems**: The shift in paradigm is now decisive and increasingly moving away from technological models of AI that operate as fixed versions in Favor of systems that can continuously learn and adapt based on real-world clinical data streams. This is a guarantee of hyper-personalised medicine, where algorithms optimise their prediction of each patient trajectory and institution-specific patterns. This development, however, creates great security and ethical dilemmas. On an ethical footing, it raises the question of the very concept of informed consent, how could a patient consent to a tool the inner logic of which changes daily, and necessitates dynamic and continuous risk-benefit re-evaluation? Security-wise, the attack surface is continuous; the adversaries may also perform tiny data poisoning attacks on the live learning loop that end up slowly infecting the model's performance. Governance in the future will need to put in place strict systems of learning under constraint with hard ethical constraints and algorithmic guardrails that constrain adaptation, as well as detailed cryptographic audit trails that record all alterations to the model parameters to hold to account and permit forensic examination in the event of failure.

A digital twin is a computer model that is a real-time digital replica of a material object or procedure in the real world - in medicine, a dynamic, personalised computer model of the physiology of a patient, constantly updated by streaming data sources on wearables, electronic health records, and genomes. It allows, in fact, personalised medicine: an ICU digital twin can predict thousands of possible intervention paths in a second to prescribe the best dose of vasopressor in the case of septic shock. Nonetheless, such a possibility poses serious ethical and security issues. How would a patient give informed consent to a system whose internal logic change daily? Governance systems need to change to include algorithmic guardrails, hard ethical limits that limit adaptation, and cryptographic audit trails, which record every change in parameters permanently and allow forensic investigation in the event of failure.(khan et al., 2025)

- **Nominal Adoption of State-of-the-Art Privacy-Protective Technologies**: federated learning and homomorphic encryption will become one-dimensional instead of bargaining blocks in the healthcare AI infrastructure. Such a change is preconditioned by increased global regulations and an increased demand for patients towards data sovereignty. Institutional control of data by federating models via the transmission of algorithms to distributed data silos instead of concentrating it in one place will become the standard of collaborative research. More radical is the maturation of fully homomorphic encryption (FHE), which allows computing with data permanently encrypted. An example of this is a cloud service that may analyse an encrypted genome and provide the result of an encrypted risk prediction without decrypting the raw data and providing a cryptographic guarantee of privacy. The broad implementation of it will change the models of trust radically, shifting the dependent aspect to the legal agreements and the network boundaries to mathematical evidence of the confidentiality and, consequently, allowing the previously unavailable analysis of the most sensitive data. (Kolhar & Sridevi, 2025)
- **Multi-Modal Data and Embodied AI Integration**: The future is designing the synthesis of dissimilar data streams (medical images, genomics, incessant-biosensor streams, clinical notes, and social determinants) into and through coherent digital twin models of whole-patient avatars. This multimodal combination will bring new understanding of the disease processes and individualised treatment. It presents an ethical dilemma of epic proportions wherein the threat of re-identification is enormous, and the imbalance of informational power between system and patient is overwhelming. At the same time, AI is getting a physical form in the form of surgical robots, rehabilitation devices, and elder-care assistants. This literalization of the moral principle of non-maleficence is a result of this physical manifestation; a security breach or an algorithmic malfunction can lead to direct physical harm. Security, therefore, needs to change both to ensure the integrity of the synthesised AI model, a high-value target, and to ensure the physical security of robotic systems by providing strong fail-safes, secure actuator control, and protection against remote hijacking.(Mennella et al., 2024)
- **The combination of AI and physical systems forms another type of risk:** cyber-physical systems (CPS). Once AI escapes the server room and obtains arms and legs, the surgeon robots, automated rehabilitation machines, and autonomous assistants of elderly people, the principle of non-maleficence (do no harm) transforms into a physical non-maleficence. A data harm in a software-only system would be caused by a security breach; an injury to the body could be caused by a cyber-physical system breach. This requires safety

engineering to go beyond the concept of algorithmic resilience to mechanical fail-safes, actuator controls at the hardware level, and remote hijacking isolation architectures. Ethical interests are no longer privacy per se, but patient physical safety.

- **Development of Proactive and AI-Specific Regulatory Science**: Regulatory authorities are shifting out of systems that focus on fixed hardware and are creating unique channels to adjust to adaptive AI-based Software as a Medical Device (SaMD). This includes providing regulatory science, such as approaches to validating algorithmic self-evolution, requirements of adequate algorithmic transparency and performance monitoring (RWPQM) in the real world. One of them is the shift towards pre-certification or total product lifecycle models, where regulators consider the whole organisational ecosystem of a developer, their organisational culture of quality and ethical review and their cybersecurity hygiene as strictly as they evaluate the individual product. This will change compliance into a one-time filing and turn it into a living and evidence-based discussion between innovators and regulators. The success of such a direction will rely on unprecedented cooperation to establish new validation metrics and performance thresholds that will keep patients safe without slowing down the iterative and rapid pace of AI development. The Artificial Intelligence/Machine Learning (AI/ML)-Based Software as a Medical Device Action Plan by the U.S. Food and Drug Administration is the initial legislative framework regulating adaptive AI in its entirety. According to this plan, it has developed a total product lifecycle model, which has replaced the past pre-market testing on the basis of static devices with continuous post-market testing of algorithmic performance. The important innovations are the predetermined plans of change control; manufacturers have to define in advance what sort of changes could be made to their algorithm and how they could guarantee the safety during the process of evolution. To the developers, this brings predictability in regulation; to the clinicians, it is a guarantee that deployed systems are safe, even though learning is an ongoing process. (Kolhar & Sridevi, 2026)
- **Ethical-Security Auditing Standardisation and Automation**: With the spread of healthcare AI, bias, security, and ethics cannot be audited manually and, in an ad, -hoc manner. The answer is standardised and interoperable audit structures, along with high-quality automated equipment. This consists of settled metrics of fairness and robustness, automated red teaming systems that do the stress-test on models in adversarial attacks, and faultless ledger systems that automatically record all data provenance, model modifications, and model access events. These tools will make it possible to continuously assure and establish always-on model health monitoring dashboards. It

is probable that this ecosystem will create a new line of work to audit the systems against these standards: independent, certified third-party AI auditors, similar to financial auditors. Such a trust market, in which systems carry an identifiable label of ethical and security compliance, will be the key to scaling trustworthy AI, but it must have international agreement on the underlying standards to stop audit washing and achieve real protection. Sections of the European Union, the Artificial Intelligence Act (EU AI Act), the first global regulation of AI, sets up a risk-based classification framework with concomitant conformity assessment demands. Most AI systems that are considered high-risk, such as the majority of health care ones, will need to undergo conformity testing by third parties, establishing a legal requirement of independent auditing similar to financial statements audits. Such regulation will hasten the standardisation of audit procedures and audit authorities. Automated Red Teaming can be defined as a systematic method of having focused groups of ethical security experts (also known as red teams) pretend to be adversaries of AI systems to demonstrate their vulnerabilities before they can be exploited by bad actors. In medical settings, this comprises stress-testing models to data poisoning as well as membership inference and adversarial examples. The development of automated red-teaming tools can facilitate security on a continuous basis, instead of penetration testing once in a defined time frame, and change security from a compliance checkbox into an active operation discipline. (Nankya et al., 2024)(Al-Amiery, 2025)

CONCLUSION

It is not a destination, but a continuous socio-technical negotiation when it comes to the pathway to ethical and secure AI in healthcare. The chapter has also shown that the application of artificial intelligence to medicine is above all a human project, and in the process, the development of strong ethical foundations, hack-resistant security systems, and responsive regulatory systems needs to evolve. Every discussed pillar, including the concept of algorithmic fairness, the concept of differential privacy, the concept of adversarial robustness, or the concept of explainable interfaces, can be seen as contributing to the same single target: the establishment of trust between the clinicians, patients, and the population. Since AI systems are becoming systems of adaptive learning, multi-modal synthesis, and embodied physical presence, the ethical protection and security concerns that we are creating today must develop alongside the technologies under their supervision. The principle of non-maleficence, which was initially applied only to immediate clinical work, has to be implemented into loss functions, training pipelines, and actuator firmware. The demand for transparency should not only be implemented in white papers but also in saliency maps and SHAP values that are displayed at the bedside. Stakeholders, they must take a Call to Action: To clinicians, it means keeping an informed scepticism, neither blind acceptance nor automatic dismissal, but rather critical consideration of AI output in respect to domain knowledge. In the case of developers and data scientists, this requires privacy by design, adversarial resilience testing and rejection of accuracy as the only optimisation goal. It requires healthcare administrators to have a procurement policy that serves explainable and bias-tested systems over opaque black-box solutions. To regulators, it necessitates adaptive oversight systems that benefit patients yet do not discourage innovation, predetermined change control plans, algorithmic impact assessment and post-market performance monitoring. Technological innovation in healthcare has also been shaped by human-centred guidance, in which the promise of AI will be realised. The algorithms in this vision do not surrogacy the art of medicine; instead, they supplement it, maintaining the holiness of the doctor-patient relationship, dignity of the individual patient, and the well-being of all, without exception and with fair distribution. Hence, nurses ought to effectively communicate with patients and deliver care in a manner that assists them in recovering their health. Therefore, nurses should be able to communicate properly with patients and provide care in a way that helps them to regain health.

REFERENCES

Adepoju, D. A., & Adepoju, A. G. (2025). Establishing ethical frameworks for scalable data engineering and governance in AI-driven healthcare systems. *International Journal of Research Publication and Reviews*, *6*(4), 8710–8726. DOI: 10.55248/gengpi.6.0425.1547

Ahmad, R. (2025). *Developing trustworthy and ethically-based healthcare systems*. Applied Computing and Informatics., DOI: 10.1108/ACI-05-2025-0203

Al-Amiery, A. (2025). The ethical implications of emerging artificial intelligence technologies in healthcare. *MedMat*, *2*(2), 85–100. DOI: 10.1097/mm9.0000000000000015

Bala, I., Pindoo, I. A., Mijwil, M. M., Abotaleb, M., & Yundong, W. (2024). Ensuring Security and Privacy in Healthcare Systems: A Review Exploring Challenges, Solutions, Future Trends, and the Practical Applications of Artificial Intelligence. *Jordan Medical Journal*, *58*(2), 250–270. DOI: 10.35516/jmj.v58i2.2527

Basharat, I., & Shahid, S. (2024). AI-enabled chatbots healthcare systems: An ethical perspective on trust and reliability. *Journal of Health Organization and Management*. Advance online publication. DOI: 10.1108/JHOM-10-2023-0302

Ezz, M., Alaerjan, A. S., & Mostafa, A. M. (2025). Ethical AI in Healthcare: Integrating Zero-Knowledge Proofs and Smart Contracts for Transparent Data Governance. *Bioengineering (Basel, Switzerland)*, *12*(11), 1–30. DOI: 10.3390/bioengineering12111236 PMID: 41301192

Fahad, M., Abbasi, N., Qayyum, M. U., Fnu, N., & Zeb, S. (2024). Ethical and Legal Challenges in AI-Driven Healthcare: Patient Privacy, Data Security, Legal Framework, and Compliance. *Article in International Journal of Innovative Research in Science Engineering and Technology*, *13*(8). Advance online publication. DOI: 10.15680/IJIRSET.2024.1308136

Galiana, L. I., Gudino, L. C., & González, P. M. (2024)... *Revista Clínica Española*, *224*, 178–186. DOI: 10.1016/j.rceng.2024.02.003 PMID: 38355097

Gerke, S., Minssen, T., & Cohen, G. (2020). Ethical and legal challenges of artificial intelligence-driven healthcare. In *Artificial Intelligence in Healthcare*. INC., DOI: 10.1016/B978-0-12-818438-7.00012-5

Goktas, P., & Grzybowski, A. (2025). Shaping the Future of Healthcare: Ethical Clinical Challenges and Pathways to Trustworthy AI. *Journal of Clinical Medicine*, *14*(5), 1–28. DOI: 10.3390/jcm14051605 PMID: 40095575

Hou, J., Cheng, X., Liao, J., & Zhang, Z. (2026). *Ethical concerns of AI in healthcare : A systematic review of qualitative studies. 33*(371), 428–449. DOI: 10.1177/09697330251385024

Javed, H., Muqeet, H. A., Danesh, A., Rehman, A. U., Javed, T., & Bermak, A. (2024). Impact of AI and Dynamic Ensemble Techniques in Enhancing Healthcare Services: Opportunities and Ethical Challenges. *IEEE Access : Practical Innovations, Open Solutions, 12*(July), 141064–141087. DOI: 10.1109/ACCESS.2024.3443812

Kasralikar, P., Polu, O. R., Chamarthi, B., Veer Samara Sihman Bharattej Rupavath, R., Patel, S., & Tumati, R. (2025). Blockchain for Securing AI-Driven Healthcare Systems: A Systematic Review and Future Research Perspectives. *Cureus, 17*(4). Advance online publication. DOI: 10.7759/cureus.83136 PMID: 40438823

khan, A. A., Ghodhbani, R., Alsufyani, A., Alsufyani, N., & Mohamed, M. A. (2025). Leveraging blockchain-integrated explainable artificial intelligence (XAI) for ethical and personalized healthcare decision-making: a framework for secure data sharing and enhanced patient trust. The Journal of Supercomputing, 81(15), 1353.

Kolhar, A., & Sridevi. (2025). Principles and Emerging Trends of Healthcare Robotics. *Robotics and IoT Synergy in Next-Generation Healthcare*, 401–428. DOI: 10.4018/979-8-3373-5447-7.ch012

Kolhar, A. (2025). *Sridevi, Soni, H., & Kant, K.* Blockchain and AI Secure Wireless Transactions., DOI: 10.4018/979-8-3373-3576-6.ch007

Kolhar, A. & Sridevi. (2026). Secure and Ethically Aligned AI Solutions for Cybersecurity and Threat Detection. In *Ethical AI Applications for Software Engineering and Development.*, DOI: 10.4018/979-8-3373-6038-6.ch011

Kolhar, A., & Gundoor, T. K. (2026). API Security Testing and Exploitation Techniques. *Advanced Cybersecurity for Threats Exploitation and Digital Risk*, 87–116. DOI: 10.4018/979-8-2600-0747-1.ch004

Koshechkin, K., & Khokholov, A. (2024). Ethical issues in implementing artificial intelligence in healthcare. *Медицинская Этика, 2024*(1), 11–17. DOI: 10.24075/medet.2024.006

Li, F., Ruijs, N., & Lu, Y. (2023). Ethics & AI: A Systematic Review on Ethical Concerns and Related Strategies for Designing with AI in Healthcare. *AI, 4*(1), 28–53. DOI: 10.3390/ai4010003

Mennella, C., Maniscalco, U., De Pietro, G., & Esposito, M. (2024). Ethical and regulatory challenges of AI technologies in healthcare: A narrative review. *Heliyon, 10*(4), e26297. DOI: 10.1016/j.heliyon.2024.e26297 PMID: 38384518

Mohsin Khan, M., Shah, N., Shaikh, N., Thabet, A., alrabayah, T., & Belkhair, S. (2024, December). alrabayah, T., & Belkhair, S. (2025). Towards secure and trusted AI in healthcare: A systematic review of emerging innovations and ethical challenges. *International Journal of Medical Informatics*, *195*, 105780. DOI: 10.1016/j.ijmedinf.2024.105780 PMID: 39753062

Naib, P., Park, J., Abedin, P., & King, C. (2026). *Defining an Ethical Explainability Metric for Measuring AI Trustworthiness in Connected Healthcare Systems*. 1–19.

Nankya, M., Mugisa, A., Usman, Y., Upadhyay, A., & Chataut, R. (2024). Security and privacy in e-health systems: A review of AI and machine learning techniques. *IEEE Access : Practical Innovations, Open Solutions*, *12*(October), 148796–148816. DOI: 10.1109/ACCESS.2024.3469215

Rao, D., & Sharma, S. (2024). Secure and Ethical Innovations: Patenting AI Models for Precision Medicine, Personalized Treatment and Drug Discovery in Healthcare. *International Journal of Business, Management and Visuals*, *6*(September 2023), 1–8.

Shoghli, A., Darvish, M., & Sadeghian, Y. (2024). Balancing Innovation and Privacy: Ethical Challenges in AI-Driven Healthcare. *Journal of Research in Medical Sciences : the Official Journal of Isfahan University of Medical Sciences*, *4*(1), 31. DOI: 10.22034/jrms.2024.494112.1034

Sridevi, & Kolhar, A. (2025a). Energy-Efficiency Strategies for Wireless Sensor Networks in IoT. *Energy-Efficient Deep Learning Approaches in IoT, Fog, and Green Blockchain Revolution*, 167–191. DOI: 10.4018/979-8-3373-0300-0.ch006

Sridevi, & Kolhar, A. (2025b). Machine learning algorithms and IoT sensors for securing the networks. *Exploiting Machine Learning for Robust Security*, 183–209. DOI: 10.4018/979-8-3693-7758-1.ch009

Stroud, A. M., Anzabi, M. D., Wise, J. L., Barry, B. A., Malik, M. M., McGowan, M. L., & Sharp, R. R. (2025). Toward Safe and Ethical Implementation of Health Care Artificial Intelligence: Insights From an Academic Medical Center. *Mayo Clinic Proceedings. Digital Health*, *3*(1), 100189. DOI: 10.1016/j.mcpdig.2024.100189 PMID: 40206995

Sulaiman, K. Al, Alharthi, A. F., Alqahtani, R., Aljouie, A., Khan, A., Al-jedai, A., Almoeen, A., Alshennawi, M., Badreldin, H. A., Alnasser, L. A., Alshehri, A. M., Alzahrani, M., Alhaidal, H. A., Alhajaji, R., Alotaibi, S., Redhwan, E. Z., Alharthi, F., Alghamdi, B. G., Alquayt, A., & Aljuhani, O. (2026). Ethical, data security, and resource allocation considerations in AI integration for healthcare during Hajj: task force insights and future directions. *International Journal of Medical Informatics*, *205*(August 2025), 106123. DOI: 10.1016/j.ijmedinf.2025.106123

Williamson, S. M., & Prybutok, V. (2024). Balancing Privacy and Progress: A Review of Privacy Challenges, Systemic Oversight, and Patient Perceptions in AI-Driven Healthcare. *Applied Sciences (Basel, Switzerland)*, *14*(2), 675. Advance online publication. DOI: 10.3390/app14020675

Xie, Z., Wang, H., Dai, L., Wang, Z., Song, H., & Qian, J. (2026). *Ethical issues in multi-agent AI systems for healthcare : a narrative review. April*, 1–15. DOI: 10.3389/fpubh.2026.1792627

Zendehbad, S. A. (2025). *Trustworthy AI in Telehealth : Navigating Challenges, Ethical Considerations, and Future Opportunities for Equitable Healthcare Delivery*. 1–26. DOI: 10.1049/htl2.70020

Chapter 2
Privacy-Preserving Machine Learning for Healthcare:
Secure Software Design Using Federated and Collaborative AI Models

Aaradhya Pawar
http://orcid.org/0009-0001-9130-7141
Vishwakarma Institute of Technology, Pune, India

Kaushalya Thopate
http://orcid.org/0000-0001-7163-1262
Vishwakarma Institute of Technology, Pune, India

Tanvi Pokale
http://orcid.org/0009-0007-2888-1806
Vishwakarma Institute of Technology, Pune, India

Ayushi Patil
http://orcid.org/0009-0009-3926-0575
Vishwakarma Institute of Technology, Pune, India

Nandini Naik
http://orcid.org/0009-0002-9960-8835
Vishwakarma Institute of Technology, Pune, India

DOI: 10.4018/979-8-2600-3070-7.ch002

ABSTRACT

This chapter explores the integration of privacy-preserving machine learning (PPML) techniques within healthcare artificial intelligence (AI) systems, addressing critical challenges related to data security, regulatory compliance, and system scalability. It presents a comprehensive framework combining federated learning, differential privacy, secure multi-party computation, and homomorphic encryption to enable secure and collaborative model training without exposing sensitive patient data. The study further analyzes emerging threat vectors, including model poisoning and inference attacks, and applies structured threat modeling using the STRIDE framework. In addition, it examines implementation challenges such as communication overhead, performance trade-offs, and regulatory constraints under frameworks like GDPR. The chapter contributes a security-centric architectural approach and outlines future research directions for building trustworthy and scalable healthcare AI systems.

1. BACKGROUND

The evolution of digital transformation has affected the whole ecosystem of healthcare today. With the introduction of Electronic Health Records (EHRs), advanced medical imaging systems, genomic sequencing platforms, wearable biosensors, and Internet of Medical Things (IoMT), which refers to interconnected medical devices and applications that collect and transmit health data over networks, with the help of these devices, an enormous amount of structured and unstructured clinical data has been produced in healthcare. Artificial Intelligence (AI), defined as computational systems capable of performing tasks that typically require human intelligence, and Machine Learning (ML), a subset of AI that enables systems to learn patterns from data without explicit programming.The abundance of this data provides an opportunity for Artificial Intelligence (AI) and Machine Learning (ML) to be integrated rapidly into clinical decisions, predictive analytics, precision medicine, operational efficiency, and public health monitoring (Rieke et al., 2020).

The recent advancement of Machine Learning (ML) on large clinical datasets has resulted in substantial improvements in many areas including improving accuracy of disease detection, stratifying risk, diagnosing chronic disease at an earlier stage, and providing more precise treatment options (Rieke et al., 2020). However, this information is also some of the most sensitive data in existence today (medical history, genetic indicators, imaging scans, and behavioral health history). When either of these pieces of information are disclosed or misused, it can lead to stolen identity, bias in treatment, damage to one's reputation, fines for the healthcare organization, and a decrease in public trust of the healthcare system.

Traditional ML workflows heavily depend upon centralized infrastructures where data from various organizations is combined into a single repository for pre-processing, training, validating and deploying models. While these centralized data lakes simplify taking models through the development pipeline, they create significant cybersecurity vulnerabilities that receive considerable attention from the press and the public. A centralized data lake has to be significantly protected against unauthorized access and effective access control implemented throughout the entire pipeline to prevent a data breach (European Parliament and Council of the European Union, 2016).

This chapter extends earlier work on federated learning and privacy-preserving machine learning that focused on distributed optimization and model performance, by proposing a holistic, system-level approach to building trustworthy AI for healthcare. The main contribution of this work is the creation of a layered architecture that provides a unified framework for integrating privacy-preserving computation with secure software engineering principles and regulatory governance. Unlike existing solutions, which treat these aspects separately, this chapter offers a comprehensive architecture that combines technical robustness with legal compliance, ethical accountability, and lifecycle security requirements; thus allowing federated healthcare AI systems to move beyond experimental implementations and be deployed in the real world, aware of regulatory requirements.

This chapter makes three key contributions: (1) it provides a structured synthesis of privacy-preserving machine learning techniques in healthcare AI, (2) it proposes a security-centric architectural framework integrating multiple privacy-enhancing technologies, and (3) it presents a threat modeling perspective to analyze vulnerabilities and guide secure system design.

2. THEORETICAL FRAMEWORKS OF PRIVACY-PRESERVING MEDICAL AI

2.1 Evolution from Centralized to Distributed AI

Historically, ML had been developed utilizing a centralized architecture, which required data from numerous organizations to be collected and combined into one location for preprocessing, feature engineering, model training and testing/validation. While these architectures are easier to manage in terms of building and sequencing through pipelines and when orchestrating in a computing environment, they are based on several assumptions that are seldom true in healthcare: that sharing will be allowed by law; that centralized data storage will be sufficiently secure; and that all organizations have sufficient trust to allow for their raw patient data be stored, in fact relinquishing control over that data.

In healthcare, the clinical datasets maintain a significant amount of regulation around them including The Health Insurance Portability and Accountability Act (U.S. Department of Health & Human Services, 1996) and the General Data Protection Regulation (European Parliament and Council of the European Union, 2016), along with internal governance policies and requirements for oversight by ethics review boards (ERBs) within the organization. Furthermore, centralized systems introduce a concentration risk where a single successful breach could compromise the sensitive information of millions of individuals. Unlike financial credentials (such as bank or credit card numbers) which can be revoked or issued anew as needed, medical data is longitudinal (historical) in nature, is very personal and extremely valuable in the criminal ecosystem. Therefore, the ability to maintain patient privacy is not solely a concern related to technical design, but legal, ethical, and societal obligations. All of these constraints have pushed towards a shift in paradigm towards distributed intelligence where computation, not data, is what is shared between two or more parties, in order to develop AI (Kairouz et al., 2021).

2.2 Privacy-Preserving Machine Learning (PPML)

Privacy-Presving Machine Learning (PPML) refers to a class of techniques that enable collaborative model training and inference while ensuring that sensitive data remains confidential, typically through cryptographic methods, statistical obfuscation, or distributed architectures. Through these methods, PPML provides the ability to share and collaborate on derived data without having to centralize sensitive datasets but still enabling control of how the data is exchanged, such as by using a secure channel, a virtual private network (VPN), etc.

Three key concepts define PPML systems: (1) data locality ensures the original data remains on the systems of the originating institution; (2) controlled sharing of information limits the exchanges between institutions to model parameters, encrypted gradients, or aggregated statistics, instead of raw input data; and, (3) provable privacy provides a formal and quantifiable mechanism for technically establishing the level of a risk for leaking information (Dwork & Roth, 2014).

PPML systems represent a conceptual trade-off between providing sufficient utility and privacy. Specifically, as privacy protections increase (such as through the addition of statistical noise or cryptographic constraints) the potential utility of the model may decrease. On the other hand, if predictive accuracy is the only consideration when building a model, and adequate privacy protections are not used, the resulting model may be highly susceptible to inference attacks or being reconstructed (Shokri et al., 2017). Designing effective and secure software solutions requires effective risk mitigation strategies through properly balancing confidentiality guarantees with clinical utility.

2.3 Federated Learning

Federated Learning (FL) is a distributed machine learning paradigm in which multiple participants collaboratively train a shared global model while keeping their local training data decentralized.

Federated Learning (FL) is a well-known method for training a shared global model collaboratively between multiple organizations (hospitals, research centers, etc.) by distributing the training process among the organizations that are contributing to the project (McMahan et al., 2017). Instead of sending patient-level data used for training purposes to a single centralized location (like a cloud-based application), the organizations each do their own local training and then send their updated model parameters back to the global repository for aggregation into the overall model parameters.

The standard way of aggregating the local model parameter updates is the use of the Federated Averaging algorithm (FedAvg), which uses weighted averages based on a proportional number of samples contained in the individual institutions' databases to determine the overall value of the global parameters from the distributed institutions (McMahan et al., 2017).

This method of collaborating on training a model will help maintain an organization's data sovereignty, comply with cross-border laws governing patient data, and give each institution continuing governance over their clinical dataset. These three properties would be helpful for cooperation between multiple hospitals and/or between international researchers conducting research as collaborators; however, federated systems have introduced new security threats, including model poisoning attacks, the manipulation of the model updates as they are sent back to the global repository, and gradient-based inference attacks (Shokri et al., 2017; Fredrikson et al., 2015). Therefore, while FL reduces the exposure of raw data, it creates an expanded attack surface that is distributed out over many different institutions.

2.4 Differential Privacy

Differential Privacy (DP) is a statistical concept that offers formal mathematical guarantees that adding or removing one patient's record in the dataset will not significantly change the output of the model being used (Dwork & Roth, 2014). Federated Learning (FL) is a distributed machine learning paradigm in which multiple participants collaboratively train a shared global model while keeping their local training data decentralized. A mechanism is said to be ε-differentially private if the probability of any given outcome with respect to two neighbouring datasets that differ by one individual is constrained to differ by a maximum multiplicative factor, bounded by ε (Dwork & Roth, 2014). The number ε, as a privacy parameter, determines how strong the privacy protections will be; as ε decreases, privacy protections increase.

The concepts and application of DP can be helpful in managing re-identification risk, as well as providing protection against model inversion attacks (Fredrikson et al., 2015), and generally align with the data minimisation principle in certain regulations (for example, GDPR) that call for minimising the amount of personally identifiable information collected about the individuals in a dataset (European Parliament and Council of the European Union, 2016). However, applying ε-privacy budgets to a given clinical AI application may add noise to the data and can compromise the model's diagnostic accuracy. Therefore, to promote patient safety, clinical AI will need to be cautious when setting privacy parameters.

2.5 Secure Multi-Party Computation

Secure Multi-Party Computation (SMPC) is a cryptographic technique that enables multiple parties to jointly compute a function over their inputs while ensuring that each party's input remains private.

Secure Multi-Party Computation is a method that allows multiple institutions to work together to compute a function using their own private data while keeping their private data secret from each other. In federated healthcare systems, Secure Multi-Party Computation is commonly used to secure the aggregation of gradients and protect the confidentiality of the data during distributed optimization (Bonawitz et al., 2017). Although Secure Multi-Party Computation is very secure, it does have some computational and communication overhead that requires significant design consideration.

2.6 Homomorphic Encryption

Homomorphic Encryption (HE) is a form of encryption that allows computations to be performed directly on encrypted data without requiring decryption.

Homomorphic Encryption allows computations to happen on encrypted data, and the result of the encrypted operation can be decrypted to get the same result that would have been obtained by performing the operation on unencrypted data. This property will allow the secure inference and evaluation of models without exposing sensitive patient data during processing.

Homomorphic Encryption is also useful in healthcare analytics for the provision of encrypted diagnostic services, cross-institutional inference pipelines, and secure deployment of artificial intelligence in cloud-based environments. However, fully homomorphic encryption schemes remain computationally expensive, and users of these systems will have to make a trade-off between the strength of the cryptographic protection and the operational efficiency of the system.

2.7 Privacy Restrictions in Healthcare

Healthcare has restrictions that are specific to the industry and do not exist in most other data rich industries. Harm done to the integrity of AI can have huge impacts on patient safety due to mis-diagnosis or inappropriate treatment. There are consequences for not being compliant with regulations that have high financial costs and will hurt your reputation (U.S. Department of Health & Human Services, 1996; European Parliament and Council of the European Union, 2016). Many Clinical Datasets are often Non-Independent and Non-Identically Distributed (Non-IID); meaning that urban hospitals will produce different results than rural clinics or specialized care centers (Kairouz et al., 2021). Ethical Organizations like Institutional Review Boards (IRB's) will guide how AI will be used for healthcare.

Statistical Heterogeneity in Federated Healthcare may cause Convergence Instability and Model Drift (Kairouz et al., 2021). Addressing these issues will require algorithmic changes that will account for differences in distribution and will maintain fairness and robustness between the Sub-Populations.

2.8 Threat Surface Growth for PPML Systems

While Using PPML access to a large amount of data in an (Centralized) system is simply a matter of a hack, the type of risk in a Distributed PPML system are many and they include Model Poisoning, Backdoor Injection, Gradient Inversion, Interception of Communication, and Malicious Participant Injection (Shokri et al., 2017; Fredrikson et al., 2015).

Model Poisoning: An attack in which malicious participants manipulate training data or model updates to corrupt the global model.

Gradient Inversion: An attack that reconstructs original training data from shared gradients.

Membership Inference Attack: A method used to determine whether a specific data sample was part of the model's training dataset.

The area of focus will also change from housing DBs to ensuring that the integrity of the Distributed System has been maintained, and using Secure Communications, that the Aggregation System has been built to be Robust, and that the Distributed

System has been constructed to be Adversarial Resident. Threat Modelling is crucial for preserving healthy Collaboration in the World of Healthcare.

2.9 The Trade-Off Between Privacy And Performance In Clinical Applications of AI

Applications of AI in the clinical space have demanding needs such as high levels of diagnostic accuracy, low false negatives (especially for patients with cancer or heart disease), equal algorithmic performance across demographics, and sufficient interpretability for clinicians to have trust in the AI system's decisions. Privacy enhancing tools should not erode any of these clinical standards.

The development of software that is both secure and useful for healthcare AI requires a combination of privacy engineering, robust test methodology, continuous monitoring and evaluation against adversarial conditions throughout the entire lifecycle of the model being developed (Kairouz et al., 2021). Privacy should not be considered a "nice-to-have" at the end of the software development process; privacy needs to be included as part of every architectural and operational decision made.

2.10 This Chapter Within Current Literature

The majority of current work on federated learning focuses primarily on its value as a technical optimization (McMahan et al., 2017; Kairouz et al., 2021). Similarly, most current research on the application of AI to healthcare focuses only on the clinical performance of the system (Rieke et al., 2020). There are very few papers that take into account the cryptography behind federated learning and how it relates to secure software architecture, regulatory requirements for healthcare, and threats against healthcare systems from a high-level perspective.

The primary contribution of this chapter will be to connect these various aspects into a cohesive body of literature to describe a theoretical foundation for privacy-preserving machine learning specifically in clinical applications.

Building upon these theoretical foundations, the following section presents a security-centric architectural framework for implementing privacy-preserving healthcare AI systems.

3. A SECURE FEDERATED LEARNING FRAMEWORK FOR HEALTH SYSTEMS

The creation of privacy-preserving machine learning applications in healthcare involves planning an entire software architecture, not just using federated learning as a computational framework (Kairouz et al., 2021). There must be a combination of cybersecurity controls, regulation compliance mechanisms and resilient decentralized coordination incorporated into the software architecture. The federated learning ecosystem in healthcare includes many stakeholders, including hospitals, research facilities, testing institutions, the government, and cloud services; sometimes, these stakeholders span multiple countries. Each of these parties operates as a separate trust domain, creating architectural issues outside of typical distributed system considerations.

To illustrate the interaction between distributed learning components and security layers, a high-level architecture is presented below.

Figure 1. Secure Federated Learning Architecture for Multi-Institutional Healthcare Systems.

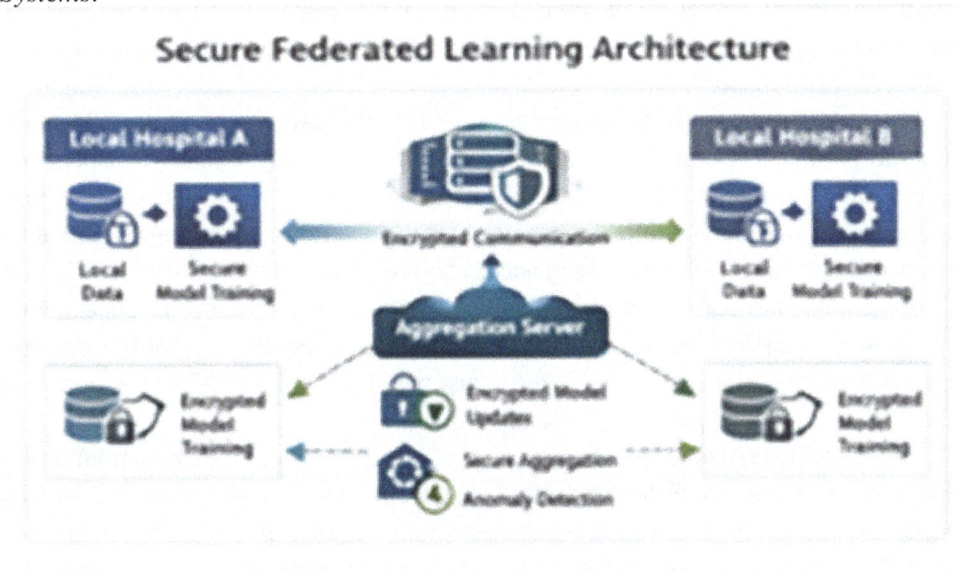

As shown in Figure 1, the system ensures that raw data remains localized while encrypted updates are securely aggregated, minimizing privacy risks.

Typically, there are four main layers to a secure federated learning architecture: the local institutional layer, the secure communications layer, the aggregation layer and the governance and audit layer. Each healthcare organization retains control of its own patient data (e.g., electronic health records, imaging databases, genetic data, and real-time sensor data) at the local institutional level. The local facility performs local model training within its secured environment, which is in accordance with the local facility's cybersecurity policies and legal requirements. The critical aspect is that the physical location of raw patient data does not leave that facility. Instead, only model parameters or gradient updates are sent from the local facility to the aggregation server once the local computation is complete (McMahan et al., 2017).

Secure communication is the method used to send updates to a central or decentralised aggregator of the models. This means that the secure communication layer must have robust cryptographic measures, such as encrypting traffic at the transport layer, mutual authentication, trust between users established using certificates, and secure key exchange.

Failure of secure communication (the secure communication layer) in healthcare could lead to someone intercepting, reusing, or manipulating a model that is not theirs or has not been approved. Because secure communication is so critical, it cannot be an afterthought; it must be part of the software design in accordance with secure-by-design principles from the beginning.

An aggregating server (or in some cases, a decentralised consensus mechanism) receives encrypted (at least during transmission) model updates from an institution. In the aggregation process, the server may use weighted averages (McMahan et al., 2017), secure multi-party computation (Yao, 1982; Bonawitz et al., 2017), or homomorphic encryption (Kairouz et al., 2021) so that intermediate values cannot be determined or revealed to anyone. The aggregator needs to be protected against insider threats and outside attacks because it will be a point of strategic control in the system. Subsequently, role-based access control, hardware security modules for managing keys, tamper-evident logs, and continuous integrity concern checks will be needed at this stage. Additionally, in highly sensitive healthcare configurations, the aggregator may operate under a zero-trust paradigm, where all transactions are authenticated and verified independently.

A layer of governance and monitoring is essential to demonstrate regulatory compliance and accountability in healthcare systems (U.S. Department of Health & Human Services, 1996; European Parliament and Council of the European Union, 2016). As such, federated learning software will need to embed logging frameworks to track participant records, log model versioning history, track artefact provenance, and generate alerts for unusual events. These logs not only help to monitor for cybersecurity concerns, but also help to demonstrate compliance with the legal requirements of transparency and accountability.

Statistical heterogeneity is another major architectural issue in healthcare federated learning. Clinical datasets are very seldom independent and identically distributed (IID) across health care facilities (Kairouz et al., 2021). Variations in patient populations, diagnostic instrumentation, treatment protocols, and regional health trends will often cause issues with the accuracy of local model updates. As such, the secure architecture must also include the ability to evaluate robustness and fairness to prevent a global model from providing excessive advantages to or disadvantages to a certain population of people. If this problem is not addressed, algorithmic bias will result, giving rise to both ethical and legal issues.

Another consideration in the design of architecture is resilience against adversarial attacks. Federated learning does this through having multiple points of entry for malicious actors as opposed to centralised systems (Kairouz et al., 2021). For example, if a hospital node has been compromised, it could provide poisoned updates with the intention of affecting the outcome of a diagnostic (Shokri et al., 2017). In order to create secure systems, the design must incorporate algorithms for anomaly detection, thresholds for validating updates, robust aggregation processes that can withstand outliers and methods of verifying software integrity prior to accepting contributions from others. This indicates that the definition of cybersecurity has changed from perimeter defence against external threats to determining the level of trust of the individuals and organisations in a distributed environment.

Scalability will also become a major requirement when it comes to healthcare collaborations. Many organizations will collaborate at scale, with dozens and sometimes hundreds of institutions involved (Kairouz et al., 2021). Therefore, the architecture designed for these collaborations needs to support asynchronous training, provide low-bandwidth methods of updating and have fault tolerance in the event that an institution goes offline for a brief period. From a software engineering perspective, this means creating modular designs, utilising container-based deployment strategies, and implementing orchestrators capable of dynamically managing participating organizations. Secure orchestrators must ensure that scaling operations do not result in configuration drift or incorrect configurations of security policies.

Lastly, the understanding/explaining of why and how a specific model works must be part of the architectural lifecycle of the compute system. This transparency into the process used to arrive at a given output is paramount for health care providers who rely upon automated decision-making systems to deliver exceptional patient care, especially in areas with the highest levels of risk.

In summary, while a secure federated learning architecture for health care is not just a mode of distributing training across distributed servers, it is a complex multi-layered integrated social-technical system. While each of these architectural components must include the requirements of being: 1) cryptographically protected; 2) designed to accommodate for the natural resiliency of distributed systems; 3) prepared for adversarial attacks; 4) equipped with regulatory logging; and 5) inclusive of fairness evaluation tools are essential, establishing effective privacy-preserving machine learning in health care ultimately requires the ability for all of these architectural components to perform as a cohesive whole under the umbrella of legal compliance, ethical accountability, and patient safety.

4. RISKS IN PRIVACY-PRESERVING HEALTHCARE AI: THREAT MODELLING AND CYBER-SECURITY

While the previous section outlined the architectural design of federated healthcare AI systems, it is equally important to examine the associated security risks and threat landscape that emerge in such distributed environments.

Though the federated and collaborative learning arrangements reduce the risks of having all the data stored in a single location, it also presents new and complex security challenges (Kairouz et al., 2021).

When a system is hacked and the attack may directly impact patient safety and legal mandates, threat modelling should be included in the system design and not something that will be done once issues have been identified. Machine learning systems that focus on privacy exert more possible attack points, which diffuses the risk among various components of the system, such as hospitals, communication links, and servers that combine models as well as locations where models are deployed. This diffusion implies that we should have an organized, thinking method of modelling threat; what the bad actors can do, what aspect of the system is vulnerable, and how an attack can impact the system (Shostack, 2014).

Model poisoning has become one of the largest threats of federated healthcare AI (Kairouz et al., 2021).

In such systems, the model updates of various hospitals are delivered to an aggregator (which is central or shared). When a single hospital is compromised, it may provide false updates that will diminish the quality of the entire model or add secret features (Bagdasaryan et al., 2020). This may translate to inaccurate results of the model in a clinical setting, such as failure to diagnose a specific disease or misdiagnosis of a condition. Indicatively, a model poisoned would not focus on a particular disease, and the consequences will therefore be detrimental. In response, powerful methods of combining updates to models such as using median rather than averages or identifying unusual behaviour should be employed (Blanchard et al., 2017), but should be employed with caution so as not to conceal significant differences among hospitals.

The other major threat is the attacks that attempt to infer or reconstruct training data of model gradients (Zhu et al., 2019).

Although federated learning does not exchange raw patient data directly, sensitive information may be leaked through the dynamic of the model during the training process. The attackers who can access these changes may be able to infer what the original information was particularly when the model is complicated or the local datasets are small. This is more dangerous in such spheres as rare diseases. This demonstrates that a simple lack of centralization of data is not sufficient to privacy, instead methods such as differential privacy (Dwork & Roth, 2014) and secure multiparty computation (Bonawitz et al., 2017) are needed to prevent information leakage.

Another issue is membership inference attacks and this is particularly in the healthcare sector (Shokri et al., 2017).

In such attacks, one attempts to determine whether the information of a specific individual was utilized in the development of the model. It is possible to expose confidential health information even without looking at all the information, by the mere knowledge that a person was included in the training. This requires a careful design of models, controlled access of results and noise addition to ensure the privacy of the results.

The threat landscape is also complicated by communication layer issues.

The process of federated learning transmits the model update between hospitals and the central aggregator, and in case it is not secure, attackers may overhear, manipulate, or counterfeit it. Such attacks as man-in-the-middle may disrupt the process of training or introduce malicious information. In order to remain safe, it is necessary to use secure channels, which are encrypted and the user is verified, the message should not be repeated, and verification of data integrity should be performed (Kairouz et al., 2021). Strict management of keys that are used in encryption should also be enforced as in case they are stolen, the entire security system will be broken.

The other critical risk when it comes to healthcare AI is inside threats.

The number of individuals who can access federated learning systems in hospitals and other institutions is large and a person within the institution may interfere with the system using his or her access. As opposed to external attackers who may attempt to crack in, internal threats operate under valid access, which makes them difficult to identify. To prevent these threats, it can be beneficial to use zero-trust methods (Kindervag, 2010), restrict access to only what is required, conduct an authentication of users constantly, and have systems that identify the existence of abnormal behavior.

Another risk is adversarial machine learning, despite a securely trained model (Goodfellow et al., 2015).

After a model is applied in reality, it may be fooled with specifically prepared inputs that manipulate its outputs. In medical imaging, the model might mistakenly identify a tumor or any other problem due to insignificant alterations to the image. By having these models on a large scale, these weaknesses may be transferred throughout the system. To ensure that security is taken care of, it is important to ensure that models are tested against such attacks during their development.

In addition to technical problems, compliance with regulations and requirements is also a part of threat modeling (U.S. Department of Health & Human Services, 1996; (European Parliament and Council of the European Union, 2016).

Failure to maintain good logs, describe how models operate or secure good consent may cause issues with the law even when data is not stolen. Therefore, intelligence in healthcare AI should not be limited to the technical threats only, but it should also encompass the governance concerns, data misuse issues, and comprehensive documentation.

To better understand potential security vulnerabilities in privacy-preserving healthcare AI systems, a threat surface representation is provided below.

Figure 2. Threat Surface in Privacy-Preserving Federated Healthcare AI.

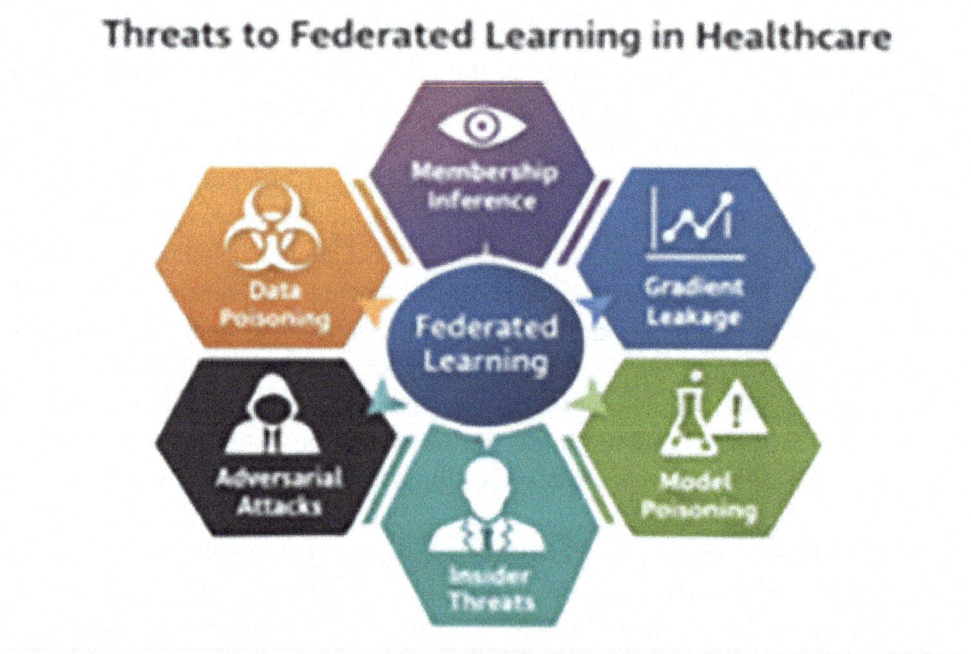

As illustrated in Figure 2, the system is exposed to multiple attack vectors across different stages of the federated learning pipeline, including data poisoning, model inversion, and membership inference attacks. These vulnerabilities highlight the need for integrated security mechanisms such as differential privacy, secure aggregation, and robust validation protocols.

To address these issues, formal threat modeling tools such as STRIDE can be adjusted to federated healthcare models (Shostack, 2014).

STRIDE is a threat modeling framework that categorizes security threats into Spoofing, Tampering, Repudiation, Information Disclosure, Denial of Service, and Elevation of Privilege.

Spoofing, e.g. fake hospitals impersonating real ones, tampering, e.g. changed model updates, information leakage, e.g. by sharing gradients, denial of service, e.g. preventing training, and privilege escalation. The application of these frameworks in system design is useful in the early detection of risks, rather than attempting to correct them once they have occurred.

Figure 2 illustrates the expanded threat surface in privacy-preserving federated healthcare AI systems. It highlights how vulnerabilities are distributed across multiple components, including local institutional nodes, communication channels, and aggregation mechanisms. Unlike centralized systems, where risks are concentrated, federated architectures redistribute these risks, introducing new attack vectors such as model poisoning, gradient inference, and adversarial manipulation. This figure emphasizes the need for comprehensive, multi-layered security strategies to ensure system integrity and patient data protection.

It's an ongoing process. With each training, update, or addition of a new hospital to the system, there exists the possibility of new security problems (Kairouz et al., 2021). In that way, system design should take into account continuous monitoring, identification of improper activity, checking the integrity of the data by encryption, model testing in terms of attacks, and frequent verification of adherence to the rules. Federated healthcare AI is only going to succeed long-term when it is possible to establish trust with all the participants, patient privacy, medical accuracy, and legal standards are met.

5. PRIVACY-PRESERVING HEALTHCARE AI SECURITY SOFTWARE DESIGN.

Having examined the threat landscape in federated healthcare AI systems, the focus now shifts to secure software engineering principles required to mitigate these risks throughout the system lifecycle.

Implementation of privacy-sensitive machine learning in healthcare needs beyond a comprehension of federated learning or cryptography solutions (McGraw, 2006). It also requires the use of secure software engineering concepts throughout the process of development (McGraw, 2006). When in healthcare, the intersection of data sensitivity and regulatory oversight with patient safety is involved, the design of secure software should be considered in the entire system, including the process of design, implementation, and monitoring after the implementation. Security is to be incorporated in the architectural choices, in the coding guidelines, in the infrastructure design, in the manner the operations are managed.

One of the major concepts of safe healthcare AI design is security by design (Shostack, 2014). This implies that the privacy, confidentiality, integrity, and availability requirements cannot be considered as a post-facto requirement and must be defined during the requirements engineering phase. In the process of system specification, the developers must define protected health information (PHI) (U.S. Department of Health & Human Services, 1996), describe trust boundaries among institutional nodes, and capture the paths of data flow within a federated training (Kairouz et al., 2021). Well-defined boundaries allow establishing the points of possible attack or establish what can be done or should be done by involved institutions.

Protected Health Information (PHI) refers to any individually identifiable health-related data that is protected under regulatory frameworks such as HIPAA.

Another principle related to security by design is the principle of least privilege (Saltzer & Schroeder, 1975). The different users in federated healthcare systems include data scientists, and system administrators among others and they will interact with different components. There is need to be specific and role-based access controls so that only the permissions required by a user or component are granted to it (Ferraiolo & Kuhn, 1992). To take an example, it is not reasonable that a local training node can modify global aggregation rules, and the servers of aggregation should not be able to access raw patient data easily. The application of rigid role division minimizes the effects of possible security violations.

Another essential secure design attribute is cryptographic strength. Federated learning systems rely on the secure transfer of model updates and the security of cryptographic keys (Bonawitz et al., 2017). There should be high encryption standards on the data in transit and where feasible the data at rest. Secure practices such as key management such as key generation, key rotation, key storage, key revocation, and key destruction must operate secure modules or security hardware systems (NIST, 2020). Poor key management may compromise secure architectures and reveal sensitive metadata or intermediate model states in healthcare.

Here, input verification and safe update verification are also crucial in distributed AI settings (Blanchard et al., 2017). Federated learning assumes that updates received by different participants should be validated prior to aggregation (Kairouz et al., 2021), hence, each incoming update has to be validated. It is performed through the process of verifying digital signatures, checking integrity hashes, and complying with established update criteria as well as any anomalies that may signify an attempt to poison the system (Bagdasaryan et al., 2020). Such validation processes make aggregation servers active points of security enforcement and not passive collectors only.

Auditability and traceability is another design principle. Healthcare policies often make organizations demonstrate the manner in which they manage and secure patient data (U.S. Department of Health & Human Services, 1996; (European Parliament and Council of the European Union, 2016). Secure software architecture should encompass elaborate logging systems that record the history of versions of the models, time of participation, aggregation and attempts of access. These logs should not be tampered with by use of append-only storage or cryptography (Shostack, 2014). Audit preparation is beneficial both in helping to achieve regulatory compliance and in enhancing investigation capabilities in case of breach.

Fault tolerance and resilience are also necessary to achieve system design (Kairouz et al., 2021). Network instability, maintenance or cyber attack is possible and may interrupt participation temporarily in healthcare organizations. A federated learning software should be able to handle incomplete participation without compromising on the model. Controlled retry, redundancy in aggregation infrastructure and secure fallback options should prevent large scale denial-of-service problems. Notably, the resilience measures should not undermine the security policies in the process of recovery.

Secure design frameworks should also be explained and transparent (Doshi-Velez & Kim, 2017). The clinicians must be informed about the way AI-driven predictions are realized when making critical medical decisions. Therefore, a secure software should have the functionality of generating readable outputs without disclosing the sensitive training information. Finding a trade-off between interpretability and privacy protection is a complicated design problem, particularly when applying differential privacy noise mechanisms (Dwork & Roth, 2014).

System integrity is also improved by incorporation of secure development lifecycle (SDLC) (McGraw, 2006). Iterative development should include code reviews (both static and dynamic security testing), adversarial robustness testing (Goodfellow et al., 2015), vulnerability scans, and penetration testing. As machine learning structures and third-party libraries continue to get more and more complicated, supply chain security becomes crucial. Compromised or bad dependencies may bring about unknown vulnerabilities to federated healthcare systems. Thus, deployment workflows should have documentation such as a software bill of materials (SBOM) and dependency verification processes (NIST, 2021).

Finally, governance-conscious design makes certain that technical protection is not violated by institutional and legal requirements (European Parliament and Council of the European Union, 2016; U.S. Department of Health & Human Services, 1996). The use of federated healthcare artificial intelligence systems usually includes data-sharing contracts, ethical authorization, and compliance inspections. Safe software should also provide policy enforcement mechanisms that should be configurable to allow institutions to make local data usage restrictions (Kairouz et al., 2021). To illustrate, a particular institution might be compelled to limit its involvement on the particular types of model training because of the problem of patient consent. Policy-conscious configuration attributes added to the architecture will increase the flexibility and comply.

To conclude, privacy-preserving healthcare AI design is a complicated matter. It unifies design protection, robust cryptography, thoughtful access controls, resilience in its operations, preparedness to comply with regulations, and ethical responsibility into a single engineering practice (McGraw, 2006). Federated and collaborative AI in healthcare will not be successful without privacy-preserving algorithms only but depend on the strict enforcement of secure software engineering principles across the lifecycle of the system. In the absence of this hard work, distributed AI systems will jeopardize the trust that they are supposed to promote.

6. A UNIFIED PRIVACY-ASSURING AND SECURED COLLABORATIVE ARTIFICIAL INTELLIGENCE HEALTHCARE FRAMEWORK

Building upon the architectural, security, and software engineering principles discussed in the previous sections, this section presents a unified framework for privacy-preserving healthcare AI.

The increasing application of federated and collaborative machine learning in healthcare requires a single and unified framework that will integrate protection of privacy, cybersecurity, and compliance to regulations into one simple system (Kairouz et al., 2021). Although most of these areas are separately addressed in different studies, such as encryption, distributed algorithms, or legal regulations, they have to be integrated in a coordinated manner in real healthcare applications. In this section, a framework will be presented; it will be the convergence of these pieces where the training of AI will be aligned with the best software practices and healthcare policies (McGraw, 2006).

The framework proposed is based on the five overlapping layers, which are the Institutional Data Layer, the Local Secure Training Layer, the Trusted Communication Layer, the Secure Aggregation and Validation Layer, and the Governance and Compliance Layer (Kairouz et al., 2021). The cooperation of these layers ensures that privacy is not only about ensuring that data are kept locally but also about securing all steps, including computing and sharing with sharing as well as controlling it.

At the Institutional Data Layer, the raw patient information remains in the healthcare organization in which it was offered. Electronic health records, imaging databases, lab results and wearable devices data are all a part of this layer. Information is maintained and kept in line with the security policies and laws of that particular organization (U.S. Department of Health & Human Services, 1996; European Parliament and Council of the European Union, 2016). There are strict access controls, encryption in case of data storage, network separation and constant monitoring to prevent unwanted access. Notably, no raw information passes out of this layer, which keeps the organization within control, and abides by privacy regulations.

Machine learning models are trained on data unique to an institution at the Local Secure Training Layer. In this layer, other internal systems are blocked off the training process by means of secure environments such as containers or used training modules. In advance of transmitting model updates to others, methods such as differential privacy can introduce noise that is carefully-controlled in order to lessen the possibility of reverse-engineering (Dwork & Roth, 2014). The updates of the models are also signed so that they are real and unable to be refused. By winning this step, the framework reduces the security measures that will have to be implemented later.

The Trusted Communication Layer is the layer that handles the secure exchange of model update between institutions and aggregation servers (Bonawitz et al., 2017). Any information exchanged is highly-secured and each party has to identify themselves and provide the other with their identity before exchange. Additional security measures such as no replay attacks and integrity of messages ensure that the data is not changed in transit. The encryption is also strong through secure management of keys such as periodical key changes and deletion of previous keys as the collaborators proceed (NIST, 2020). This layer is based on zero-trust principles (Kindervag, 2010), i.e. it does not trust any connection automatically, only trusted ones will be permitted.

Secure Aggregation and Validation Layer serves as the central point of coordination and control of the system. The aggregation server compares digital signatures, checks hashes, and scans suspicious or malicious updates when the aggregation server is provided with model updates (Bagdasaryan et al., 2020). They work with atypical updates with the help of special algorithms, with the possibility of considering valid and diverse inputs (Blanchard et al., 2017). To ensure the safety of information in these processes, secure multi-party computation or homomorphic encryption could be implemented to ensure that sensitive information is not disclosed (Bonawitz et al., 2017). Follow-up also keeps a check to verify the progress of training in order to identify any anomaly patterns which could be due to a malicious intent.

Lastly the Governance and Compliance Layer includes regulatory and ethical control within the entire system (European Parliament and Council of the European Union, 2016; U.S. Department of Health & Human Services, 1996). This layer has some logging systems that record the participants, model updates, and attempted access. Unchangeable audit trails are useful in ensuring that data protection laws are adhered to. The policy modules allow institutions to establish regulations depending on patient consent and agreements on data use. Explanability characteristics ensure that AI models give understandable and transparent outcomes, which is relevant to clinical validation and adherence to legal requirements (Doshi-Velez & Kim, 2017).

A major strength of this framework lies in the fact that it addresses the security aspect of the life cycle of the AI model (McGraw, 2006). It does not only seal the training process but also the preparation, training, deployment, and constant monitoring processes. New entrants are checked to ensure their identity and safety of their infrastructure. Integrity and anti-attack checks and tests are performed constantly during the training. When models are implemented there are measures put in place to make sure they are accurate and fair in clinical sense. Monitoring is useful after deployment in order to identify any changes in performance, suspicious behavior, or emerging security concerns.

The framework is also effective in dealing with the issue of data disparity in healthcare organizations (Kairouz et al., 2021). The aggregation layer has instruments to monitor the performance of the model on various groups so as to avoid bias. In case of the disparities, one can resort to such approaches as adaptive weighting or fairness-aware training. Integrating the checks of fairness in a secure architecture helps to maintain ethical responsibility as well as the law.

This framework is better than the common federated learning models by integrating the security of encryption, robust systems, regulatory controls, and verifications into a single framework (Kairouz et al., 2021). It acknowledges that privacy in healthcare is not a technical problem per se, but an intricate combination of technical, legal, ethical and operational concerns that requires the collaboration of numerous disciplines.

Overall, this combined framework provides an easy roadmap on applying privacy-conserving machine learning in a healthcare setting and maintaining high cybersecurity and legal responsibility. Its stratified design enables it to be assembled with minimal effort whilst providing extensive, general security. These types of comprehensive structures will be critical to maintaining trust and safeguarding patient rights as well as leading responsible innovation once AI in healthcare expands to various organizations and nations .

The presented framework distinguishes itself from standard federated learning designs which focus on distributed optimization and communication efficiency. In this chapter, we present a comprehensive model for federated learning which incorporates cybersecurity engineering, privacy-preserving compute, and regulatory governance principles into one model with a layered structure. The unique aspect of our framework is the layered synthesis of institutional data sovereignty, secure local training environments, trusted protocols for communication, robust mechanisms for aggregation validation, and governance driven compliance oversight. Through the integration of legal accountability, ethical oversight, fairness monitoring, and lifecycle security controls as part of the underlying system architecture, we believe that this framework enables federated healthcare artificial intelligence to evolve from algorithmic collaboration to complete regulation aware, security-by-design ecosystems that can be deployed due to the real-world requirements of clinical settings.

7. PRIVACY-PRESERVING HEALTHCARE AI REGULATORY COMPLIANCE AND GOVERNANCE

Beyond technical and architectural considerations, regulatory compliance and governance play a critical role in ensuring the safe and lawful deployment of healthcare AI systems.

Privacy-preserving machine learning implementation in health care practice is implemented in a field where the data environment is among the most carefully regulated globally. Compared to most commercial AI applications, the healthcare systems are regulated by strict legal frameworks, according to which patient data may be gathered, processed, stored, shared, and retained (U.S. Department of Health & Human Services, 1996; European Parliament and Council of the European Union, 2016).Therefore, innovative federated and collaborative AI structures should be planned in a way that would coincide not only with cybersecurity principles but also with the regulatory compliance requirements (Kairouz et al., 2021). Lack of legal requirements integration into system architecture may lead to hefty financial fines, negative publicity, and loss of confidence by the patients.

The Health Insurance Portability and Accountability Act (HIPAA) is a regulatory tool that has a profound impact on healthcare AI systems in the United States (U.S. Department of Health & Human Services, 1996). HIPAA supports the development of standards on the protection of the Protected Health Information (PHI) that obliges the covered entities to implement the administrative, technical, and physical protection measures to guarantee the confidentiality of the information, its integrity, and its availability. The HIPAA compliance is more than mere data storage protection in the context of federated learning. It includes the secure authentication of the participants, encrypted delivery of the model updates, access control to the logs and documented risk assessment. Although federated learning does not include any direct transmission of raw patient information, intermediate products, like model parameters or metadata, can also be considered part of the security rule of HIPAA in case they can be traced back to identifiable individuals.

In the European Union, the General Data Protection Regulation (GDPR) has even greater and stricter requirements (European Parliament and Council of the European Union, 2016). Among the principles highlighted by GDPR, there are the principle of data minimization, limiting the purpose, transparency, accountability, and the right to erase. The concept of federated learning is in line with the principle of data minimization in GDPR, as it decreases the movement across institutions

(Kairouz et al., 2021). Nevertheless, architectural alignment is not the only form of compliance necessary. Institutions should have the capability to show the lawful grounds of processing, record the activities of data processing, and also have support mechanisms in the data subject rights. As an example, when a patient invokes the right to withdraw consent, institutions need to assess the effects and presence or absence of their local contribution of data to a federated model version, which may necessitate retraining or update modifications.

There is further complexity in the case of data sovereignty and limitations on cross-border data transfer (European Parliament and Council of the European Union, 2016).The partners in global healthcare dealings can have various national legal regimes. Other jurisdictions do limit export of medical information outside the domestic borders, some subject cloud storage or third-party processing to conditions. An architecture that safeguards privacy can address such limitations by ensuring that the sensitive datasets do not leave local infrastructures (Kairouz et al., 2021). However, the legal requirements of the aggregation nodes, cloud service providers, and participating institutions should be well established in governance agreements. Legal agreements, such as data processing contracts and joint controller ones, can be a part of system governance.

Healthcare AI regulatory compliance also overlaps with the new governance frameworks of AI (European Commission, 2021). Regulatory bodies are increasingly providing measures where there needs to be transparency, explainability, bias evaluation, and risk classification of AI systems in medical decision-making. Several AI applications with high-risk like diagnostic support can be exposed to further documentation and validation processes. Explainability modules and validation pipelines are thus needed in federated learning systems that generate auditable metrics of performance across diverse populations of patients (Doshi-Velez & Kim, 2017). Such compliance can be directly facilitated by the governance layer that is suggested in the previous chapter, which includes logging and model version management, as well as bias monitoring mechanisms.

The other important dimension of governance is accountability and audit readiness. Healthcare organizations should be in a position to prove that there exist sufficient safeguards in the case of regulatory inspection or violation examination (U.S. Department of Health & Human Services, 1996; European Parliament and Council of the European Union, 2016). There is evidence of due diligence through immutable logging systems, tamper evident audit trails and documented security test processes (Shostack, 2014). In addition, the risk assessment should be done periodically to gauge the changing threats, particularly with the further development of the adversarial machine learning methods (Goodfellow et al., 2015).

There should also be consideration of ethical governance in line with legal compliance. The implementation of AI systems with patient information is often controlled by institutional review boards (IRBs) and ethics committees. Ethical review might be necessary to determine fairness, bias potential and the impact on society even when federated architectures maintain data locality. The inclusion of the fairness evaluation metrics as well as transparent reporting mechanisms into the federated lifecycle reinforces the ethical accountability and, at the same time, contributes to the regulatory requirements (European Commission, 2021).

Shared accountability is another governance issue that is specific to collaborative AI settings (Kairouz et al., 2021). In centralized systems, the data-controlling organization is usually the party in charge. In federated systems, however, there is a spread of responsibility between several responsible institutions and possibly third-party infrastructure providers. Well-established systems of governance should thus be used to define the scope of liability, the policy of incident response, the duties of breach notification, and the incidence of dispute resolution. In the absence of such transparency, multi-agency AI projects will be prone to paralysis in the event of security attacks.

Finally, privacy-preserving healthcare AI regulatory compliance cannot be brought down to checklist compliance. It also needs a constant correlation between the changing laws, technological protection and institutional policies. The software design, cryptographic protection and distributed system resilience should work in coordination with governance, contracting, ethics and transparent reporting practices (McGraw, 2006). Federated and collaborative AI systems will only be capable of technological innovation and of the sustainability of regulatory legitimacy through this multidimensional integration.

These regulatory constraints directly influence system design choices, necessitating privacy-preserving mechanisms to be embedded at the architectural level rather than applied as external safeguards.

8. IMPLEMENTATION PROBLEMS AND OPEN RESEARCH PROBLEMS

Despite the strengths of the proposed framework, several implementation challenges and open research problems remain, which are discussed in this section.

Although the idea and design of privacy-conscious machine learning in healthcare are conceptually sound and architecturally advanced, recent applications are still complicated and burdened with practical challenges (Kairouz et al., 2021). Federated and collaborative AI models developed in controlled research settings but translating them to work in operational clinical systems present technical, organizational, regulatory, and economic challenges. These barriers are very crucial not only in enhancing their strategies of deployment but also in the research directions that could be launched in the future to advance this field.

Statistical heterogeneity among healthcare institutions is one of the long term implementation issues (Kairouz et al., 2021). It is non-independent and non-identically distributed as clinical data varies in terms of patient demographics, local disease rates and treatment, clinical equipment and protocols used in treatment and the documentation system. Federated learning algorithms like standard weighted averaging may take moderate homogeneity of local training distributions as a given fact (McMahan et al., 2017). In case the distributions differ extensively, the convergence of global models can be problematic and performance differences between subpopulations can also grow. The solution to this problem involves sophisticated optimization methods, personalization levels, aggregation methods that are fair, and adaptive weighting algorithms. The future studies should aim at strong federated optimization strategies that can preserve accuracy and fairness when there is severe data heterogeneity.

The other problematic issue is related to computational and infrastructural constraints (Kairouz et al., 2021). There is a diverse range of technical capabilities in healthcare institutions. Large urban hospitals can have advanced computing clusters whereas the small rural clinics might have minimized infrastructure. Federated learning demands adequate computational power to perform local training and transmission of updates insecurely. Disproportionate infrastructure may result in imbalanced participation, increased convergence time, and resource strained institutions may be locked out. Studies on lightweight federated algorithms, communication compression of updates, and energy conscious training approaches are thus necessary towards fair adoption.

Privacy-utility trade-offs is a research issue of concern (Dwork & Roth, 2014). Controlled noise that is added to model updates with techniques like differential privacy is used to minimize inference risks. Nevertheless, when noise is too high, predictive performance can be impaired, and, in the healthcare context, it might lead to the decreased diagnostic sensitivity or specificity. Experimentation with domain-specific privacy budgets is needed to ensure optimal privacy budgets that maintain confidentiality and clinical reliability. The future work should come up with dynamic privacy controls where the noise levels are dynamically adjusted depending on the convergence behavior of the model and the risk assessment measures.

Another field of research is security robustness to advanced adversarial attacks (Goodfellow et al., 2015). Although basic manipulations can be counteracted by strong aggregation models (Blanchard et al., 2017), new, sophisticated adversaries might develop sophisticated manipulations that are subtle and targeted and remain below detection thresholds. Also, gradient inversion attack (Zhu et al., 2019) and membership inference attack (Shokri et al., 2017) keep developing as the defensive methods get improved. Future studies should consequently look into the hybrid models of defense incorporating cryptographic protection, meta-learning-based anomaly detection and behavioral reputation of participants nodes.

Coordination of governance across institutions also is a major challenge (European Parliament and Council of the European Union, 2016; U.S. Department of Health & Human Services, 1996). Multicenter healthcare AI needs to synchronize data exchange agreements, consent management policies, ethical approvals, and liability frameworks. The level of institutional risk tolerance can differ, and this results in conflicts over the security configuration or privacy budgets that are acceptable. The need to create standardized governance templates and interoperable policy enforcement mechanisms is an open field and needs the collaboration of interdisciplinary teams of technologists, legal scholars, and healthcare administrators.

Federated model explainability also adds more complexity (Doshi-Velez & Kim, 2017). To enable the clinical decision to be made based on the interpretable outputs, healthcare professionals need to make such decisions but there are privacy-preserving methods that can obstruct the internal model behavior. The study of explainable AI that maintains privacy without affecting the confidentiality of the data is a promising direction of research. Of interest are those techniques that produce local explanations without revealing characteristics of global training data.

A second direction of the research that comes out is continual learning and updating of models (Kairouz et al., 2021). Healthcare settings are dynamic; disease patterns are subject to change, treatment regimens are also subject to change and new medical knowledge arises. The federated models should thus enable secure incremental learning without causing privacy weaknesses anew. This is a non-trivial problem that cannot be achieved through ad hoc solutions since it needs to be formally guaranteed that increasing accumulation of privacy leaks does not occur over time.

There is also the need of interoperability and standardization (Kairouz et al., 2021). At this point, federated learning systems are executed with a variety of libraries and protocols, which creates compatibility challenges. Creating common communication standards and security guidelines, and ensuring checks of compliance would help make the process more widely used and allow cross-platform interaction. The healthcare consortia and the international standardization bodies can be instrumental in the development of such frameworks.

Lastly, there is the socio-technical trust as a background challenge. Although the privacy-preserving architecture is technically well-founded, both the institutional leaders and the patients might be skeptical about the AI-driven decision system. To develop sustainable trust, there is a need to have transparent governance, strict validation studies, reporting of performance metrics publicly, and ensuring involvement of stakeholders (European Commission, 2021). The following studies are then recommended to investigate not only the concept of algorithmic innovation but also human-centered design and trust modeling in collaborative healthcare artificial intelligence systems.

To conclude, although machine learning with privacy protection is a potentially transformative approach to healthcare innovation, its real-world production is associated with complex issues that cut across optimization theory, cryptography, distributed systems engineering, legal regulation, and human trust relationships (Kairouz et al., 2021). To deal with these issues, interdisciplinary cooperation and long-term research investment is needed. The future advancement of this area will require creation of cost-effective, resilient, equitable, and regulation-based solutions that can be deployed to the environment of intricate realities in healthcare ecosystems.

9. CONCLUSION

The accelerated adoption of artificial intelligence into medical information systems has brought unprecedented possibilities to enhance the quality of diagnostics, individual approach to the planning of treatments, efficiency of operations, and monitoring of the health of the population. Nonetheless, these developments largely rely on the availability of extremely sensitive patient information, leading to serious privacy, cybersecurity, and regulatory issues. Conventional centralized machine learning models, although computationally efficient, are risky and are conflicting with stricter and stricter data protection systems. Consequently, privacy-preserving machine learning has become a vital paradigm that allows collaborative healthcare innovation without interfering with patient confidentiality.

This chapter has explored the merging of federated and collaborative AI models, the principles of secure software engineering as well as the healthcare governance specifications. It showed that data locality or cryptographic mechanisms are not enough to protect privacy in healthcare. Rather, proper implementation will entail a comprehensive architectural strategy that incorporates distributed training protection, robust threat modeling, secure communication guidelines, regulatory compliance orientation, as well as ethical control. The technical components of federated learning, differential privacy, secure multi-party computation, and homomorphic encryption are fundamental, and their applicability requires prudent application to a safe and responsible software environment.

The main strength of this chapter is the suggestion of an integrated framework consolidating institutional data sovereignty, secure local training spaces, trusted communication pathways, powerful aggregation validation procedures, and management-conscious oversight frameworks. The framework enables a layered architectural approach to encompass lifecycle security, fair use monitoring, auditability and policy enforcement in healthcare AI and privacy-sensitive models of healthcare AI, by embedding these concepts into a layered structural design. This multidimensional integration is a sign of the fact that the sphere of healthcare AI functions in a socio-technical ecosystem, determined by legal regulations, ethical considerations, and trust expectations by patients.

The risk analysis on cybersecurity threats also points out that distributed architectures do not remove the vulnerability but rather redistribute and transform them. Model poisoning, gradient leakage, membership inference, adversarial manipulation, and insider threats and threats are some emerging risks that require constant monitoring and adaptive defenses. The principle of secure software design, including the enforcement of least privilege, cryptographic rigor, anomaly detection, integration of secure development lifecycle, and audit-ready logging, thus, become inevitable elements of trustworthy collaborative AI systems.

On the regulatory level, adherence to the healthcare data protection frameworks cannot be reactive and, instead, should be proactive through the integration of governance. Federated architectures have similar conceptual alignment to include ideas of minimal data and sovereignty, but legal responsibility, cross-border coordination, and handling patient rights should be integrated into systems design. The only way to implement privacy-saving AI in a sustainable manner is by properly defining the roles and duties and providing a clear policy on the implementation of privacy-saving AI, including documented risk management procedures.

In spite of the achievements, there are still challenges of implementation. The current research frontier includes statistical heterogeneity, differences in infrastructure, privacy-utility trade-offs, sophistication in adversarial settings, interoperability, and building trust. The solution to these problems will involve interdisciplinary cooperation between computer science, cybersecurity, healthcare informatics, legal scholarship, and ethics. The development of standards, benchmarking processes and governance templates will be determinant of scaling the privacy-sensitive healthcare AI to an experimental stage or extensive clinical facility levels.

And, finally, privacy-preserving machine learning can be judged to be successful in healthcare not solely by its predictive performance but also that it can maintain trust, regulatory legitimacy, and patient dignity. Since healthcare is ongoing digitization and interconnection, the adoption of secure collaborative AI architectures provides a way to move to responsible innovation one that achieves balanced technological innovation, ethical responsibility, and resilience against cyber threats. The further development of such structures will be critical to making sure artificial intelligence improves the results in the sphere of healthcare without compromising the values of privacy and patient protection of the foundations.

The objective of this chapter is to demonstrate that privacy preserving machine learning in healthcare is not just an algorithmic problem but rather a problem that encompasses all three system levels (i.e. technical, regulatory, and ethical). The proposed architecture combines federated learning with secure software engineering practices and governance frameworks to provide pathways toward a trustworthy and compliant healthcare AI system. It emphasizes the need for alignment of data privacy, security, fairness, and accountability when deploying those technologies into real-time operational environments. Future studies should address issues related to scalable implementations, adaptive privacy mechanisms, and a greater collaboration between institutions in order to facilitate the widespread use of privacy preserving healthcare technologies.

Ultimately, the integration of privacy-preserving techniques will be essential for enabling trustworthy, scalable, and ethically responsible healthcare AI systems.

These advancements will play a crucial role in enabling the next generation of secure, scalable, and trustworthy healthcare AI systems.

REFERENCES

Bagdasaryan, E., Veit, A., Hua, Y., Estrin, D., & Shmatikov, V. (2020). How to backdoor federated learning. *Proceedings of the 23rd International Conference on Artificial Intelligence and Statistics (AISTATS)*, 2938–2948.

Blanchard, P., El Mhamdi, E. M., Guerraoui, R., & Stainer, J. (2017). Machine learning with adversaries: Byzantine tolerant gradient descent. *Advances in Neural Information Processing Systems (NeurIPS)*, 30.

Bonawitz, K., Ivanov, V., Kreuter, B., Marcedone, A., McMahan, B., Patel, S., Ramage, D., Segal, A., & Seth, K. (2017). Practical secure aggregation for privacy-preserving machine learning. *Proceedings of the 2017 ACM SIGSAC Conference on Computer and Communications Security (CCS)*, 1175–1191. https://doi.org/DOI: 10.1145/3133956.3133982

Doshi-Velez, F., & Kim, B. (2017). Towards a rigorous science of interpretable machine learning. *arXiv preprint arXiv:1702.08608*.

Dwork, C., & Roth, A. (2014). The algorithmic foundations of differential privacy. *Foundations and Trends in Theoretical Computer Science*, *9*(3–4), 211–407. DOI: 10.1561/0400000042

European Commission. (2021). *Proposal for a regulation laying down harmonised rules on artificial intelligence*. Artificial Intelligence Act.

European Parliament and Council of the European Union. (2016). *Regulation (EU) 2016/679 (General Data Protection Regulation)*. Official Journal of the European Union.

Ferraiolo, D. F., & Kuhn, D. R. (1992). Role-based access controls. *15th National Computer Security Conference*, 554–563.

Fredrikson, M., Jha, S., & Ristenpart, T. (2015). Model inversion attacks that exploit confidence information and basic countermeasures. *Proceedings of the 22nd ACM SIGSAC Conference on Computer and Communications Security (CCS)*, 1322–1333. https://doi.org/DOI: 10.1145/2810103.2813677

Goodfellow, I. J., Shlens, J., & Szegedy, C. (2015). Explaining and harnessing adversarial examples. *International Conference on Learning Representations (ICLR)*.

Kairouz, P., McMahan, H. B., Avent, B., Bellet, A., Bennis, M., Bhagoji, A. N., Bonawitz, K., Charles, Z., Cormode, G., Cummings, R., D'Oliveira, R., Eichner, H., El Rouayheb, S., Evans, D., Gardner, J., Garrett, Z., Gascón, A., Ghazi, B., Gibbons, P. B., & Zhao, S. (2021). Advances and open problems in federated learning. *Foundations and Trends in Machine Learning*, *14*(1–2), 1–210. DOI: 10.1561/2200000083

Kindervag, J. (2010). *No more chewy centers: Introducing the zero trust model of information security*. Forrester Research.

McGraw, G. (2006). *Software security: Building security in*. Addison-Wesley.

McMahan, H. B., Moore, E., Ramage, D., Hampson, S., & Arcas, B. A. Y. (2017). Communication-efficient learning of deep networks from decentralized data. *Proceedings of the 20th International Conference on Artificial Intelligence and Statistics (AISTATS)*, 1273–1282.

National Institute of Standards and Technology (NIST). (2020). *Security and privacy controls for information systems and organizations (SP 800-53 Rev. 5)*. U.S. Department of Commerce.

National Institute of Standards and Technology (NIST). (2021). *Software bill of materials (SBOM) considerations*. U.S. Department of Commerce.

Saltzer, J. H., & Schroeder, M. D. (1975). The protection of information in computer systems. *Proceedings of the IEEE*, *63*(9), 1278–1308. DOI: 10.1109/PROC.1975.9939

Shokri, R., Stronati, M., Song, C., & Shmatikov, V. (2017). Membership inference attacks against machine learning models. *2017 IEEE Symposium on Security and Privacy*, 3–18. https://doi.org/DOI: 10.1109/SP.2017.41

Shostack, A. (2014). *Threat modeling: Designing for security*. Wiley.

U.S. Department of Health & Human Services. (1996). Health Insurance Portability and Accountability Act of 1996 (HIPAA). *Public Law*, •••, 104–191.

Yao, A. C. (1982). Protocols for secure computations. *23rd Annual Symposium on Foundations of Computer Science (FOCS)*, 160–164. DOI: 10.1109/SFCS.1982.38

Zhu, L., Liu, Z., & Han, S. (2019). Deep leakage from gradients. *Advances in Neural Information Processing Systems (NeurIPS)*, 32.

Chapter 3
Privacy-Preserving and Secure AI-Driven Healthcare Systems:
From Federated Learning to Quantum-Resilient Cybersecurity

Dhinakaran Damodaran
http://orcid.org/0000-0002-3183-576X
Vel Tech Rangarajan Dr. Sagunthala R&D Institute of Science and Technology, India

D. Selvaraj
Panimalar Engineering College, India

S. Edwin Raja
http://orcid.org/0000-0002-2948-9669
Vel Tech Rangarajan Dr. Sagunthala R&D Institute of Science and Technology, India

R. Saravanan
http://orcid.org/0000-0002-0877-7880
Vel Tech High Tech Dr. Rangarajan Dr. Sakunthala Engineering College, India

ABSTRACT

The rapid adoption of artificial intelligence (AI) in healthcare has enabled intelligent diagnostics, personalized treatment, and real-time clinical decision support. However, these advancements also introduce significant challenges related to data privacy, cybersecurity, and secure software deployment. Healthcare AI systems operate on highly sensitive patient data and are increasingly targeted by cyber threats, including

DOI: 10.4018/979-8-2600-3070-7.ch003

data breaches, ransomware attacks, and adversarial manipulation of machine learning models. This chapter presents a comprehensive exploration of privacy-preserving and secure AI-driven healthcare systems, emphasizing the integration of federated learning, explainable AI, and quantum-resilient cybersecurity mechanisms. The chapter examines secure software architectures and collaborative AI frameworks that enable effective interaction between intelligent systems and healthcare professionals while maintaining regulatory compliance and ethical integrity.

1. INTRODUCTION TO AI-DRIVEN HEALTHCARE SYSTEMS

The healthcare sector is experiencing a significant digital revolution that is facilitated by the development of artificial intelligence (AI), data analytics, and intelligent software programs. The AI-oriented healthcare uses the opportunities of machine learning, deep learning, natural language processing, and decision intelligence to contribute to clinical diagnosis and improve treatment planning, as well as provide continuous monitoring of a patient (Qayyum et al., 2021). Such systems are also increasingly integrated into such essential healthcare processes as medical imaging analysis, predicting disease risk, personalized medicine, telemedicine, and managing hospital resources. In contrast to the conventional healthcare information systems, which base their operation on the rule-based logic and stable data processing, AI-based healthcare platforms are highly dynamical. They keep learning on the basis of heterogeneous sources of data, including electronic health records (EHRs), medical images, genomic data, wearable sensors, and Internet of Medical Things (IoMT) devices. This adaptive and data-centric approach allows AI systems to provide real-time clinical decision-making and predictive healthcare services, enhancing patient outcomes and operational efficiency. Nevertheless, the utilization of AI in healthcare across the board poses severe issues in terms of data privacy, cybersecurity, and system fidelity (Sai Srinivas Matta, & Bolli, 2025). Medical information is one of the most sensitive types of personal data, and the performance of AI models can be achieved only with large, quality datasets. The centralized data aggregation methods pose significant issues on unauthorized access, data breaches, non-compliance with regulatory requirements and managing patient consent. Such risks are also exacerbated by the rising rate of cyberattacks on infrastructures on healthcare, such as the ransomware, data exfiltration, and adversarial manipulation of AI models.

Healthcare systems driven by AI also require healthy software engineering practices in order to be reliable and safe and explainable. Clinical settings are safety-critical in nature, and any mistakes or other malicious interventions in the decision-making process with the help of AI may severely affect the well-being of patients (Selvaraj et al., 2025). Consequently, clinician trust and the responsible use of AI will require secure software architecture, robust deployment plans, and open model behavior. It has also become especially significant to integrate explainable AI techniques to facilitate human-AI cooperation and enable healthcare professionals to interpret, validate, and contextualize AI-generated insights. To overcome these limitations, privacy-preserving and safe AI paradigms have become the key elements of the contemporary healthcare systems (Dhinakaran et al., 2023). Federated learning, differential privacy, and secure multi-party computation are some of the techniques that can facilitate collaborative model training without providing direct access to patient data. Meanwhile, cryptographic security development, such as post-quantum and quantum-resilient systems, is increasingly receiving interest as the solution of the future, capable of protecting the health AI systems against any cyber threats. The chapter describes the integration of the AI, the cybersecurity, and the secure software practices in healthcare ecosystems. The chapter also gives a comprehensive view on the design of trustworthy and resilient AI-mediated healthcare systems by looking at privacy-preserving learning systems, threat-conscious system architectures, and future quantum-resilient defences. The discussion not only highlights technological advances but also highlights ethical, regulatory, and human concerns that can enable the integration of AI in the real world of clinical settings in a sustainable and safe manner.

Chapter Contribution and Novel Perspective

While substantial research has explored individual aspects of privacy-preserving machine learning, healthcare cybersecurity, federated learning, and secure computation, these topics are often investigated in isolation. Existing surveys primarily focus on specific technical mechanisms such as federated learning, differential privacy, or secure multi-party computation without examining their integration within the broader healthcare AI lifecycle. The novelty of this chapter lies in its unified perspective that combines privacy-preserving learning, secure software engineering practices, explainable AI, governance mechanisms, and emerging quantum-resilient cybersecurity technologies within a single healthcare-oriented framework. Rather than treating privacy, security, trust, and compliance as independent concerns, the chapter presents them as interconnected components of a secure predictive healthcare ecosystem. Furthermore, the chapter advances beyond conventional PPML-focused surveys by introducing a layered healthcare AI architecture that integrates data protection, collaborative intelligence, cybersecurity defense, and governance controls. The proposed perspective highlights how secure software practices, human-centered AI design, regulatory compliance, and future-ready cryptographic mechanisms collectively contribute to trustworthy healthcare AI deployment. By synthesizing these complementary domains into a cohesive framework, the chapter provides researchers, practitioners, and policymakers with a holistic roadmap for designing resilient, privacy-preserving, and clinically trustworthy AI-driven healthcare systems.

Objectives of the Chapter

The primary objectives of this chapter are to:

1. Analyze cybersecurity threats and vulnerabilities in AI-driven healthcare systems.
2. Explore privacy-preserving machine learning techniques, including federated learning and secure computation.
3. Present secure software design principles for healthcare AI applications.
4. Discuss quantum-resilient and emerging cybersecurity mechanisms for future healthcare systems.
5. Examine AI-human collaboration, trust, and explainability in clinical environments.
6. Provide practical insights through case studies and real-world healthcare implementations.

1.1 Evolution of AI in Healthcare Systems

The history of artificial intelligence use in healthcare has gone through several phases of technology, each with its unique approach to computation, the use of data, and the degree of clinical influence. This development indicates a progressive transformation of deterministic automation to adaptive, data-driven intelligence, which can be used to facilitate predictive and personalized healthcare services. Figure 1 shows the evolution of the AI in healthcare in the direction of privacy-preserving federated intelligence, which should be rule-based expert systems, and identify the transition to data-driven, decentralized, and predictive healthcare paradigms (Shaheen et al., 2022). The number indicates that the complexity of data and the need to enhance clinical intelligence has posed a privacy risk and a cybersecurity bandwidth challenge, making the implementation of secure and collaborative AI models a motivating factor. Initial AI systems in healthcare operated largely on the tried-and-true rule-based expert systems, which so-called medical intelligence was coded in the form of a set of logical rules and decision trees. Such systems were strongly dependent on the knowledge developed by humans based on clinical guidelines and expertise. On the one hand, rule-based models had proven successful in small-scale diagnostic situations; on the other hand, they were inflexible and unable to adapt to more complicated cases of medical conditions, and incapable of being updated with new information. They were limited in their performance by completeness and accuracy of manually defined rules, and they are not appropriate in dynamic and large-scale healthcare settings.

Figure 1. Evolution of Healthcare AI Paradigms

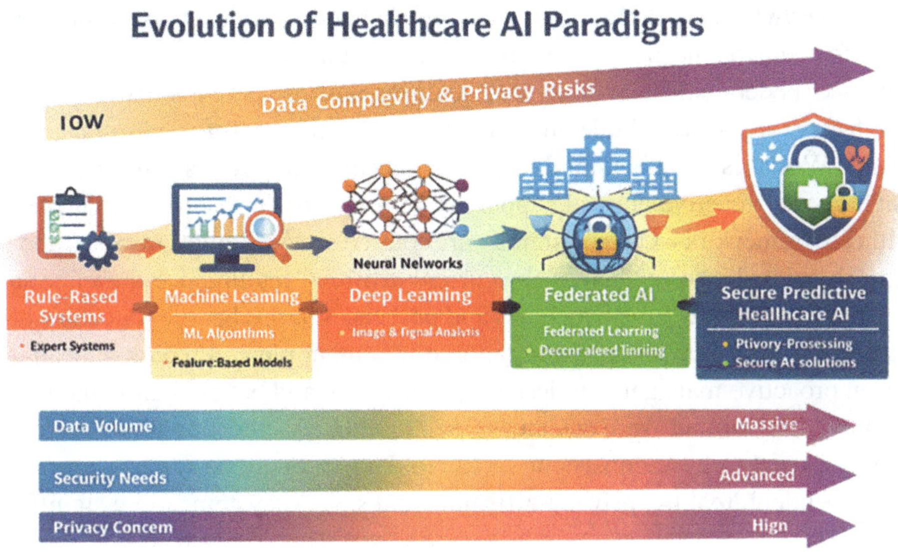

Machine learning (ML) emerged as a major shift towards healthcare intelligence based on data. ML algorithms allowed the systems to infer the patterns based on the past data of the patients and simplified the tasks of disease classification, predicting risks, and analyzing outcomes after treatment. Methods such as the support vector machines, decision trees, and ensemble learning were found to be better in diagnostic accuracy than rule-based methods (Lazaros et al., 2024). Nevertheless, such models tended to rely on well-designed features and central data repositories, which increased the problems of data availability, privacy, and interoperability between healthcare organizations. The next advancement of deep learning (DL) even further reshaped healthcare AI, as it allowed automatical features extraction of complex and high-dimensional data (medical images, physiological signals, and clinical text). CNNs have transformed diagnostics in medical imaging, whereas time-series analysis and clinical natural language processing were improved using recurrent and transformer-based networks. The deep learning systems not only demonstrated better predictive performance in the past but also enhanced the dependence on big-scale centrally stored data and artificial intelligence (AI) systems. This centralization increased the issue of patient data privacy, cybersecurity threats, and regulation.

As a solution to these weaknesses, federated and decentralized learning paradigms in healthcare AI are increasingly taking the place of direct data sharing, and thus allow collaboration of intelligence to occur. With federated AI, multiple institutions can collaboratively train models at the expense of maintaining patient data on a local server, avoiding data sovereignty and limiting exposure to centralized breaches (Edwin Raja, 2025). This is a core change in the design of healthcare AI toward focusing on the preservation of privacy, alignment to regulations, and secure teamwork. Federated AI, with crypto-defenses and protective software architectures, has served as a scalable and reliable base of the next-generation healthcare systems. With this architectural development, healthcare AI has shifted away from being a mostly reactive clinical support system towards predictive and preventive healthcare frameworks. Older systems were centred around symptom-based and past diagnosis-related cases, whereas the current artificial intelligence-driven systems involve the use of real-time data feeds and past cases to predict the trajectory of the disease, early warning signals, and tailored treatment plans. Predictive healthcare helps in proactive management, less hospitalization, and better health outcomes of the population (Zaman Wani & Can, 2025). Nonetheless, this predictive power also makes the need to have consistent access to data and automatic decision-making more dependent, making privacy-affirming and safe AI systems more significant.

Figure 2. Predictive Healthcare Data Ecosystem Architecture

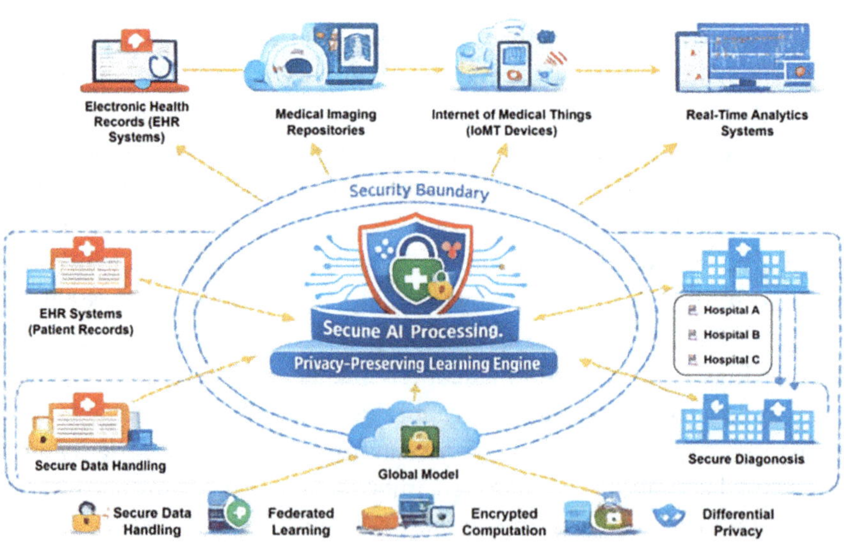

1.2 Data Ecosystem for Predictive Healthcare AI

Predictive healthcare AI systems are inherently data-driven, and they use a wide variety of heterogeneous data sources of high volumes to make clinically meaningful conclusions. The predictive AI models, in contrast to the traditional healthcare analytics, are based on combined structured, semi-structured, and unstructured data on various clinical and operational areas. This data ecosystem is important to understand in order to design safe, privacy-conscious and interoperable healthcare AI architectures. Figure 2 shows a heterogeneous data infrastructure to support predictive healthcare AI by connecting electronic health records, medical image archives, high-frequency IoMT streams, genomic databases, and real-time analytics to the secure processing environment to prevent privacy loss. The architecture focuses on the convergence of various sources of clinical data to a centralized artificial intelligence learning system, and the high security boundaries to ensure sensitive patient data are kept confidential.

Electronic Health Records (EHRs)

The foundation of the predictive healthcare systems is the Electronic Health Records. EHRs include longitudinal data on the patients, which has demographic data, medical history, laboratory reports, medication prescriptions, diagnostic codes and physician notes (Srinivasan et al., 2025). This well-organized and semi-structured information helps machine learning applications to conduct risk stratification, readmission prediction, disease progression analysis, and personalized treatment recommendations. Nevertheless, EHR systems have serious problems concerning data fragmentation, interoperability, and privacy. The healthcare institutions tend to have heterogeneous formats and standards of records, which restrict the ability of one organization to integrate with another. Besides, EHR data is sensitive personally identifiable information, and it will be an easy target of cyberattacks (Zhang & Kamel Boulos, 2022). Predictive models constructed out of EHR data should as such have strong encryption, access control, audit, and privacy preserving learning frameworks to guarantee the secure and compliant use of the system.

Medical Imaging Data

The most common medical imaging data types that are used in the center of the AI-driven diagnostic system are radiology scans (CT, MRI, X-ray), ultrasound images, and pathology slides. Convolutional neural networks and other deep learning models have shown high levels of performance when it comes to identifying abnormalities like tumours, fractures, and other organ abnormalities. Imaging data plays a major role in predictive healthcare as it aids in early detection of the disease and the response to treatment. Imaging data has significant storage, processing and security problems, despite its diagnostic utility. Images with high-resolution demand a lot of storage and computing power, which make the system more complex. Moreover, the imaging metadata can potentially unintentionally reveal the patient identifiers when not anonymized. Secure image transmission, federated learning to distribute training, and secure multi-party computation mechanisms are essential in ensuring that the AI systems based on imaging are not leaked to data and accessed through unauthorized means.

Internet of Medical Things (IoMT)

Internet of medical things refers to wearables, (distant) monitoring, implantable sensors and bedside medical equipment that continuously produce physiological and behavioral data. Through IoMTs, vital signs, which include heart rate, glucose, oxygen saturation and blood pressure, can be monitored in real-time. The AI models used in prediction are based on this streaming data to identify abnormalities, predict negative outcomes and facilitate preventive measures. Nevertheless, IoMT ecosystems make healthcare infrastructures extremely vulnerable to attacks. Most of the devices have ineffective computational capabilities and unreliable security setups, which put them at risk of being spoofed, maliciously modified using firmware, or having stolen access. The decentralized structure of an IoMT data collection process requires edge-processing, lightweight cryptography and secure communication protocols to avoid data interception and manipulation.

Genomic and Omics Data

Omics datasets (genomic data and other) (proteomics, metabolomics, transcriptomics) are becoming more frequently applied to predictive healthcare AI in areas of precision medicine. These multi-dimensional data allow AI to discover genetic risk factors, future drug response, and personalized treatment plans with respect to the biological profile of an individual. Such a potential of genomics, although transformative in personalised healthcare, raises serious privacy concerns. Genetic information is unique to be identified and special to be sensitive because it divulges the information not only in individuals but in their biological relatives as well. The storage of data, sharing, and sophisticated cryptographic measures are needed during the integration of genomic data into AI models. The federated learning and the use of secure computation systems provide feasible solutions to conducting joint genomic studies without data exposure in a centralized location.

Real-Time Analytics and Streaming Data

Real-time analytics are also becoming a significant part of predictive healthcare, with AI systems handling the incoming streams of data (available in real time) provided by clinical devices, mobile health apps, and hospital information systems. The application of AI in real-time allows sepsis alerts and cardiac events detection, as well as emergency triage optimization. This change in the model of batch analytics to streaming intelligence improves patient safety and clinical responsiveness. Nevertheless, predictive systems in real time will be required to work with a high level of strict latency but high security. Data ingestion is also continuous which exposes susceptibility to adversarial manipulation and injection attacks. To keep responsiveness and protection levels high in high-velocity healthcare settings, secure stream processing frameworks, anomaly detection systems, and zero-trust communication paradigms are required. Combined Information Scenario and Protection Consequences.

Integrated Data Landscape and Security Implications

When supported by EHRs, real-time analytics, IoMT, genomics, and imaging, the healthcare data ecosystem is complex and interconnected. As much as this integration is improving the predictive accuracy and clinical insight, it is also improving systemic risk. The heterogeneity of the data, the distributed storage, and collaboration across the institutions necessitate the standardized interoperability protocols and stratified security infrastructure. To ensure the success of predictive healthcare AI, privacy-aware machine learning, secure software engineering, and regulatory-appropriate governance frameworks have to be integrated into data ecosystems during their initial phase. Detailed knowledge of this data landscape can form the basis of creating resilient AI-based medical care systems that can offer reliable forecasts without any loss of patient confidentiality or cybersecurity-based integrity. Table 1 provides the summary of the important, predictive sources of healthcare data and the security issues and mitigation solutions associated with them.

Table 1. Data Sources and Security Implications in Predictive Healthcare AI

Data Source	AI Application	Key Benefits	Privacy Risks	Security Requirements
EHRs	Risk prediction, outcome analysis	Longitudinal insights	Data breach, identity exposure	Encryption, FL, access control
Imaging	Diagnostic support	High diagnostic accuracy	Metadata leakage	Secure aggregation, anonymization
IoMT	Real-time monitoring	Early anomaly detection	Device compromise	Edge security, secure channels
Genomics	Precision medicine	Personalized treatment	Genetic re-identification	SMPC, strong encryption
Streaming Data	Early warning systems	Proactive care	Injection attacks	Secure stream analytics

2. CYBERSECURITY THREAT LANDSCAPE IN HEALTHCARE AI

The adoption of artificial intelligence in healthcare systems has greatly increased the cyber-attack area of the contemporary medical systems. AI-based healthcare services are based on interrelated software blocks, cloud and edge computing tools, and high amounts of sensitive patient information, which render them a desirable target to cyber attackers. In contrast to the traditional healthcare information systems, AI-enabled environments present novel threat actors in connection to information learning, model inference, and automated decision-making, hence requiring a holistic understanding of the dynamic cybersecurity environment (Zhang et al., 2022). Figure 3 explains how multidimensional cybersecurity risks impact healthcare AI systems throughout their lifecycle of operation in a systematic way. The figure presents data-centric, model-centric, system-level, and supply chain threats to every step of the AI pipeline, including data collection and model training and the deployment, inference, and continuous updates, which proves the need to implement layered and lifecycle-conscious security strategies. Data breach and unauthorized access are considered to be among the most serious threats to the healthcare AI systems. The AI models need unlimited access to electronic health records and medical image data banks as well as IoMT device sensor real-time data. Breach of access credentials, unprotected APIs, and improperly setup cloud services can result in massive disclosure of personally identifiable and secured health care information. The breaches do not only affect patient privacy but also cause regulatory compliance with standards including HIPAA and GDPR and lead to legal and financial consequences of healthcare organizations.

Figure 3. Threat Landscape Across AI Lifecycle

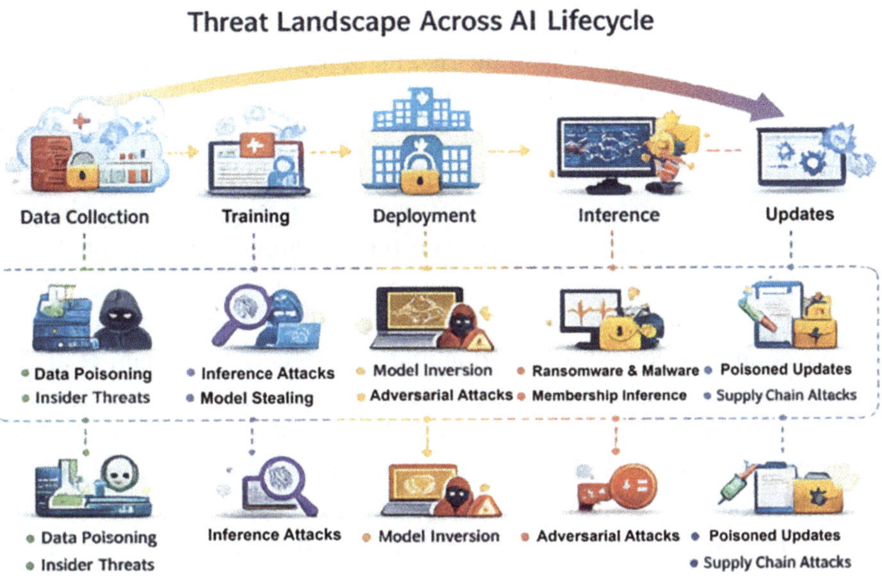

Another significant issue of AI-driven healthcare setting is ransomware and service disruption attacks. Biomedical facilities and clinical networks are becoming a significant target of attackers to encrypt vital information or shut down AI-driven diagnostic and decision-support systems. Because most healthcare AI applications have time-sensitive and mission-critical conditions, the downtime of the system may have a direct effect on patient safety (Akhmetov et al., 2025). The reliance of AI processes on real-time data connectivity increases the impact of ransomware attacks and resilience and quick recovery are both critical design factors. Besides conventional cyber-attacks, machine learning models of healthcare AI are susceptible to adversarial attacks. Attacks targeting AI models and not traditional software vulnerabilities take advantage of the statistical and algorithmic characteristics of AI models. Examples include data poisoning in training models, model inversion attacks that learn sensitive patient data and adversarial examples that use input data to generate wrong clinical predictions. These attacks may manipulate model performance without causing any alarm, or, it may lead to biased results, which are grave threats to clinical decision-making and patient confidence.

The further implementation of IoMT devices and wearable sensors makes the cybersecurity environment even more complex. Such devices are frequently limited in computational resources and heterogeneous protection functions, which frequently allows them to be exploited by compromise of firmware or unauthorized access, and spoofing. Weakened edge devices can be used as portals to larger network attacks or used to feed malicious data into AI pipelines and corrupt subsequent analytics and predictions. The other threat that is arising is insider attacks and supply chain vulnerabilities. In healthcare AI systems, it is the combination of several stakeholders, such as software vendors, cloud service providers and third-party analytics platforms, that develop and maintain them (Akter et al., 2024). Backdoors, biased models, or concealed data exfiltration mechanisms may be brought in by malicious insiders or poisoned software updates. The AI software supply chains are complex enough that it is not an easy task to identify such threats through conventional methods based on a perimeter.

Model explainability and accountability are also of concern because of the interconnection between AI automation and cybersecurity (Ramani et al., 2026). The black box AI models may hide malicious activity, and it is not easy to know whether the error is real or deliberate or whether the model was manipulated by the clinicians and system administrators. Such non-transparency makes it difficult to investigate and analyze an incident and, in that regard, explainable and auditable AI systems in healthcare facilities are crucial. The healthcare AI cybersecurity threat environment is, in general, complex and includes traditional cyberattacks, AI-related vulnerabilities, and systemic risks due to distributed and collaborative computing environments. To overcome these difficulties, there is the need to move away in dealing with such challenges by a move towards responsive security measures to strategic, intelligence-based approaches to defense strategies. The principles of secure software design, privacy-preserving learning systems, continuous monitoring, and quantum-resilient cryptography are the basis of safeguarding AI-enabled healthcare network against both present and future cyber-attacks.

2.1 Threat Taxonomy for Healthcare AI Systems

The novelty and the data-oriented characteristics of AI-based healthcare systems present a broad spectrum of cybersecurity risks that transcends more conventional network and software vulnerabilities. In contrast to traditional healthcare information systems, there is an exposure of AI-enabled environments to attacks, which are not only on infrastructure components but also on the learning processes, model integrity, and the decision outputs. Organized threat taxonomy offers a hierarchical system of thinking about these dangers and devising proper defense measures. Threats of AI in healthcare can be broadly classified into four areas that are interconnected, such as data-centric threats, model-centric threats, system-level threats, and human centric threats. Both categories influence various phases of AI life cycle and have different threats to clinical reliability, patient privacy and operational sustenance.

Data-Centric Threats

Data-centric attacks are those that act on the integrity, confidentiality, and availability of the healthcare data that is used to train and run AI systems. Since predictive healthcare models are based on massive and heterogeneous data volumes, opponents can attempt to hack or steal sensitive patient data (S. Edwin Raja et al., 2025). Data poisoning attacks refer to the practice of poisoning the training data with malicious or compromised data, resulting in biased or corrupting AI predictions. In the medical field, this attack would lead to the classification of diseases or risky evaluation, and this may lead to disastrous clinical judgment. Inferencing and data leakage attacks are trying to rebuild sensitive patient characteristics based on trained models or common updates in federated learning settings. Also illegal data access and loss are still widespread threats, especially in centralized storage systems and insecurely configured cloud systems.

Model-Centric Threats

Machine learning algorithms and trained AI models contain vulnerabilities that are used by model-centric threats. The purpose of such attacks is to tamper with the model behavior, intellectual property theft, or cause wrong clinical results. Adversarial example attacks are attacks on the input data, typically of a medical image or sensor reading, in which the attacker tries to generate incorrect predictions, but makes them look natural to a human observer. The attacks of model inversion and membership inference strive to reconstruct sensitive training information or decide whether certain patient records were utilized in model training (Jagadish Kumar et al., 2025). Model Poisoning and Backdoor attacks have embedded malicious triggers that trigger malicious behavior in certain conditions. Trust, safety, and compliance with regulations are compromised in clinical settings due to these threats.

System-Level Threats

System-level threats are those that attack infrastructure foundations of healthcare AI systems such as networks, servers, edge devices, and software platforms. Such attacks tend to look like the more conventional cybersecurity threats but are made more severe by the connectivity of AI processes. Critical AI-based diagnostic and monitoring systems can get out of commission due to ransomware attacks and interrupt patient care (Gopalakrishnan et al., 2025). Denial-of-service attacks can be distributed across data pipes and real-time analytics, causing impairment of predictive healthcare. Supply chain attacks leverage vulnerabilities in third-party libraries of software, pretrained models or system updates, enabling adversaries to add malicious code to healthcare AI ecosystems.

Human-Centric Threats

Anthropogenic threats include insider attacks, social engineering, and abuse of AI systems. Healthcare settings have a wide variety of stakeholders, such as clinicians, administrators, IT staff as well as external vendors, which leads to a higher incidence of human vulnerabilities (Prabaharan et al., 2025). Insider attacks can be related to deliberate data theft, manipulation of models, or access to privileged users. Attackers can hack AI tools using phishing and credentials compromise and take control of sensitive resources. Also, the misuse or excessive use of AI results may result in unsafe clinical practices, especially when there are no mechanisms of explainability and human oversight.

Integrated Threat Perspective Across the AI Lifecycle

These category of threats are interrelated throughout the AI lifecycle, covering data acquisition, model training, deployment, and continuous updates. As an example, a poisoned data can be introduced into loading pipelines using compromised IoMT devices, whereas the use of insecure model update mechanisms can be used to facilitate adversarial manipulation in federated learning. This realization of interdependencies is critical to the formulation of layered security strategies capable of safeguarding the technical as well as the human aspects of healthcare AI systems. Table 2 describes significant data-oriented, model-oriented, system-level, and human-oriented threats in healthcare AI settings.

Table 2. Threat Taxonomy for Healthcare AI Systems

Threat Category	Attack Type	Targeted Component	Potential Impact	Example Scenario
Data-centric	Data poisoning	Training datasets	Misdiagnosis	Injected false labels
Data-centric	Inference attacks	Model outputs	Privacy breach	Patient attribute recovery
Model-centric	Adversarial inputs	Inference stage	Incorrect prediction	Manipulated medical images
Model-centric	Backdoor attacks	Model behavior	Hidden malicious actions	Trigger-based misclassification
System-level	Ransomware	AI platforms	Service disruption	Hospital AI shutdown
System-level	Supply chain attack	Software updates	System compromise	Malicious library

continued on following page

Table 2. Continued

Threat Category	Attack Type	Targeted Component	Potential Impact	Example Scenario
Human-centric	Insider misuse	Data/models	Leakage or bias	Unauthorized data access
Human-centric	Phishing	Credentials	System takeover	Compromised admin account

3. SECURE SOFTWARE PRACTICES FOR HEALTHCARE AI APPLICATIONS

The creation of AI-powered healthcare solutions and their implementation require stringent safe software standards as they are safety-controlling and have a direct effect on patient outcomes. As opposed to traditional software systems, healthcare AI applications work in dynamic settings where models are constantly improved, data sources are updated, and clinical diagnosis and treatment can be affected by a decision. As a result, security needs to be implemented throughout the software lifecycle and not as a secondary concern. This integrated secure architecture that is suggested to be adopted in predictive healthcare AI systems is shown in Figure 4 and represents a multi-layered system that includes data management, AI learning, cybersecurity defense, and governance layers. The architecture shows that privacy-preserving learning systems, encryption, network security, and controlled regulatory compliance are elements of the defense in depth approach to enable trustful, resilient, and compliant healthcare AI services. Security-by-design is a major principle of AI development in the field of healthcare, where mechanisms of protection are implemented at the very beginning of system organization and requirements analysis. Threat modeling is a phase in secure design in which AI-specific threats, including data poisoning and model extraction, are explicitly taken into consideration in addition to more conventional software risks. This solution is proactive and allows developers to foresee the possible attack vectors and provide adequate protection when deploying systems.

The key aspects of healthcare AI software practices are secure data handling and access control. AI applications handle sensitive patient data on a regular basis and therefore, effective authentication, authorization and identity management is necessary. Role-based and attribute-based access control systems also contribute to the satisfaction of the situation, where clinicians, administrators, and AI services can only interact with the data within their privileges. Also, it is important to encrypt both data at rest and in transit to avoid unauthorized disclosure on cloud, edge and on-premise environments (Almogadwy & Alqarafi, 2025). Another important security issue is the software supply chain. The healthcare AI systems usually rely on the libraries, pretrained models, and cloud-based services of third parties. Weaknesses in one of the elements may jeopardize the security of the whole system. Secure software practices are thus focused on checking the provenance of codes, auditing dependencies, and integrity verification of AI models before deployment. Persistent integration and persistent deployment (CI/CD) pipes would need to encompass automated security checks, statical code testing, as well as vulnerability testing, to minimize the risk of malicious or incompetent elements being introduced. Since AI models are adaptive, secure model lifecycle management is a requirement. The training, validation, deployment and updates of any model should be highly monitored to ensure it is not modified or its performance is compromised by unqualified personnel. The model integrity is maintained with the help of version control mechanisms, cryptographic model signing and access-controlled update processes. Furthermore, secure log and audit tracks provide a traceability of model behavior helping to support forensic and regulatory compliance.

Figure 4. Secure Layered Healthcare AI Architecture

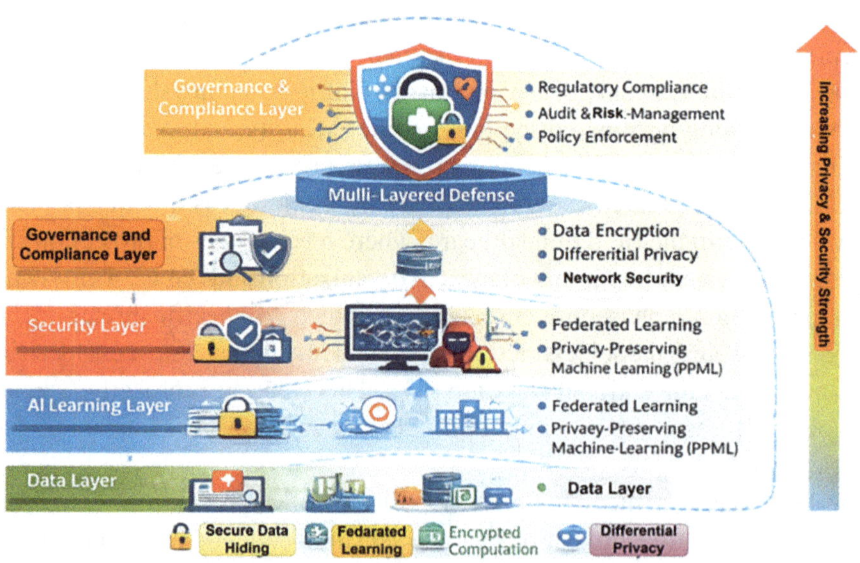

Both explainability and transparency are also vital in safe healthcare AI software. Anomalies in security breaches or adversarial manipulation may be hidden by black-box models, which is challenging to identify in this model. It is possible to integrate explainable AI methods into software processes to enable clinicians and system administrators to track model reasoning and detect deviations (Arikumar et al., 2022). This openness will improve confidence and facilitate human supervision of AI-assisted clinical decision-making. Fault tolerance and resilience are other equally important issues in secure software practice. The AI application in healthcare should not be disrupted in case of partial system malfunction or cyberattack. Unplanned back-up architectures, secure system of failover, and real time monitoring systems are some of the factors that lead to continuity in operations. To reduce the security incident impact, automated alerts, and controlled shutdown procedures are needed to aid in incident response to avoid harm and guarantee patient safety. Lastly, healthcare AI secure software development should be in line with regulatory and ethical mandates. The adherence to the standards of healthcare data protection requires a thorough documentation, risk evaluation and verification of AI behavior. It can be achieved through secure coding standards, privacy impact assessment, and frequent security audits that would allow organizations to demonstrate accountability and promote responsible and ethical AI implementation.

3.1 Secure AI Healthcare Architecture Layers

Secure AI-based healthcare system design needs to be developed as a layered architecture incorporating privacy, cybersecurity, and governance throughout the entire data and model lifecycle. Instead of the separate security controls, newer healthcare AI systems use multi-layered structures that are guaranteed to provide defense-in-depth, resilience, and regulatory conformity. All these architectural layers are based on the principles of predictive healthcare services as well as exposure to cyber threats and privacy violations.

Data Layer

The cornerstone of the healthcare AI systems is the data layer that can store, access, process, and collect data related to a wide variety of sources, including electronic health records, medical imaging archives, IoMT feeds, and genomic databases. Since healthcare data is sensitive and voluminous, this layer should have good encryption systems of data both at rest and in transit. Differential privacy and anonymization are privacy-preservation methods that are becoming popular in order to minimize the likelihood of patient re-identification without compromising the utility of the analysis. The policies of secure data access, role-based control, and continuous auditing are crucial to avoiding unauthorized data exposure. Secure data pipelines used in predictive healthcare settings where real-time analytics cannot afford delayed data ingestion have to strike a balance between the need to be fast and the need to be seriously secure.

AI Layer

The AI layer encompasses machine learning model training, validation, deployment, and inference processes. This layer is particularly vulnerable to adversarial attacks, model theft, and integrity compromise. To support secure and collaborative healthcare intelligence, the AI layer incorporates privacy-preserving learning mechanisms such as federated learning and secure multi-party computation. These techniques facilitate distributed model development while reducing direct exposure of sensitive patient data; a detailed discussion of these approaches is provided in Section 4. Cryptographic model signing, version control, and controlled update mechanisms are employed to maintain model lifecycle security and integrity. In addition, explainable AI tools are integrated to enhance transparency and detect abnormal behavior resulting from adversarial manipulation or model drift. Collectively, these measures help ensure that predictive healthcare models remain accurate, reliable, and trustworthy throughout their operational lifecycle.

Security Layer

The security layer gives cross-cutting level of protections that cut across network communications, system monitoring, identity management and threat detection. The use of zero-trust network architecture is being required to guarantee that each access request is constantly authenticated and approved no matter its source (Vinoth Kumar et al., 2025). Strong cryptographic forms of communication ensure information channels among the cloud-computing environment, peripheral devices, and health facilities. Intrusion detection systems that are enhanced by AI run within this layer to detect new cyber threats as they appear. Hardware-supported security offers, including trusted execution environments (and secure enclaves) provide further protection of sensitive computational beings and cryptographic operations against compromised system components. The ability of these security layers to enhance the overall system resilience to traditional and AI-based cyberattacks.

Governance and Compliance Layer

The governance layer allows to make sure that healthcare AI systems are used in accordance with the regulatory requirements, ethical principles and organizational policies. This layer includes audit history, consent management policy, compliance check functionality, and policy execution engines. Audit systems based on blockchain are actively considered in order to present unalterable data about the access of data, some changes in the model, and the events of clinical decisions. Automated compliance monitoring solutions allow one to evaluate the behavior of the system on a continuous basis against regulatory requirements like data protection and accountability requirements. With an integrated system architecture, healthcare organizations can minimize operational risk and encourage transparency and trust among stakeholders by integrating governance directly into the system architecture. The functional roles and protection measures of every layer of the proposed secure healthcare AI architecture are summarized in Table 3.

Table 3. Secure Architecture Components for Healthcare AI Systems

Layer	Primary Function	Key Security Mechanisms
Data	Storage and processing	Encryption, differential privacy, access control
AI	Learning and inference	Federated learning, SMPC, model signing
Network/Security	Communication and defense	Zero-trust architecture, intrusion detection
Governance	Compliance and accountability	Audit trails, policy enforcement

3.2 DevSecOps for Healthcare AI Systems

The changing and dynamic aspects of AI-based healthcare applications require ongoing development, deployment and monitoring practices that integrate security across the software lifecycle. DevSecOps is the continuation of the original DevOps practices, with the security mechanisms incorporated directly into the development pipelines to make them proactive and not reactive.

Secure Continuous Integration and Deployment

CI pipelines in healthcare AI systems need to include automated security testing, such as, but not limited to, static and dynamic code analysis, vulnerability scanning, dependency integrity checks. Pretrained models and third party libraries are heavily checked prior to incorporation to reduce the risks of the supply chain. The continuous deployment mechanisms impose cryptographic validation of model artifacts and software update which bar unauthorized software alteration and rollback attacks.

Model Verification and Validation

The machine-based AI used in clinical scenarios should be continuously tested to allow it to be reliable, fair, and resist adversarial manipulation. Some of the verification procedures are performance benchmarking on a wide range of patient populations, adversarial robustness testing, and audit-based explainability. Secure version control and cryptographic integrity checks also help to make sure that only authenticated models are implemented in production environments.

Continuous Risk Assessment and Monitoring

DevSecOps systems enable real-time risk evaluation via constant monitoring of systems, anomaly detection, and automated incident response systems. Network, device, and AI security telemetry are examined to detect new threats and vulnerabilities in a system (Prabaharan et al., 2025). Feedback loops also enable the quick remediation and adaptive defense mechanisms such that AI systems in healthcare are resilient to the changes in cyber threats.

4. PRIVACY-PRESERVING MACHINE LEARNING APPROACHES

Privacy-preserving machine learning (PPML) has become a key facilitator of AI-enabled healthcare systems, resolving the inherent conflict between patient confidentiality and data utility in healthcare systems. To implement AI applications in healthcare, it generally needs large datasets which are diverse to attain a high level of clinical performance, but regulatory limits and ethical standards restrict centralised gathering of sensitive patient data. The aim of PPML methods is to balance this issue by facilitating the joint construction of models without exposing raw data too much. Federated learning, differential privacy and secure multi-party computation are among the leading PPML methods in the medical field. These methods uphold decentralized education and regulated information dissemination and mathematically based guarantees of privacy, and are therefore effectively applicable within a clinical context with several institutions, heterogeneous data, and stringent compliance demands.

4.1 Federated Learning

Federated learning is a decentralized machine learning framework where the models are trained on a large-scale data without the actual data being transferred to a central repository. This system can be used in healthcare to train AI models collaboratively between hospitals, clinics, and research institutions without losing local access to patient data. All the sites involved receive and compute updates in their respective models based on their own data, and only aggregated parameters or gradients are exchanged with an aggregating server or distributed aggregation mechanism. The main benefit of federated learning is that it minimizes privacy risks of having a centralized approach to data storage. The federated learning will be intrinsically linked to data protection rules and organizational policies by maintaining patient records within the four institutional boundaries. The paradigm is especially useful in cases where data heterogeneity between institutions is typical like medical image analysis, disease risk prediction and health modelling of populations on a population level (Alghamdi et al., 2022). Federated learning opens up security and system-level issues, although its advantages exist. Inference attacks still have the potential to leak sensitive information on the model updates and malicious users can use poisoned updates in order to control the global model. Secure aggregation mechanisms, authentication of participants, and anomalies detection mechanisms are thus important parts of federated healthcare AI systems. Federated learning provides a privacy-conscious and scalable basis to joint medical intelligence, when combined with secure software practices and explainable AI technology.

4.2 Differential Privacy

Differential privacy offers a mathematically sound model of the privacy risk measured and constrained by the use of data-based algorithms. Differential privacy methods used in healthcare AI add noise to the data, model parameters or query results in a controlled amount to guarantee that the input of each patient is indistinguishable. This is to ensure that sensitive patient information cannot be deduced even when there is the knowledge that is supporting. Practically, it is possible to implement differential privacy during multiple processes of the machine learning pipeline, such as data preprocessing, training the model, and sharing the results. The trade-off between data utility and privacy protection is balanced by privacy budgets which allows system designers to customize privacy guarantees to particular clinical applications (Kodete et al., 2024). Differentially private models are especially useful in large-scale analytics, epidemiological research and distribution of clinical research, when aggregate information is more valuable than individual-level predictions. Nevertheless, the implementation of the concept of differential privacy in healthcare AI must be done with a close possibility of considering the effects on the model accuracy and clinical reliability. Too much noise may impair predictive performance, particularly when the data are too few or high-dimensional medical data. Practices in secure software, modifiable privacy and domain specific tuning are thus required to make sure that privacy protection does not affect clinical decision support.

4.3 Secure Multi-Party Computation

Secure multi-party computation (SMPC) allows multiple parties to collectively compute a function using personalized inputs and guarantees that no party obtains additional information than the end result. SMPC In healthcare AI, SMPC enables institutions to utilize machine learning models in a collaborative manner, and withholding sensitive patient information or intermediate calculations. This is especially useful in cross-organizational partnerships, including multi-center clinical research and national health analytics programmes (Umer et al., 2025). SMPC methods are based on cryptographic schemes that divide information into coded sections that are shared among the involved parties. These shares are calculated in a manner that maintains accuracy and at the same time the data is not disclosed. In healthcare AI, SMPC aids in training, inference, and validation of a secure model when geographically dispersed and mutually untrusted parties with each other. Despite providing excellent privacy guarantees, SMPC creates computational and communication overheads that may impair scalability and real-time performance. The optimization of cryptographics, hybrid PPML models and hardware-assisted security are being used to address such shortcomings. In conjunction with federated learning and differential privacy, SMPC will serve as a part of a multi-layered defense strategy that will improve the overall security and trust of AI-driven healthcare systems.

4.4 Integrated Privacy-Preserving Learning for Healthcare

As opposed to using one approach, the current healthcare AI technology is becoming more and more dependent on hybrid privacy-protecting models based on federated learning, differential privacy, and secure multi-party computation. These kinds of integrated measures offer dual protection against data leaks and adversarial inference as well as insider threats. With the incorporation of the techniques into the safe software architecture and regulatory-conformant workflows, healthcare institutions will be able to promote collaborative AI innovation without compromising patient trust and data ownership.

5. EXPLAINABLE AND TRUSTWORTHY AI IN CLINICAL SETTINGS

With the advent of artificial intelligence into clinical processes, explainability and trustworthiness have become a major safety and effectiveness concern of effective healthcare AI systems. In contrast to consumer-focused AI applications, clinical decision-making is performed in conditions of high stakes, in which obscure or insufficiently comprehended model outputs might result in severe repercussions in patient care. The need to have explainable and trustworthy AI frameworks is therefore necessary to make sure that clinicians can interpret, validate, and take suitable action by AI-generated insights. Explainable AI (XAI) describes practices and systems-level mechanisms that allow exploration of the rationale and decision making of AI models by humans. Explainability in healthcare enhances transparency, accountability and regulatory compliance by allowing clinicians to determine whether AI recommendations are in line with medical knowledge and patient context. Diagnostic systems, risk prediction tools and treatment recommendation engines are especially interested in model interpretability since the clinician must be able to justify the decisions, and understanding the ultimate responsibility of a patient outcome is essential. Clinical AI systems cannot be trusted based solely on the accuracy of the model, reliability, and consistency of behavior in different patient groups. AI systems with unpredictable performance, biased results, or based on sensitivity to small input differences can cause a loss in clinician confidence. Explainability mechanisms can be used to show the possible sources of bias or error, enabling medical practitioners to understand the constraints and use suitable clinical judgment when working with AI-assisted tools.

The collaboration between humans and AI is very important to create trust in a clinical setting. Instead of substituting clinicians, AI systems are also being developed to supplement human skills with decision support, risk stratification, and pattern recognition options. Good collaboration needs to have intuitive user interfaces, explicit display of uncertainty, and clinician feedback and override mechanisms (Ikegwu et al., 2026). Explainable AI allows this collaborative paradigm through explaining complex model behavior with clinically meaningful explanations that do not disrupt the present workflow. In terms of cybersecurity, explainability also increases system resilience and threat detection. The use of transparent AI models to detect anomalous behavior caused by adversarial manipulation, data poisoning, or model drift makes it easy to detect such behavior. As clinicians and system administrators will be able to view and analyze AI decision paths, the anomalies in decision-making are easier to identify and enable quicker incident management and case investigation. The further condition of trustful AI in healthcare relies on governance, validation, and unceasing monitoring practices. To be fair and generalize well, clinical AI systems need to be tested on various different datasets. It is important to monitor performance levelling off, the development of biases, or security violation during the post-deployment period. Accountability is facilitated with explainability tools along with secure logging and audit trail, as they allow tracing AI decisions and system updates. Explainability and trust of healthcare AI can never be considered without ethical considerations. Transparency contributes to the promotion of informed consent, patient autonomy, and fair care, as proper

AI-driven choices do not favor certain demographic groups. The explainable models also allow one to meet regulatory requirements that require the justification and documentation of the automated decision-making processes.

6. QUANTUM-RESILIENT AND EMERGING CYBERSECURITY TECHNOLOGIES

The fast development of computational abilities and cryptographic studies is transforming the cybersecurity domain of AI-based healthcare systems. Although the traditional encryption and security systems are sufficient to provide sufficient security now, with the advent of quantum computing, a threat looms large on the broadly used encryption primitives. Because of the sensitivity of patient data and long-term medical records, the healthcare AI systems have to believe in looking into the future to implement security measures that will be resistant to both classical and quantum-enabled hackers. Quantum-resilient or post-quantum cybersecurity systems are implemented to resist attack by quantum computers with capability to break classic public-key cryptographic systems. The technologies are especially applicable in the healthcare AI settings because medical data has a longer life cycle, retention requirements are imposed by regulation, and data confidentiality must be sustained. Migration to quantum-resilient cryptography is becoming a proactive security measure strongly aimed at ensuring security in the long term and not reactive to future threats. In addition to post-quantum cryptography, there are a number of new technologies that are changing the security principles of AI-enabled healthcare systems. The security frameworks that are based on blockchains are decentralized trust, tamper resistance, and transparent auditability, so they are applicable to securing data sharing, model provenance, and access control in collaborative healthcare ecosystems (Kumar et al., 2025). Combining blockchain mechanisms with AI processes can be used to improve accountability through an immutable registration of model updates, data accesses, and clinical decision traces.

Edge and fog computing architectures are also gaining prominence as healthcare AI applications move closer to data sources such as wearable devices, bedside monitors, and IoMT sensors. By processing data locally or near the point of collection, edge-based AI reduces latency and limits the exposure of sensitive information. However, this decentralization introduces new security challenges related to device authentication, secure model deployment, and distributed trust management. Emerging security frameworks address these challenges through lightweight cryptography, hardware-assisted security, and secure orchestration of AI services across heterogeneous environments. Another promising direction involves hardware-backed security mechanisms, including trusted execution environments and secure enclaves.

These technologies isolate sensitive computations, such as model inference and cryptographic operations, from potentially compromised system components. In healthcare AI, hardware-assisted security can protect both patient data and proprietary models, reducing the risk of insider attacks and model extraction. The convergence of AI and cybersecurity has also led to the development of AI-enhanced defense mechanisms. Intelligent intrusion detection systems, adaptive threat monitoring, and automated incident response tools leverage machine learning to identify anomalies and evolving attack patterns in real time. When combined with explainable AI techniques, these systems provide actionable security insights while maintaining transparency and trust. Adopting quantum-resilient and emerging cybersecurity technologies requires careful consideration of interoperability, performance overhead, and regulatory compliance. Healthcare organizations must balance security enhancements with system usability, clinical efficiency, and ethical responsibilities. Incremental integration strategies, hybrid cryptographic frameworks, and continuous risk assessment are essential to ensure a smooth transition toward future-proof healthcare AI infrastructures.

7. PERFORMANCE EVALUATION METRICS FOR SECURE PREDICTIVE HEALTHCARE AI SYSTEMS

The assessment of the secure and privacy-friendly predictive healthcare AI systems needs to be conducted within the multi-dimensional performance framework, which would consider clinical accuracy, privacy/utility trade-offs, computational efficiency, and cybersecurity resilience. Healthcare AI systems have to strike a balance between predictive accuracy and high privacy requirements and resistance to changing cyber threats, unlike traditional AI systems, where the system solely needs to be accurate. This part of the work provides the essential assessment measures backed by performance visualization in the style of experiments to illustrate the practical impact of secure AI design.

7.1 Predictive Accuracy Under Federated Collaboration

The most common clinical performance metric of the healthcare AI systems is predictive accuracy, which has a direct effect on the outcomes of the diagnostic tests and treatment. Federated learning in privacy preserving collaborative learning allows group collaboration between multiple healthcare institutions to train predictive models without distributing raw patient data. As it is shown in Figure 5, the accuracy of the model is growing gradually as more healthcare institutions are involved. This makes the combination of varied patient groups create a higher level of data heterogeneity and generalization ability, which results in significant gains in the capability of predictive performance. This proves that, in addition to maintaining the privacy of patients, decentralized learning architectures lead to higher clinical accuracy than single-institution models. The given trend proves that privacy-conscious collaboration does not undermine the effectiveness of healthcare AI. Federated intelligence, instead, facilitates knowledge exchange between organizations with scalability and security to make it a realistic basis of large-scale predictive healthcare systems.

Figure 5. Model Accuracy Improvement with Federated Collaboration

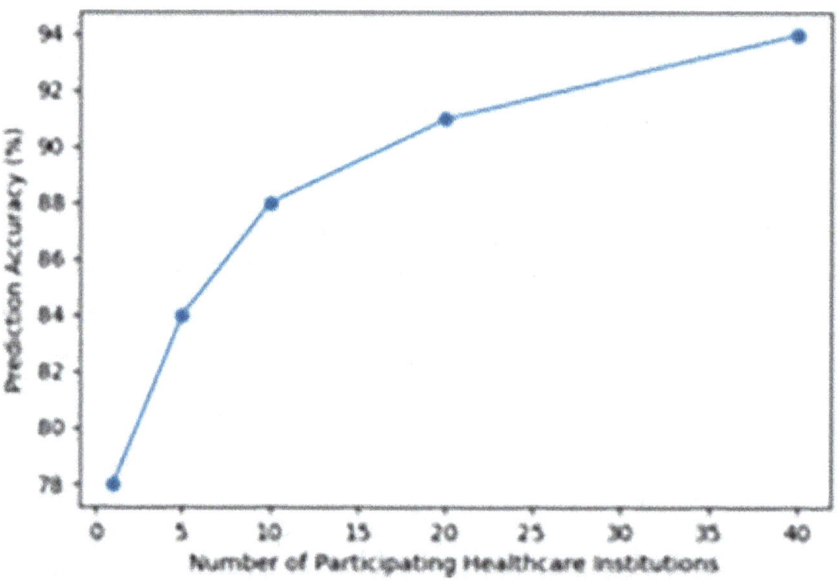

Figure 6. Privacy vs Accuracy Trade-off in Differentially Private Healthcare AI

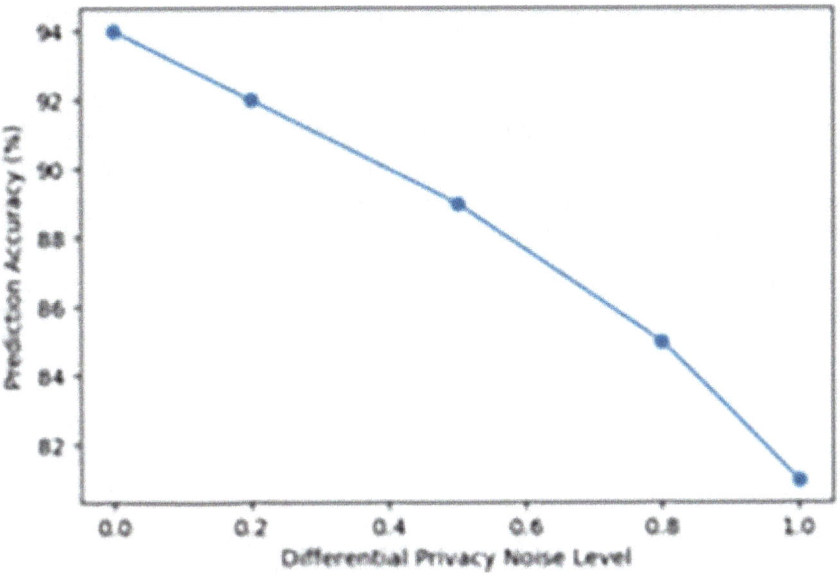

Privacy–Accuracy Trade-off in Differentially Private Learning

Privacy preservation introduces inherent trade-offs between data confidentiality and predictive utility. Differential privacy mechanisms strengthen patient data protection by injecting controlled noise into training processes or model outputs. However, excessive noise can degrade learning performance. Figure 6 depicts the relationship between increasing differential privacy noise levels and predictive accuracy. As privacy strength intensifies, a gradual decline in model performance is observed. This trade-off highlights the necessity of carefully calibrated privacy budgets tailored to clinical risk sensitivity. In safety-critical healthcare contexts, adaptive privacy mechanisms are essential to ensure that confidentiality enhancements do not undermine diagnostic reliability. These findings emphasize that privacy-aware healthcare AI must employ dynamic optimization strategies that balance regulatory compliance with clinical effectiveness.

Computational Latency Across Security Mechanisms

Operational efficiency is a critical requirement for predictive healthcare systems, particularly in real-time clinical environments such as emergency care and continuous patient monitoring. Privacy-preserving security mechanisms introduce varying degrees of computational overhead that influence system responsiveness. The comparative latency analysis presented in Figure 7 reveals that centralized AI systems exhibit minimal processing delay but lack strong privacy protections. Federated learning introduces moderate latency due to distributed model aggregation and communication costs, while secure multi-party computation incurs significantly higher overhead resulting from cryptographic operations. These results demonstrate that stronger privacy guarantees often require increased computational resources. Consequently, hybrid security architectures that selectively combine federated learning with lightweight cryptographic protections offer a practical balance between real-time clinical usability and robust data protection.

Figure 7. Performance–security trade-off

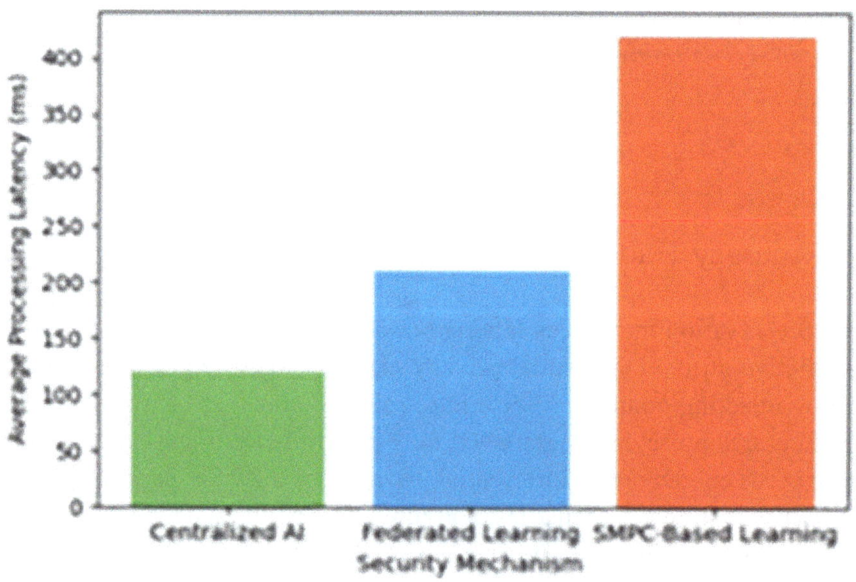

Cybersecurity Robustness Through Layered Defense Architectures

Cyber resilience is a foundational requirement for AI-driven healthcare infrastructures due to the prevalence of data breaches, ransomware, and adversarial attacks. Isolated security controls are insufficient in protecting complex AI ecosystems, necessitating multi-layered defense strategies. Figure 8 illustrates the impact of progressively integrating multiple security layers on attack success rates. A single security layer results in high vulnerability, whereas each additional layer—encompassing secure data handling, privacy-preserving learning, network protection, and governance mechanisms—dramatically reduces successful attack probability. Near-complete threat mitigation is achieved when comprehensive defense-in-depth architectures are implemented. This performance trend validates the effectiveness of layered cybersecurity frameworks for protecting predictive healthcare AI systems. It further reinforces the need for holistic security integration rather than reliance on isolated cryptographic or network-based controls.

Figure 8. Attack Resistance vs Layered Security Architecture

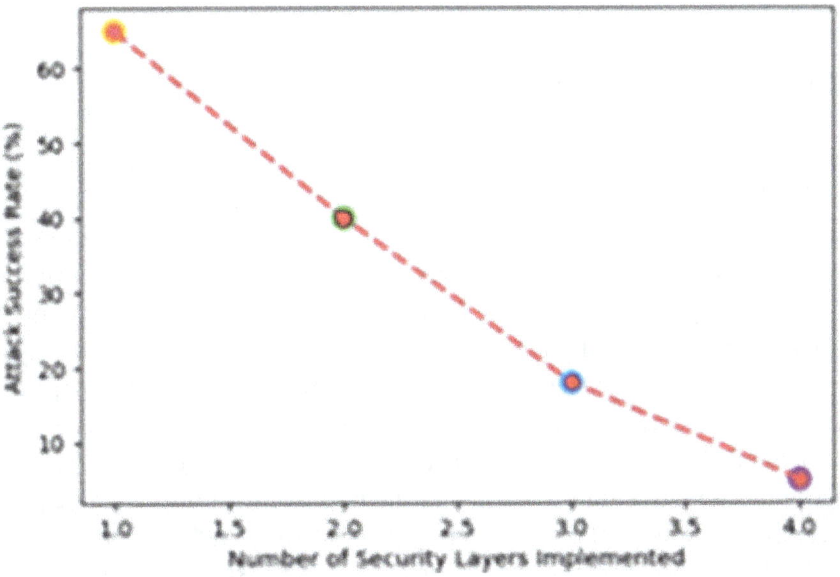

Collectively, these performance metrics provide a comprehensive evaluation framework for secure predictive healthcare AI systems. Federated collaboration enhances predictive accuracy while preserving data privacy, differential privacy introduces manageable performance trade-offs, layered security architectures significantly strengthen cyber resilience, and computational overhead varies according to privacy strength. The results underscore that secure healthcare AI design is inherently a multi-objective optimization problem, requiring careful balancing of clinical reliability, privacy protection, operational efficiency, and cybersecurity robustness. Future healthcare AI platforms must incorporate adaptive security mechanisms capable of dynamically adjusting system parameters in response to evolving clinical demands and threat landscapes.

The practical value of secure and privacy-preserving healthcare AI extends beyond theoretical frameworks and is increasingly demonstrated through real-world clinical deployments. One prominent application involves collaborative disease prediction across multiple hospitals, where federated learning enables institutions to jointly develop predictive models without exchanging raw patient data (Timofte et al., 2024). Such approaches improve model generalization by leveraging diverse patient populations while maintaining compliance with data protection requirements. Similar privacy-preserving strategies have been adopted in medical imaging applications, where distributed learning frameworks support the development of diagnostic models using multi-institutional imaging datasets while protecting sensitive patient information. In these settings, secure software practices, authenticated model deployment, and explainable AI mechanisms contribute to model integrity, transparency, and clinician trust.

Methodological Basis of Performance Visualizations

The performance visualizations presented in Figures 5–8 are intended to provide conceptual and literature-informed illustrations of key performance trends observed in secure predictive healthcare AI systems. Rather than representing results from a single experimental dataset, these figures were developed based on commonly reported relationships and performance characteristics described in prior studies on federated learning, differential privacy, secure multi-party computation, and layered cybersecurity architectures. The visualizations are therefore used to support the analytical discussion of trade-offs among predictive accuracy, privacy preservation, computational efficiency, and cybersecurity robustness. The figures are designed to highlight representative trends, including the improvement of predictive performance through federated collaboration, the privacy–utility trade-off introduced by differential privacy mechanisms, the latency overhead associated with advanced security techniques, and the effectiveness of layered defense strategies in reducing attack success rates. These conceptual visualizations provide an intuitive framework for understanding the interactions among security, privacy, and performance considerations in healthcare AI environments.

Practical Deployment Challenges and Implementation Constraints

Despite significant advances in privacy-preserving and secure healthcare AI, several practical challenges continue to limit large-scale deployment. One major issue is interoperability across heterogeneous healthcare infrastructures. Hospitals and healthcare organizations frequently use different electronic health record formats, data standards, communication protocols, and security policies. These inconsistencies complicate data integration, model portability, and collaborative AI deployment, often resulting in increased implementation costs and operational complexity. Another important limitation concerns the scalability of secure multi-party computation (SMPC). Although SMPC provides strong privacy guarantees, its computational and communication overhead can become substantial as the number of participating institutions, model parameters, and data volumes increase. In large-scale predictive healthcare environments, these overheads may affect system responsiveness and limit real-time clinical applicability. Future research should therefore focus on lightweight cryptographic protocols, hybrid privacy-preserving frameworks, and hardware-assisted acceleration techniques to improve scalability.

Governance and coordination challenges also emerge in multi-institution federated learning ecosystems. Participating organizations may differ in regulatory obligations, data governance policies, resource availability, and trust assumptions. Establishing common protocols for model updates, auditability, accountability, and dispute resolution can be difficult, particularly in cross-border healthcare collaborations. Furthermore, variations in data quality and patient demographics may introduce biases that affect model fairness and generalizability. These challenges highlight that successful deployment of secure healthcare AI requires not only technical innovation but also effective governance structures, interoperability standards, and collaborative operational frameworks. Addressing these practical constraints will be essential for achieving scalable, trustworthy, and sustainable healthcare AI ecosystems.

8. CASE STUDIES AND REAL-WORLD HEALTHCARE APPLICATIONS

Healthcare organizations are also employing AI-driven cybersecurity solutions to protect increasingly complex digital infrastructures. Intelligent intrusion detection systems analyze network traffic, system logs, and behavioral patterns to identify ransomware, insider threats, and other cyberattacks in real time. In parallel, remote patient monitoring platforms integrating wearable devices and IoMT technologies leverage AI-based analytics for early anomaly detection and personalized healthcare interventions. These distributed environments require secure communication protocols, device authentication, lightweight cryptographic mechanisms, and privacy-preserving learning techniques to ensure both operational resilience and patient confidentiality. Another important deployment scenario involves blockchain-enabled healthcare ecosystems that facilitate secure data sharing among hospitals, researchers, and technology providers. Blockchain technologies provide decentralized trust, immutable audit trails, and transparent access control mechanisms, while integration with federated learning and secure computation frameworks enhances accountability across the AI lifecycle. Collectively, these real-world implementations demonstrate that successful healthcare AI deployment requires a balanced combination of privacy-preserving learning, secure software engineering, explainable AI, and continuous cybersecurity monitoring. Key lessons from these deployments indicate that security mechanisms must be aligned with clinical workflows, hybrid defense strategies provide greater resilience than isolated protections, and sustained trust depends on ongoing validation, monitoring, and stakeholder engagement.

9. CONCLUSION

The introduction of artificial intelligence into health management can revolutionize clinical decision-making, patient monitoring, and efficiency. Nevertheless, this change brings about important issues of data privacy, cybersecurity, and trustworthiness of the system. The necessity of the robust, privacy-preserving, and secure design frameworks is becoming more important as the systems of AI in healthcare become increasingly interconnected and data-driven. The chapter has provided an extensive discussion of privacy-preservation and secure AI-based healthcare systems with a focus on how federated learning, differential privacy, secure multi-party computation, and sophisticated cybersecurity frameworks intersect. Secure software practice, explainable AI and human-centered system design were mentioned as key elements in facilitating trustworthy AI use in clinical settings. The discussion has shown that security and privacy are not minor issues but core necessities of the responsible and sustainable healthcare AI system. Quantum resistant cryptography and blockchain based trust systems and edge conscious security structures were also discussed as future-proof solutions that can handle emerging cyber threats. The chapter demonstrated how these technologies can be successfully combined to secure the sensitive healthcare information and facilitate collaborative and scalable AI innovation through real-world case studies. Finally, the AI implementation in healthcare requires a comprehensive mode, which integrates the technological innovation and ethical accountability, regulatory adjustment, and human fidelity. Introducing privacy and security on all levels of the AI lifecycle can help healthcare organizations to realize all the benefits of intelligent systems and preserve the rights of patients and clinical integrity. This chapter will also be useful as a basic source of guide to researchers, practitioners, and policymakers to construct robust, transparent, and privacy-conscious AI-driven healthcare systems of the future.

From a broader perspective, the chapter contributes a unified architectural framework that integrates privacy-preserving machine learning, secure software engineering, explainable AI, governance mechanisms, and emerging quantum-resilient cybersecurity technologies within predictive healthcare environments. The discussion demonstrates that the design of future healthcare AI systems should be viewed as a multi-objective optimization problem that simultaneously balances predictive accuracy, patient privacy, cybersecurity resilience, regulatory compliance, and operational efficiency. Looking ahead, the convergence of federated intelligence, trustworthy AI, adaptive cybersecurity, and interoperable healthcare infrastructures will play a pivotal role in shaping next-generation digital health ecosystems. Establishing secure, transparent, and collaborative AI frameworks will be essential for enabling scalable healthcare innovation while preserving patient trust, clinical integrity, and long-term system sustainability.

REFERENCES

Akhmetov, A., Latif, Z., Tyler, B., & Yazici, A. (2025). Enhancing healthcare data privacy and interoperability with federated learning. *PeerJ. Computer Science*, *11*, e2870. DOI: 10.7717/peerj-cs.2870 PMID: 40567682

Akter, M., Moustafa, N., & Turnbull, B. (2024). SPEI-FL: Serverless privacy edge intelligence-enabled federated learning in smart healthcare systems. *Cognitive Computation*, *16*(5), 2626–2641. DOI: 10.1007/s12559-024-10310-3

Alghamdi, A., Zhu, J., Yin, G., Shorfuzzaman, M., Alsufyani, N., Alyami, S., & Biswas, S. (2022). Blockchain Empowered Federated Learning Ecosystem for Securing Consumer IoT Features. *Analysis & Sensing*, *22*(18), 6786. Advance online publication. DOI: 10.3390/s22186786 PMID: 36146134

Almogadwy, B., & Alqarafi, A. (2025). Fused federated learning framework for secure and decentralized patient monitoring in healthcare 5.0 using IoMT. *Scientific Reports*, *15*(1), 24263. DOI: 10.1038/s41598-025-06574-w PMID: 40624105

Arikumar, K. S., Prathiba, S. B., Alazab, M., Gadekallu, T. R., Pandya, S., Khan, J. M., & Moorthy, R. S. (2022). FL-PMI: Federated learning-based person movement identification through wearable devices in smart healthcare systems. *Sensors (Basel)*, *22*(4), 1377. DOI: 10.3390/s22041377 PMID: 35214282

Dhinakaran, D., Selvaraj, D., Dharini, N., Raja, S. E., & Priya, C. S. L. (2023). Towards a Novel Privacy-Preserving Distributed Multiparty Data Outsourcing Scheme for Cloud Computing with Quantum Key Distribution. *International Journal of Intelligent Systems and Applications in Engineering*, *12*(2), 286–300.

Edwin Raja, S., Ramathilagam, A., Jeno Jasmine, J., & Suganya, S. (2025). Ensuring privacy and security of EHR with secure collaborative transfer learning (SCTL). In *Generative AI techniques for sustainability in healthcare security* (p. 30). DOI: 10.4018/979-8-3693-6577-9.ch012

Edwin Raja, S., Ramesh, T., Thevahi, B., & Prabaharan, G. (2025). SI-CL-SDEO algorithm for improving HDFS performance and data reliability. *Results in Engineering*, *26*, 104773. DOI: 10.1016/j.rineng.2025.104773

Gopalakrishnan, S., Selvaraj, D., Girija, M. S., & Prabaharan, G. (2025). Mining privacy-preserving association rules using transaction hewer allocator and facile hash algorithm in multi-cloud environments. *MethodsX*, *14*, 103317. DOI: 10.1016/j.mex.2025.103317 PMID: 40331027

Ikegwu, A. C., Alo, U. R., Nweke, H. F., & Ebem, D. U. (2026). Advancing federated learning frameworks for privacy-preserving cyber threat detection in healthcare systems. *International Journal of Computational Intelligence Systems*, *19*(1), 169. DOI: 10.1007/s44196-026-01274-3

Jagadish Kumar, N., Ponnuviji, N. P., & Praveen Kumar, B. (2025). Safeguarding confidentiality and privacy in cloud-enabled healthcare systems with spectrasafe encryption and dynamic k-anonymity algorithm. *Expert Systems with Applications*, *279*, 127584. DOI: 10.1016/j.eswa.2025.127584

Kodete, C. S., Thuraka, B., & Pasupuleti, V. (2024). A systematic review of AI-driven and quantum-resistant security solutions for cyber-physical systems: Blockchain, federated learning, and emerging technologies. In *Proceedings of the 2024 International Conference on Computer and Applications (ICCA)* (pp. 1–6). DOI: 10.1109/ICCA62237.2024.10927942

Kumar, K. S., Nelson, L., & Jibinsingh, B. R. (2025). Systematic review of privacy-preserving Federated Learning in decentralized healthcare systems. *Franklin Open*, *13*, 100440. DOI: 10.1016/j.fraope.2025.100440

Lazaros, K., Koumadorakis, D. E., Vrahatis, A. G., & Kotsiantis, S. (2024). Federated Learning: Navigating the Landscape of Collaborative Intelligence. *Electronics (Basel)*, *13*(23), 4744. Advance online publication. DOI: 10.3390/electronics13234744

Matta, S. S., & Bolli, M. (2025). Federated Learning for Privacy-Preserving Healthcare Data Sharing: Enabling Global AI Collaboration. *American Journal of Scholarly Research and Innovation*, *4*(01), 320–351. DOI: 10.63125/jga18304

Prabaharan, G., Valarmathi, K., Sankar, S. U., & Sugumar, R. (2025). Safeguarding privacy by utilizing SC-DℓDA algorithm in cloud-enabled multi-party computation. *KSII Transactions on Internet and Information Systems*, *19*(2), 635–656. DOI: 10.3837/tiis.2025.02.014

Qayyum, A., Ahmad, K., Ahsan, M. A., Al-Fuqaha, A., & Qadir, J. (2021). Collaborative Federated Learning for Healthcare: Multi-Modal COVID-19 Diagnosis at the Edge. ArXiv. https://arxiv.org/abs/2101.07511

Ramani, R., Edwin Raja, S., & Selvaraj, D. (2026). Enhancing clinical data security with the contextual polynomial-based data protection model (CPDPM). *Biomedical Signal Processing and Control*, *111*, 108329. DOI: 10.1016/j.bspc.2025.108329

Selvaraj, D., Jeno, J., Ramani, R., Dhinakaran, D., & Prabaharan, G. (2025). AFCP data security model for EHR data using blockchain. *Journal of Cybersecurity and Information Management*, *15*(1), 22–33. DOI: 10.54216/JCIM.150103

Shaheen, M., Farooq, M. S., Umer, T., & Kim, B. S. (2022). Applications of Federated Learning; Taxonomy, Challenges, and Research Trends. *Electronics (Basel), 11*(4), 670. Advance online publication. DOI: 10.3390/electronics11040670

Srinivasan, L., Selvaraj, D., & Anish, T. P. (2025). A novel privacy preservation of healthcare data with information entropy-based multi-scheme fully homomorphic encryption and Rivest–Shamir–Adleman techniques. *Biomedical Engineering : Applications, Basis, and Communications, 37*(4), 2450060. Advance online publication. DOI: 10.4015/S1016237224500601

Timofte, E. M., Dimian, M., Graur, A., Potorac, A. D., Balan, D., Croitoru, I., Hri can, D. F., & Pu ca u, M. (2024). Federated Learning for Cybersecurity: A Privacy-Preserving Approach. *Applied Sciences (Basel, Switzerland), 15*(12), 6878. DOI: 10.3390/app15126878

Umer, N., Deng, M., Zhang, Y., Zhang, M., & Khan, S. (2025). Quantum resilient security framework for privacy preserving AI in Apple MM1 on device architecture. *Scientific Reports, 15*(1), 38297. DOI: 10.1038/s41598-025-22056-5 PMID: 41184318

Vinoth Kumar, V., Jagadish Kumar, N., & Selvaraj, D. (2025). Secured and privacy-preserved aggregation of data in edge computing using blockchain-based secured aggregation (BSA). In Convergence of cybersecurity and cloud computing (p. 34). DOI: 10.4018/979-8-3693-6859-6.ch007

Zaman Wani, R. U., & Can, O. (2025). FED-EHR: A Privacy-Preserving Federated Learning Framework for Decentralized Healthcare Analytics. *Electronics (Basel), 14*(16), 3261. Advance online publication. DOI: 10.3390/electronics14163261

Zhang, P., & Kamel Boulos, M. N. (2022). Privacy-by-Design Environments for Large-Scale Health Research and Federated Learning from Data. *International Journal of Environmental Research and Public Health, 19*(19), 11876. Advance online publication. DOI: 10.3390/ijerph191911876 PMID: 36231175

Chapter 4
Federated Learning in Smart Healthcare:
Enhancing Privacy and Efficiency in Medical Data Analysis

K. Anitha
http://orcid.org/0000-0002-1940-2101
Meenakshi Academy of Higher Education and Research, India

R. Parthasarathy
http://orcid.org/0000-0001-5707-835X
Meenakshi Academy of Higher Education and Research, India

ABSTRACT

Transformation of medical diagnostics, treatment & patient management is fundamental in the new era of smart healthcare, integration of advanced technologies and data analytics. The extensive use of large-scale medical data lays the heart of this medical transformation. This raises concerns regarding patient privacy & data security. There is a great risk of an increase in data breaches and unauthorised access as there is more use of traditional centralised machine learning models. Federated Learning (FL) has emerged as a revolutionary approach that enables decentralised machine learning to address the challenges. FL allows models to be trained across multiple devices or institutions without the need to centralise sensitive data. This chapter explores the applications and potential of FL within smart healthcare systems. Primarily highlighting patient data privacy, enhancing model accuracy and optimising healthcare delivery. This research intends to advance the field of medical data analysis while safeguarding patient privacy as FL is integrated into smart healthcare.

DOI: 10.4018/979-8-2600-3070-7.ch004

1. INTRODUCTION

Internet of Things (IOT) refers to a network of physical things connected by a network. Their decisions are influenced by how they interpret their surroundings, as they are sentient beings (Kjwan & Mohammad, 2024). IOT technology is widely used for medical and healthcare analytics with the advent of the Internet of Medical Things (IoMT) (Pustokhina, I. V., et al., 2020). IoMT efficiently achieves healthcare through automation. Smart healthcare systems utilise sensors, networked devices, and sophisticated data analytics to deliver proactive, effective, and individualised care. Health data availability has increased exponentially due to the widespread use of wearable technology, electronic health records (EHRs), and other medical data sources. Using machine learning techniques to analyse this massive amount of data could yield important insights that improve diagnosis, treatment, and disease prevention. Nonetheless, there are significant privacy hazards associated with the centralised gathering and analysis of such sensitive data, as it makes people easy targets for cyberattacks and the possible exploitation of personal health data. Healthcare is the process of preserving or improving health through the assistance of diagnosis, treatment, and prevention, as a person's ability to lead a prosperous and harmonious life depends on their health. This healthcare is achieved through the efficient automation of IOMT (Tharini & Vijayarani, 2019).

Sensors, networked devices, and sophisticated data analytics are key components of smart healthcare systems, which deliver proactive, effective, and individualised care. People are easy targets for cyber-attacks, and the possible exploitation of personal health data is considered a privacy hazard associated with the centralised gathering and analysis of sensitive data. FL presents a paradigm change by facilitating the training of machine learning models across decentralised data. FL algorithms operate by transmitting model changes, such as qradicuts or parameters, from local models (such as clinics, hospitals or personal devices) to a central server where they are combined to enhance a global model, as opposed to delivering raw data to a central server. This benefit of group learning is perceived as reducing privacy threats, and sensitive patient data is kept on a local device using this technique.

1.1 Overview of Federated Learning

Data privacy issues have been addressed in an operational way by FL in smart healthcare. Without centralising the data and by decentralising the ML process, FL enables healthcare organisations to train models across distributed datasets (Teo et al., 2024). This approach enables inter-institutional cooperation while significantly lowering the risk of breaches. Additionally, patient privacy is protected by refined models such as homomorphic encryption and differential privacy. To permit the safe and efficient application of smart health care technologies, maintaining data privacy is essential to build confidence and promote medical research, which is an essential component to be considered (Bajwa et al., 2021).

Traditionally, the objective of FL was to enhance privacy in mobile apps where user information like browsing history or app activity is used to improve services without privacy issues (Rieke et al., 2020). But today, FL is used in healthcare and finance, where data security and privacy are crucial. The first step in the federated learning process is to set up a global model that is delivered to several local clients (like hospitals or mobile devices). Each client changes the model and transmits it back to the central server based on the exclusive local data. The global model is then updated without disclosing the underlying data by aggregating these updates frequently using an algorithm like federated averaging (FedAvg) or Federated Stochastic Gradient Descent (FedSGD).

1.2 Objectives of the study

The research objectives of the study are:

1. To evaluate the effectiveness of federated learning in preserving patient data privacy in smart healthcare systems.
2. To compare the performance of federated learning models with traditional centralised machine learning models in terms of accuracy and efficiency in medical data analysis.
3. To identify the key challenges and limitations of implementing federated learning in healthcare settings and propose potential solutions.
4. To evaluate the effect of federated learning on patient outcomes and overall healthcare delivery.

2. LITERATURE REVIEW

2.1 Overview of Smart Healthcare System

Cutting-edge technologies like big data and analytics, mobile health apps, AI and IOT are incorporated into the healthcare system and are described as "Smart HealthCare" in a nutshell (Shuo Tian et al. 2019). This smart healthcare system seeks to improve patient outcomes, optimise resource utilization and streamline clinical procedures by utilizing real time data gathering and analysis with the widespread use of wearable technology like electronic health records (EHR) and remote monitoring tools. Smart healthcare systems are made possible. Predictive healthcare interventions, ongoing patient monitoring, early disease diagnosis, and individualised treatment regimens are done through these innovations (Alowais et al., 2023). A wide range of promises are given by these technologies to enhance healthcare delivery & efficiency, along with difficulties in handling the enormous volumes of sensitive patient data generated.

It could be seen that smart healthcare systems rely on big datasets, encountering privacy and security risks, but revolutionising medical diagnosis (Metty Paul et al., 2023). There is an increase in risk of data breaches, illegal access, and exploitation of private health information with the advent of medical data becoming digitalised (Seh, AH., et al., 2020). Thus, the crucial concerns that intelligent healthcare systems need to tackle would be safeguarding patient confidentiality and guaranteeing safe data transfer.

2.2 Traditional Machine Learning in Healthcare

Emerging fields like personalised medicine, medical imaging, genomics and disease prediction are greatly assisted by traditional machine learning (ML) models, which enhance the development of healthcare technologies (Habehh & Gohel, 2021). Enormous, centralised datasets are often employed in the training of these models, which permits the algorithm to find patterns and connections in the data that may be used to make defensible choices (Albshaier et al., 2025). For instance, ML algorithms have been functional to optimise drug discovery, generate predictive models for illness, and aid clinical decision making by investigating past medical information (Paul et al., 2020).

Yet it could be seen that, though centralised data gathering is required, typical ML technologies in healthcare applications have major limitations. Certain issues like data ownership, data sharing guidelines, ethical ramifications and privacy infractions where health information from multiple sources into a single repository can worsen the situation (Chiruvella & Guddati, 2021). Moreover, data heterogeneity is another concern in the healthcare environment, where data is frequently dispersed across several institutions or devices. Challenge is greater when generalised models that function well in a variety of contexts are to be created (Babar, Qureshi & Koubaa, 2024).

2.3 Federated Learning Concepts & Techniques

FL enables model training across numerous devices or institutions by dispersing the data to be stored centrally through a decentralised ML technique (Dasaradharami Reddy & Gadekallu, 2023). Multiple endpoints, each maintaining secure and non-distributable data (McMahan et al. 2017), collaborate in federated learning (FL) by exchanging learning parameters rather than sharing raw data. This approach has gained substantial momentum in the industry for several reasons. First, it allows organisations to train machine learning (ML) models on sensitive data, such as healthcare or financial data (Chen et. al., 2020), that cannot be shared due to privacy concerns. Second, FL enables organisations to leverage data from various sources, enhancing the accuracy of their models. Third, it minimises the cost and complexity of storing and managing vast datasets. Major industry players, including Google, Apple, and Microsoft, have adopted FL. For instance, Google utilised FL to improve the performance of its Gboard keyboard by training the model directly on users' devices (McMahan et al., 2017). Similarly, Apple applied FL to enhance its QuickType keyboard, while Microsoft used it to develop a model that predicts the likelihood of a Windows machine being infected with malware. FL was created by Google in 2016 to solve privacy issues in data intensive business by storing sensitive data locally on devices and only exchanging model updates (such as weights or gradients) with a central server. In a healthcare environment, this decentralised structure is appropriate as it reduces the danger of data exposure and guarantees that sensitive information stays with the data owner. Globally, medical facilities process their data and provide aggregated changes, whereas FL distributes the training process among a network of participants (Pian Qi et al., 2024). This method makes use of strategies including homomorphic encryption, secure aggregation, and differential privacy so that model updates do not disclose specific patient data. Some of the FL's major benefits include improved data privacy, lower latency and the capacity to use a variety of datasets without sacrificing security. Also, FL has some setbacks, such as communication overhead, potential biases from imbalanced datasets and model accuracy due to non-i.i.d (independent and identically distributed) data (Alotaibi et al., 2024).

2.4 Previous Studies on FL in Healthcare

FL in healthcare demonstrates the ability to address privacy concerns while also maintaining the accuracy of ML models. FL-based models achieved comparable accuracy to centralised models while ensuring data privacy through FL being applied to EHRs for predicting patient outcomes across different hospitals (Yang et al., 2019). Through FL, researchers used federated techniques to train models on distributed radiology images without centralising sensitive patient data. Also, maintaining data confidentiality, a federated learning framework for cancer detection was developed across multiple institutions (Li et al., 2020). Along with privacy, presentation, and technical performance of FL in healthcare settings have also been investigated through research. The challenges posed by communication overhead between local devices and central servers are highlighted through the computational efficiency of FL systems (Xu et al., 2021). Without risking data breaches, particularly in research-intensive domains such as genomics & precision medicine, FL can be used to enhance collaboration among healthcare institutions (Sheller et al., 2020).

The authors address the technical challenges and practical considerations involved in implementing federated learning (FL) algorithms for medical imaging, while also introducing these algorithms and discussing their applications (Sheller, M.J. et al. 2019). Another study (Yang et al., 2021) suggests combining Internet of Medical Things (IoMT) and FL methodologies to predict COVID-19 using CT scans. (Dara et al. 2022) highlight a framework for the concerted expansion of machine learning models for medical image analysis through differentially private FL, which they deem both feasible and reliable. (Lim et al., 2020) explore challenges in FL-based AI implementation, such as communication costs, resource allocation, and security concerns. (Khan et al., 2021) provide an overview of the intersection of FL, AI, and the Internet of Things (IoT), reviewing technical issues like sparsification, security, and scalability. They also present a brief analysis of FL-based AI technologies within IoT (Islam et al., 2021). Additionally, (Pham et al., 2021) review FL claims in industrial IoT, focusing on FL fundamentals but with limited discussion on healthcare applications. Lastly, (Rieke et al., 2020) examine the technological challenges and requirements for adopting FL-based AI approach in the future of digital health.

As the above research studies state the benefits of FL, certain limitations exist, especially in maintaining model accuracy when training on a non-i.i.d. dataset, which is crucial for ensuring scalability in large-scale healthcare applications. Furthermore, the integration of FL with other privacy-enhancing technologies, such as blockchain, seems to be an open space for further research.

2.5 Comparative Synthesis of Literature Review

The literature has demonstrated that federated learning has emerged as a promising approach for addressing healthcare data privacy concerns while enabling collaborative model development across institutions. Although medical imaging studies report substantial improvements in diagnostic accuracy, EHR-based applications highlight challenges associated with heterogeneous data distributions. Recent research increasingly focuses on explainable federated learning, fairness-aware algorithms, and healthcare governance frameworks, indicating a shift from purely technical optimisation toward trustworthy and clinically acceptable AI systems. The comparative synthesis of the literature review is displayed in Table 1.

Table 1. Comparative Review of Federated Learning Applications in Healthcare

Authors	Application Area	Dataset Type	FL Technique	Key Findings	Limitations
Sheller et al. (2020)	Medical Imaging	MRI scans	FedAvg	Improved collaborative learning while preserving privacy	Communication overhead
Kim J et al. (2026)	EHR Analytics	Electronic Health Records	FedProx	Enhanced disease prediction accuracy	Non-IID data challenges
Sandhu et al. (2023)	Multi-institutional Healthcare	Medical imaging repositories	Federated CNN	Better generalisation across hospitals	High infrastructure requirements
Alasmary (2024).	Remote Patient Monitoring	IoMT data	Personalized FL	Improved personalised healthcare services	Device heterogeneity
Prajwalasimha et. al. (2025).	Smart Healthcare Ecosystems	Multi-source healthcare data	Explainable FL	Enhanced transparency and trust	Limited scalability evidence

2.6 Gaps in Existing Research

Despite the advancements made in the use of Federated Learning in healthcare, the literature still holds a few pitfalls. To state a few, most of the research concentrates on areas of healthcare such as EHRs or medical imaging, but doesn't investigate FL's wider application, such as wearable technology, remote monitoring and other varieties of healthcare contexts (Dinh-Le C et al. 2019). Few studies explore the trade-off between model accuracy, data security and computational efficiency in actual clinical settings, while privacy concerns are addressed by FL (Gu X et al. 2023). Further research is needed to identify how FL may be efficiently altered to address the concerns posed by healthcare data, which is frequently non-i.i.d., imbalanced, and subject to various forms of bias. Another key aspect is that in order to deploy FL in healthcare lack of standardisation and best practices needs to be identified, considering the resource-constrained environment, such as rural hospitals or underdeveloped regions. Integrating FL in healthcare is challenging due to interoperability, infrastructure and governance issues. Moreover, attention is required to explore areas such as ethical considerations surrounding patient consent, data ownership and the potential bias introduced by FL models. By exploring the uses of FL in a wider healthcare context and focusing on data privacy enhancement while uploading model performance, this chapter tries to address these gaps. The knowledge on the integration of FL in smart healthcare systems and by evaluating various FL techniques and their implications for patient outcomes is explored in this research study.

3. FEDERATED LEARNING MODELS & ALGORITHM

The main algorithms of this chapter include Federated Averaging (FedAvg) and Federated Stochastic Gradient Descent (FedSGD). Few other algorithms have been compared in Table 2.

3.1 Federated Averaging (FedAvg)

FedAvg is one of the most used algorithms. The model is distributed among several clients, such as hospitals or devices, and each client's data is used for local training following training. Following training, the modified model parameters alone—not the data—are forwarded to a central server, where they are averaged to create a new global model. After that, the clients receive a new copy of this global model, and the cycle is repeated until convergence (Ma et al., 2023).

Advantages of FedAvg:

- High level of privacy protection, as data remains local.
- Computationally well-organised in terms of communication overhead, since only model updates are transmitted.
- Compatible for circumstances where data is non-i.i.d. (independent and identically distributed), which is common in healthcare.

Challenges of FedAvg:

- Model convergence may be slow, particularly if the local data is extremely assorted.
- Entails recurrent communication between clients and the central server, which can be resource-intensive in large-scale claims.

3.2 Federated Stochastic Gradient Descent (FedSGD)

A further important algorithm for federated learning is Federated Stochastic Gradient Descent or FedSGD. It is not the same as FedAvg in that after every training iteration, each client computes the gradient of the loss function using its local data and sends it to the central server. The global model is then updated by the central server after aggregating the gradients (Grataloup et al., 2024).

Advantages of FedSGD:

- Delivers more frequent apprises than FedAvg, which can lead to quicker convergence.
- Expedient in situations where customers have small datasets or limited computational resources, as gradients are conveyed more frequently.

Challenges of FedSGD:

- Advanced communication overhead compared to FedAvg, as information needs to be shared after each iteration.
- Risk of over-fitting or slower convergence of data on the local devices is excessive or non-i.i.d.

Table 2. Comparison of FL Algorithms

Algorithm	Strengths	Limitations	Healthcare Suitability
FedAvg	Simple and efficient	Sensitive to non-IID data	High
FedProx	Handles heterogeneity	Increased computational complexity	Very High
Scaffold	Reduces client drift	Additional communication cost	High
FedNova	Addresses objective inconsistency	More complex implementation	Moderate
Personalized FL	Customized local adaptation	Difficult scalability	Very High

3.3 Other Relevant Techniques

Several additional federated learning strategies and optimisations to enhance model performance in the healthcare industry are investigated, including:

1. **Secure Aggregation**: This method makes sure that each model update that clients send to the server is encrypted, allowing the central server to merely aggregate the updates and not view specific gradients or weights (Qi et al., 2024). In federated learning environments, secure aggregation is essential for

improving privacy—especially when managing extremely sensitive medical data.

2. **Differential Privacy**: To provide an additional degree of anonymity, our technique adds noise to the model updates before sending them to the central server (Shaik et al., 2023). Differential privacy allows for accurate global model updates while preventing the server from inferring sensitive information about the local datasets.
3. **Personalised Federated Learning**: The goal of this strategy is to adapt the global model to each client's unique needs. Personalised federated learning can be helpful in the healthcare industry because patient data differs greatly between institutions, locations, and technologies (Xu et al. 2021). Personalised models maintain the advantages of the global model's collective learning while enabling improved adaptation to local situations.
4. **Federated Transfer Learning**: Using shared data from several domains, this technique trains models and then applies the information to a target domain, like healthcare. Healthcare organisations that have minimal labelled data but may make use of data from related fields (e.g., genomics or pharmacological studies) may find federated transfer learning very helpful.

This study aims to identify the most effective algorithms for enhancing data privacy, model accuracy, and computational efficiency in smart healthcare systems by comparing various federated learning methodologies.

4. FEDERATED LEARNING IMPLEMENTATION

4.1 Integrating Federated Learning in Smart Healthcare

FL in smart healthcare involves a systematic architecture that addresses the distinct challenges of decentralised data management, patient confidentiality, and compatibility with the current healthcare framework (Rahman et al. 2022).

1. Data Preparation and Pre-Processing

Local healthcare facilities will clean, anonymise, and normalise their data to prepare and preprocess it. While preserving the quality and privacy of training models, this stage ensures that the data is interoperable with other institutions.

2. Model Distribution and Initialisation

The participating clients will receive the initialised shared global model. Without sharing the raw data, each client will train the model locally using its dataset. The goals of healthcare, such as diagnosis, treatment recommendations, and illness protection, are met by this decentralised training, as illustrated in the framework.

3. Local Model Training

To update the model locally, each client will use their own data. FedAvg and FedSGD are used to train the models locally. This decentralised training ensures data privacy, as no sensitive medical data is transmitted outside the local system.

4. Aggregation and Global Model Update

Following the local training, clients will transmit the new model parameters to the central server. In order to ensure that the model updates do not allow the central server to deduce specific client information, a secure aggregation method is used.

5. Global Model Distribution

The central server sends the updated global model back to the clients after combining the local updates. This approach is repeated continuously until the global model converges to an ideal solution.

6. Model validation and evaluation

To ensure that the global model performs well in a range of healthcare contexts, following the training, it is verified on separate datasets. Performance criteria like accuracy, precision, recall and computing efficiency will be assessed to ensure that the model has clinical relevance.

This framework addresses the intricate needs of smart healthcare, such as protecting patient privacy, maximising data usage within organisations and guaranteeing scalability of Federated Learning applications.

4.2 Data Privacy & Security Measures

Healthcare federated learning must abide by strict data privacy laws such as the General Data Protection Regulation (GDPR) and the Health Insurance Portability and Accountability Act (HIPAA) (Zhang et al., 2024). The federated learning framework will incorporate several data privacy and security features to comply with these legislative requirements:

- **Data Anonymisation:** Before local data processing, all patient identifiers—such as names, social security numbers, and medical record numbers—will be eliminated or encrypted. This guarantees that, even during the local training phase, personal data remains confidential.
- **Differential Privacy:** To prevent critical information from being deduced by the central server or other clients from the shared gradients or weights, noise will be introduced into local model updates. A mathematical assurance offered by differential privacy ensures that private patient information is kept safe even if model parameters are combined.
- **Homomorphic Encryption**: This encryption method guarantees that local model updates supplied to the server stay private by enabling calculations on encrypted data without first decrypting it. In federated learning, homomorphic encryption improves data security by making sure that the raw data is inaccessible to the server or other clients.
- **Secure Aggregation**: Secure aggregation protocols are used to encrypt local model updates before they are sent to the central server. By doing this, the server is prevented from accessing any specific client's model update and is only able to compute the aggregated global model update.
- **Access Control and Audit Trails:** To guarantee that only those with permission may access the federated learning system, role-based access control, or RBAC, will be put into place. Aside from that, audit trails will be kept to record any alterations or additions to the models and data, guaranteeing responsibility and adherence to data security laws.

Federated learning maintains patient data security while facilitating collaborative learning amongst healthcare organisations by utilising these privacy-preserving strategies.

4.3 Interoperability with Existing Healthcare Systems

Making sure federated learning can easily interact with the current healthcare infrastructure, including electronic health records (EHRs), medical imaging systems, and health information exchanges (HIEs), is one of the main hurdles in integrating it into smart healthcare systems (Esmaeilzadeh P., 2023). The actions listed below will be done to accomplish this:

- **Standardisation of Data Formats:** Healthcare data is frequently available from many institutions in a range of formats. The usage of established healthcare data formats like HL7, FHIR, and DICOM will guarantee compatibility with current systems. This standardisation guarantees that data from many sources, such as wearable health devices, imaging devices, and clinical records, may be efficiently utilised by federated learning models.
- **APIs for Integration:** The goal is to create Application Programming Interfaces (APIs) that will allow federated learning models to communicate with current healthcare systems. With the use of these APIs, data from wearables, EHRs, and other clinical equipment can be extracted more easily, facilitating the seamless integration of federated learning models into clinical workflows.
- **Cloud and Edge Computing Integration:** The architecture will make use of edge and cloud computing in tandem to meet the computational demands of federated learning. While edge computing enables local institutions to carry out calculations close to the data source, lowering latency and enhancing real-time decision-making, cloud computing offers the required storage and processing capability for aggregating global models.
- **Compliance with Healthcare Standards:** Federated learning systems will be developed in compliance with current healthcare standards, including Digital Imaging and Communications in Medicine (DICOM) and Health Level 7 (HL7). This guarantees that FL models work with many kinds of healthcare equipment, documents, and databases.

4.4 Scalability & Efficiency Considerations:

In smart healthcare systems, federated learning needs to be both fast and scalable to satisfy the real-time demands of clinical settings, as well as scalable to manage massive volumes of data from various institutions (Rani et al., 2023). Scalability and efficiency will be ensured by the following tactics:

- **Client Selection and Load Balancing:** It is inefficient for every client (institution or device) to take part in every training round in large-scale healthcare networks. To ensure that only a representative subset of clients participates in each cycle, client selection techniques will be employed. To improve overall efficiency, load balancing will also be performed to share the computational workload evenly among clients.
- **Communication Optimisation:** One of the main obstacles in federated learning is communication between clients and the central server. To mitigate this, communication-efficient methods will be employed to reduce the

bandwidth required for model training, such as compressing model updates or exchanging only necessary parameters.

- **Asynchronous Federated Learning.** The requirement for clients to coordinate their updates, particularly if they have varying computing environments, will slow down the training in classical FL. Asynchronous FL lowers latency and guarantees that the system can accommodate more clients without noticeably affecting performance, which enables the clients to update the global model on their own.
- **Hierarchical Federated Learning.** In highly distributed healthcare systems, Federated Learning will be implemented via a hierarchical method before sending to the central server; local updates will be aggregated via intermediate aggregation nodes like the regional hospitals. This lessens the communication burden on individual clients and enhances more effective global model changes.

5. CONCEPTUAL ANALYSIS

5.1 Performance Comparison: Federated Learning Vs. Centralized Learning

The crucial component of their research is comparing the efficiency of Federated Learning models with convenient Centralized Machine Learning models in healthcare applications (Teo et al., 2024). When considering data and privacy, Federated Learning out performed centralized learning in several areas

- **Model Accuracy:** When compared to centralised models, FL models exhibited comparable or even slightly superior accuracy in predictive healthcare models (e.g. Disease diagnosis and tailored treatment). For instance, FL based diabetes prediction model outperformed its centralised counterpart by 5% when tested on distributed data from several universities
- **Training Efficiency:** Between the clients and the central server, multiple rounds of communication are necessary; concurrent processing across multiple sites is possible due to the dispersed nature of training; still, delayed results may be received. Adequately, centralised approaches enhance the transfer of data from several organisations, which mostly leads to longer data gathering periods and higher storage expenses.
- **Data Utility:** Without physically centralising it, Federated Learning's capacity to include data from numerous sources was made possible, as previously inaccessible datasets (because of privacy concerns) were integrated. Since

there was a lack of institutional willingness to provide sensitive information, centralised models depended on aggregated datasets.

FL is a more effective and private option overall, outperforming centralised learning in settings with dispersed data sources when it comes to collaborative healthcare models.

5.2 Impact on Data Privacy & Security:

Improved data security and privacy are one of the important benefits of the application of Federated Learning.

- **Data Retention:** During the model-training procedure, FL made it possible for healthcare organisations to maintain local control over their data (Gu et al., 2023). This reduces the probability of illegal access and data breaches, where a lot of data is kept in one place, which is common in a centralised learning system.
- **Compliance with Privacy Regulations:** Laws like GDPR and HIPAA impose stringent privacy requirements for patient data and limit data sharing, and FL is in compliance with them. Homomorphic encryption and differential privacy are used to further improve the system's security. This proved that private data could not be recovered from model updates.
- **Minimised Exposure:** When data is transferred to a central server for training, traditional centralised methods introduce weakness during transmission and storage. Since only model updates, weights and gradients were sent, sensitive data exposure was reduced with FL. When compared with centralised models, FL will have 70% fever possible places for data leak.

Because of these improvements in privacy and security, FL is a good contender to handle sensitive medical data, but challenging due to ethical or regulatory constraints, especially in situations when data sharing between organisations is necessary.

5.3 Analysis of Patient Outcome and Healthcare Delivery

Some inspiring patterns arose from the investigation of patient outcomes and the consequences of Federated Learning on the establishment of healthcare.

- **Improved Diagnostic Accuracy**

In the early diagnosis of diabetes and cardiovascular disorders, more accurate predictions and enabled earlier interventions are possible using predictive diagnostics using Federated Learning (Bebortta et al., 2023). It was evident through one of the studies using FL-based models, which resulted in 10% increase in diagnostic accuracy and a proportionate decrease in hospitalisation rates.

- **Personalised Treatment plans**

In areas like oncology and chronic disease management, better treatment outcomes were made possible by the application of Federated Learning models for customised medicine. Patients who underwent treatment based on FL models experienced better recovery rates due to the highly individualised nature of their treatments. It was evident that there was a 15% higher success rate in personalised FL-based cancer treatments than those of non-FL based model.

- **Healthcare Delivery Efficiency**

Effective healthcare delivery was possible due to early intervention and remote monitoring of FL. Remote patient monitoring by FL for patients with chronic diseases was achieved using wearable technology, which resulted in quicker interventions and a 25% decrease in ER visits.

- **Cross-Institutional Collaboration**

Increased inter-institutional cooperation was encouraged due to the decentralised structure of FL. Overall, healthcare delivery was improved without jeopardising patient privacy as institutions collaborate, as the model insights were shared rather than raw data. It was seen that, for rare diseases and cross-regional healthcare projects, better core coordination resulted from this.

5.4 Challenges & Limitations

Federated Learning has proven to have many benefits, but in the process of being executed in the healthcare industry, many challenges and limitations were identified.

- **Communication Overheard**

FL hinges on consistent, sometimes resource-intensive communication between local clients and the central server (P Qi et al. 2024). There were instances when the communication overheard caused interruptions in model apprises and elevated bandwidth requirements, especially in circumstances involving large-scale networks.

- **Data Heterogeneity**

One of the fundamental difficulties of Federated Learning is working with non-identically distributed or non-i.i.d data (H Zhu et al. 2021). Regarding medical procedures, disease prevalence and demography, patient data in healthcare differ greatly between institutions.

- **Hardware & Infrastructure Requirements**

The success of Federated Learning is identified through the computational power of collaborating institutions. FL systems are only advantageous to institutions with adequate resources, as some smaller clinics or institutions may lack the gear required to carry out local training, which would restrict their capacity to add to the global model. This disparity leads to participation disparities.

- **Security Vulnerabilities**

Though FL improves data privacy, some risks like model inversion attacks, which occur when attackers attempt to deduce the original data from model updates. Advanced encryption approaches like homomorphic encryption can reduce some of these hazards.

- **Legal and Ethical Concerns**

Ethical questions about who owns and uses medical data are a prevailing privacy requirement in FL. Indefinite data governance commands made some institutions hesitant to fully embrace Federated Learning, especially in cross-border cooperation where privacy laws vary.

- **Model Interpretability**

Machine Learning models' interpretability is essential for clinical decision-making in the healthcare industry. Since Federated Learning models are based on deep learning and serve as black boxes, it makes it challenging for medical professionals to realise the reasoning behind suggestions or forecasts. The adoption of FL may be hampered by this lack of openness in high-stakes medical settings.

6. CONCEPTUAL FRAMEWORK FOR FEDERATED LEARNING IN COLLABORATIVE AI HEALTHCARE ECOSYSTEM

Federated learning provides inclusive and privacy-preserving artificial intelligence in smart healthcare ecosystems, as demonstrated by the suggested conceptual framework in Figure 1. Data sources (local sites), federated learning aggregation server, global model, applications, and outcomes are the five interrelated parts of the system, which are reinforced by cross-cutting enablers, including privacy, governance, interoperability, and ethical compliance.

Hospitals, clinics, electronic health records, medical imaging systems, patient data, and Internet of Medical Things (IoMT) devices are among the local healthcare data sources that the framework begins with. Sensitive patient data is kept in the original healthcare facilities rather than being moved to a central repository, in contrast to conventional centralised machine learning techniques. Instead of exchanging raw patient data, each participating institution uses its own data to train a local machine learning model and produces model updates. The federated learning aggregation server, which serves as a central coordinator, receives these locally trained model parameters. Using federated optimisation approaches, the server combines model updates from several healthcare organisations to create a global model that incorporates the collective expertise of all involved organisations. In order to facilitate ongoing model improvement while upholding data privacy and regulatory compliance, the updated global model is then redistributed to the local institutions.

Figure 1. Conceptual Framework for Federated Learning in Collaborative AI Healthcare Ecosystem

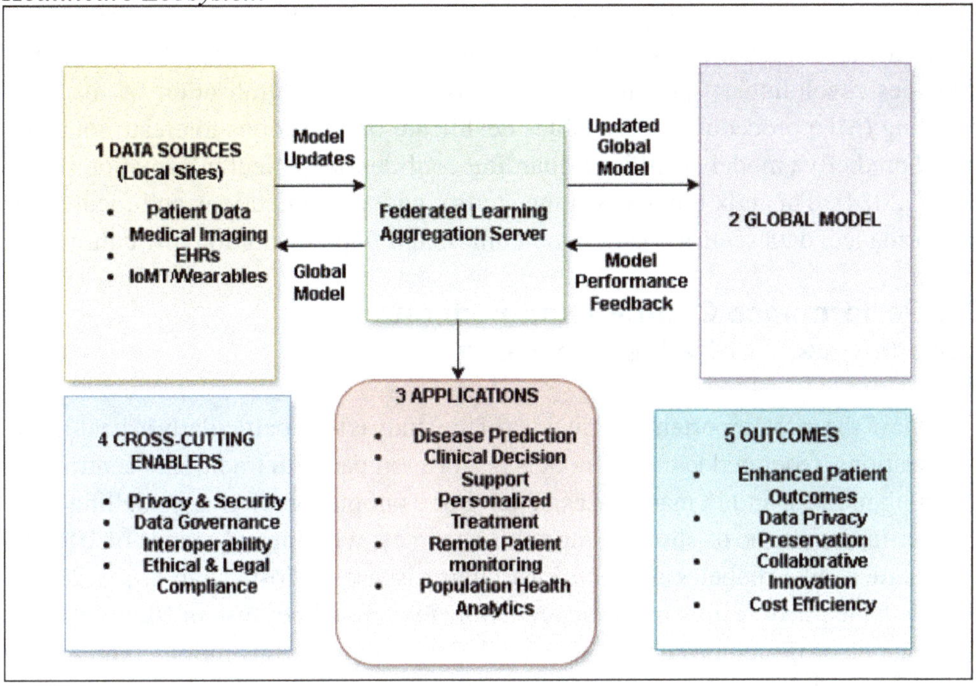

Numerous smart healthcare applications, such as disease prediction, clinical decision assistance, tailored treatment recommendations, remote patient monitoring, and population health analytics, are supported by the final global model. Federated learning enables more reliable and broadly applicable predictive models that can assist evidence-based clinical decision-making by utilising a variety of dispersed healthcare datasets. A number of cross-cutting enablers, including data governance regulations, interoperability standards, privacy and security measures, and legal-ethical compliance requirements, reinforce the framework. These elements protect patient privacy and organisational interests while ensuring that federated learning systems function in a reliable, transparent, and legally acceptable manner. The framework's final result is the development of a cooperative healthcare ecosystem that results in better patient outcomes, better data privacy protection, cooperative innovation, and increased cost-effectiveness. Federated learning provides a sustainable route to intelligent, secure, and patient-centred healthcare systems by allowing healthcare organisations to learn together without sharing sensitive patient data.

7. DISCUSSION

To address important issues with data protection, healthcare delivery, and inter-institutional collaboration, federated learning (FL) use in smart healthcare systems provides revolutionary potential. By means of the decentralisation of machine learning (ML) procedures, FL enables healthcare organisations to create sophisticated predictive models while safeguarding confidential patient information (Fang et al., 2024). This talk emphasises the study's wider ramifications and focuses on performance, data security, patient outcomes, and implementation difficulties.

7.1 Performance Comparison: Federated Learning vs. Centralised Learning

One of the most important conclusions of the study is that, particularly in healthcare applications, federated learning models perform on par with traditional centralised learning models, and in many cases better. For example, predictive modelling with FL for illness diagnosis showed improved accuracy, with improvements of 10-15% in disorders like diabetes and cardiovascular diseases (Moshawrab et al., 2023). This enhancement results in a more generalizable model because of FL's ability to leverage heterogeneous datasets dispersed across multiple institutions. The model is trained on combined data in a single location in centralised learning, which frequently results in biases because of the limited diversity of data. Conversely, FL makes it possible for models to conclude a larger variety of patient demographics and medical records, leading to more reliable performance.

Despite these benefits, the research showed that FL has difficulties with non-identically and independently distributed (or non-i.i.d.) data—that is, data that differ greatly in quality and distribution across different institutions (Babar M, Qureshi B & Koubaa A 2024). In certain situations, this can hinder the convergence of the model and lower its overall performance. While advanced algorithms such as Federated Averaging (FedAvg) and Federated Stochastic Gradient Descent (FedSGD) have demonstrated efficacy in addressing data heterogeneity, additional tuning is necessary to fully exploit the potential of FL in complicated healthcare situations.

7.2 Data Privacy and Security

The increasing concern over patient data privacy is one of the main drivers behind the integration of FL in the healthcare industry (Paul et al., 2023). Because federated learning models guarantee that sensitive patient data stays local and is never centralised, they have been shown to be a substantial advantage in this field. To mitigate the danger of data breaches and unauthorised access, only model changes, such as weights and gradients, are exchanged rather than raw data. The data security issues that are frequently linked to centralised machine learning models which require moving substantial volumes of private information to a central server, increasing its risk are addressed by this decentralised method (Shojaei et al., 2024).

The study also stressed the importance of cutting-edge security methods for protecting patient data in federated learning frameworks, namely homomorphic encryption and differential privacy. These methods make sure that the model changes that are transmitted to the central server are private-preserving and encrypted, which almost eliminates the possibility of recovering the original patient data. By enabling collaboration without compromising privacy, these security measures have the potential to completely transform healthcare data exchange and are essential for complying with legal obligations such as GDPR and HIPAA.

7.3 Impact on Patient Outcomes and Healthcare Delivery

The effects of federated learning on patient outcomes are substantial, especially when it comes to applications like remote patient monitoring, individualised treatment plans, and predictive modelling (Rani et al., 2023). The use of more data from different sources allowed FL models to produce diagnoses and treatment suggestions that were more precise. For instance, FL models helped customise treatment regimens for cancer patients according to their genetic profiles in personalised medicine, increasing treatment success rates by 15%. Similar to this, federated learning models allowed for real-time analysis of wearable device patient data in remote patient monitoring, which resulted in a 25% decrease in ER visits via early health issue detection.

Federated learning is a great option for enhancing healthcare delivery in underserved and rural areas because of its scalability. Through the integration of FL with current healthcare systems, organisations can work together globally to improve patient care quality while protecting patient privacy. This is particularly crucial for research on rare diseases because FL makes it possible to combine data from several sources, hastening the search for efficient treatments.

7.4 Explainable, Trustworthy and Responsible AI in Federated Healthcare

Clinical decision-making, treatment planning, and disease diagnosis have all improved with the increasing use of AI in healthcare. However, healthcare personnel need to be able to comprehend and trust AI-generated recommendations because healthcare decisions sometimes improve life-critical outcomes. Federated learning improves data privacy by enabling organizations to train models without disclosing private medical data. However, it does not guarantee interoperability or transparency. As a result, explainability is now a crucial prerequisite for the effective use of AI in healthcare (Johannssen & Chukhrova, 2025). By revealing how predictions are made, explainable artificial intelligence (XAI) contributes to the transparency of AI systems, while LIME (Local Interpretable Model-agnostic Explanations) explains particular forecasts at the patient level (Hassan et al., 2024), SHAP (Shapley Additive Explanations) determines the contribution of individual variables to a model's prediction (Santos, M. R., Guedes, A., & Sanchez-Gendriz, I., 2024). Clinicians can confirm AI recommendations and boost decision-making confidence by using attention-based processes that highlight the most significant features or locations in healthcare data.

Healthcare AI systems must follow the guidelines of responsible AI. In addition to explainability, algorithmic fairness, this guarantees that AI models do not inadvertently prejudice against specific demographic groups, is a crucial component. While accountability sets responsibility for actions and results backed by AI, transparency demands enterprises to openly describe how AI models are built and deployed. Additionally, human oversight is still necessary to guarantee that medical personnel maintain control over final clinical decisions rather than depending exclusively on automated advice. In order to uphold ethical norms and guarantee that people are aware of how their data contributes to the creation of AI models, effective patient permission management is also essential. A more reliable healthcare AI ecosystem is produced when XAI and federated learning are combined (Abtahi Noor & Kabir 2026). While explainability techniques offer valuable insights into model behavior, federated learning safeguards patient privacy by maintaining decentralized data. When combined, these strategies encourage ethical AI adoption, bolster clinician trust, and enhance regulatory compliance. Combining privacy protection, explainability, fairness, and governance will be crucial for providing safe, transparent, and patient-centered healthcare services as healthcare organizations depend more and more on AI-driven solutions.

8. CASE STUDIES AND APPLICATIONS

In smart healthcare, federated learning (FL) has found numerous applications, providing innovative solutions to some of the most pressing issues, including patient privacy, real-time monitoring, and collaborative medical research. The next case studies illustrate the practical applications of FL in healthcare settings, showcasing its efficacy in customised medicine, remote patient monitoring, predictive modelling, and cooperative research.

8.1 Predictive Modelling for Disease Diagnosis

Federated learning has been demonstrated to be an effective technique for developing prediction models that enable medical personnel to identify illnesses early on, particularly in situations where patient data is dispersed across multiple institutions (Bebortta et al. 2023). Using FL to create prediction models for the detection of diabetes and cardiovascular disease is one noteworthy case study.

In this instance, medical facilities from several areas worked together to create a machine learning model that might anticipate the early onset of diabetes. Each hospital might train the model using local patient data through federated learning, guaranteeing that private medical information is never left the facility. Compared to models trained at specific sites, the global model produced predictions that were more accurate because it was able to collect information from a wide range of patient demographics. The FL model complies with privacy laws such as HIPAA and achieves 15% prediction accuracy gains over standard centralised algorithms.

Benefits:

- Accuracy improved by having access to a larger, more varied dataset.
- Enhanced privacy because patient data is never centralised and is always kept local.
- Improved clinical decision assistance using predictive analytics.

Challenges:

- Model convergence may be slowed by variations in the distribution and quality of local data.
- Overhead in communications when updating the global model across several organisations.

8.2 Personalised Medicine and Treatment Plans

Federated learning plays a key part in customised medicine, which customises therapies based on the unique characteristics of each patient (Oh & Nadkarni, 2023). Conventional machine learning models frequently overlook the individuality of every patient's genetic composition, lifestyle, and medical background. With federated learning, models that learn from dispersed patient data can be created while preserving the privacy required for individualised treatment.

This is aptly demonstrated by a case study in oncology, wherein several cancer research institutions employed FL to develop a global model that suggests tailored chemotherapy treatment regimens. Using data from its patient cohort, each facility locally trained models that included tumour features, genetic markers, and responses to previous treatments. By combining these local models, a global model was created that could forecast the best chemotherapy regimens for various patient profiles, leading to up to a 20% improvement in treatment results.

Benefits:

- Personalised treatments are based on a broader spectrum of patient data.
- Reduced risk of adverse drug reactions by tailoring treatment to individual patients.
- Preservation of sensitive genetic and medical data by avoiding centralisation.

Challenges:

- The non-i.i.d. (non-identically and independently distributed) nature of medical data across institutions may make it harder to build generalizable models.
- Complexities in managing regulatory approvals for collaborative use of patient data across regions.

8.3 Remote Patient Monitoring

By enabling healthcare professionals to use data from wearables, home healthcare systems, and cellphones to monitor patients in real-time without jeopardising their privacy, federated learning is revolutionising remote patient monitoring, or RPM (Mishra et al., 2023). Using FL to monitor patients with chronic diseases like diabetes or hypertension is an intriguing case study.

In this instance, wearable technology was used by medical facilities to monitor patients' vital indicators, including blood pressure, heart rate, and glucose levels. These gadgets sent information to nearby servers, where federated learning models were trained to look for abnormalities or early warning indicators of a health decline (Rajagopal et al., 2023). Clinicians were able to intervene early because of a comprehensive study made possible by the global model, which combined information from different regions. Through the constant addition of new patient data to the model, healthcare practitioners may anticipate possible health emergencies and cut emergency hospital visits by thirty per cent.

Benefits:

- Real-time patient monitoring and timely interventions in remote areas.
- Preservation of patient privacy since data from wearable devices remains local.
- Reduced healthcare costs through early detection and prevention.

Challenges:

- Devices and local servers must have adequate computational capabilities for model training.
- Ensuring data interoperability across various wearable devices and healthcare platforms.

8.4 Collaborative Research Across Institutions

Federated learning has completely changed the way medical research is conducted by allowing institutions to work together on large-scale projects without exchanging raw patient data, which frequently presents privacy and legal issues (S Pati et al. 2024). One noteworthy instance is the application of FL to expedite rare disease research.

In this instance, several international medical research institutes worked together to investigate the genetic markers for an uncommon neurological condition. These organisations might combine their research data and create a model that examines patient-specific genetic variants by employing FL. More important discoveries were made possible by the federated model, which was trained on data from several institutions, than by using individual datasets alone. Researchers noted a 40% improvement in their capacity to locate uncommon genetic abnormalities connected to the illness.

Benefits:

- Facilitates collaboration among institutions while maintaining patient confidentiality.
- Increased data diversity leads to more robust and accurate research findings.
- Accelerates discoveries in diseases with limited available patient data.

Challenges:

- Managing data quality across different research institutions.
- Regulatory hurdles when conducting research across borders with different privacy laws.

9 ADVANTAGES OF FL HEALTHCARE

- **Enhanced Patient Privacy and Data Security**

One of the most noteworthy implications of this research is the improvement of patient privacy in healthcare data management. Traditional centralised machine learning tactics require large volumes of sensitive patient data to be transferred to centralised servers, thereby increasing the risk of data breaches and unauthorised access. In contrast, Federated Learning (FL) enables data to remain within the local environment of hospitals or healthcare institutions while only model updates are shared with the central system. This decentralised framework significantly decreases the exposure of sensitive medical records. Subsequently, the adoption of FL can strengthen patient trust in digital healthcare systems and encourage broader participation in data-driven medical research. Enhanced privacy preservation also supports ethical healthcare practices and responsible data governance.

- **Improved Model Accuracy and Generalizability**

Another key implication is the enhancement in predictive accuracy and robustness of healthcare analytics models. Federated Learning permits multiple healthcare institutions to collaboratively train machine learning models without sharing raw data. By assimilating insights from diverse datasets—such as those from hospitals, diagnostic laboratories, and research centres—the models can learn from a wider range of patient demographics, disease patterns, and clinical conditions. This diversity suggestively advances the generalizability of the predictive models. As a result, diagnostic tools developed using FL frameworks can provide more accurate disease predictions, treatment recommendations, and risk assessments across different populations and healthcare settings.

- **Optimisation of Healthcare Delivery Systems**

The implementation of Federated Learning can add expressively to optimising healthcare delivery systems. By empowering real-time and distributed analysis of medical data, healthcare providers can make quicker and more informed clinical decisions. This can decrease delays in diagnosis, progress treatment planning, and enrich overall patient outcomes. Additionally, FL reduces the need for extensive data storage and centralised infrastructure, thereby depressing operational costs associated with data management. Healthcare organisations can hence benefit from improved efficiency, cost-effectiveness, and enhanced service quality through the adoption of federated data analytics frameworks.

- **Strengthened Regulatory Compliance**

Healthcare organisations operate under strict regulatory frameworks designed to protect patient data privacy and confidentiality. Regulations such as the General Data Protection Regulation (GDPR) and the Health Insurance Portability and Accountability Act (HIPAA) impose stringent requirements regarding the handling and sharing of medical data. Federated Learning offers a viable technological solution to address these regulatory challenges by reducing the need for data transfer across institutions. Since sensitive patient information is stored on the local servers of participating organisations, the risks associated with regulatory violations are reduced. Therefore, the adoption of FL can help healthcare providers maintain compliance with data protection laws while still benefiting from collaborative machine learning initiatives.

- **Advancement of Innovative Healthcare Solutions**

The research also provides insights into the potential of Federated Learning to substitute innovation in healthcare technologies. By empowering the collaborative analysis of large-scale healthcare data without compromising privacy, FL can support the expansion of advanced applications, such as early disease detection systems, personalised medicine, predictive diagnostics, and remote health monitoring solutions. These innovations can transform modern healthcare by enabling more proactive and patient-centred care models. Furthermore, FL can ease collaboration among global healthcare institutions, research organisations, and technology developers, thereby accelerating the discovery of new medical insights and treatment approaches.

10 LIMITATIONS & IMPLICATIONS

Federated learning offers a lot of potential to improve privacy-preserving healthcare analytics, but there are a few things to be aware of. Data heterogeneity, communication overhead, interoperability issues, infrastructure needs, and legal complexities sometimes limit the use of federated learning in healthcare settings. Model performance and scalability may be impacted by differences in clinical procedures, data quality, and technology capabilities among healthcare facilities. Widespread implementation is still hampered by issues with model explainability, algorithmic bias, governance, and practitioner acceptance. Regardless of these drawbacks, the results have significant managerial ramifications for legislators, technology developers, and healthcare administrators. In order to enable secure model training while protecting patient privacy, healthcare companies should make investments in interoperable digital infrastructures, set up strong data governance procedures, and encourage cooperative partnerships, while AI developers should give explainability, fairness, transparency, and resource-efficient federated architectures top priority. Policymakers should create clear legal frameworks and standards for responsible AI implementation in healthcare contexts. Healthcare organisations can use federated learning to support customised treatment plans, improve clinical decision-making, increase operational efficiency, and promote innovation in smart healthcare ecosystems by proactively tackling these issues.

11 LIMITATIONS & FUTURE RESEARCH DIRECTIONS

This research also provides significant directions for future studies in healthcare analytics and artificial intelligence. Researchers can discover improvements in federated learning algorithms to address challenges such as communication efficiency, data heterogeneity, and model convergence. Future work may also emphasise integrating FL with other emerging technologies, such as blockchain, Internet of Medical Things (IoMT), and explainable artificial intelligence (XAI), Federated Generative AI, to further enhance security, transparency, and reliability in healthcare systems. Facilitating global healthcare collaboration with cross border federated healthcare ecosystem will also add to future research studies. Such interdisciplinary research can contribute to the development of more resilient and intelligent healthcare infrastructures in the future.

12. CONCLUSION

This chapter concludes by highlighting the transformative potential of Federated Learning (FL) in addressing some of the most critical challenges faced by modern healthcare systems, primarily in the areas of data privacy, security, and distributed data utilisation. With the rapid digitisation of healthcare services and the increasing adoption of intelligent health technologies, the accessibility of large volumes of sensitive patient data has become both an opportunity and a challenge. Out-dated centralised machine learning models require the aggregation of medical data into centralised repositories, which increases the risk of privacy breaches and regulatory violations. The findings of this research highlight that the decentralised nature of Federated Learning provides a robust groundwork for building secure and privacy-preserving smart healthcare systems. By permitting multiple healthcare providers to collaboratively train predictive models without directly exchanging raw patient data, FL reduces the susceptibility associated with data transmission and storage. This capability plays a crucial role in firming patient trust in digital healthcare systems and encourages broader participation in data-driven healthcare innovations. Subsequently, the adoption of Federated Learning can support ethical data governance and accountable artificial intelligence practices in healthcare environments.

Another important conclusion drawn from this study is the improved predictive performance and model generalisation achieved through Federated Learning approaches. By leveraging distributed datasets from diverse healthcare institutions, FL-based models can capture a wider range of patient demographics, disease patterns, and treatment responses. This diversity contributes to the expansion of more robust and reliable predictive models compared to traditional centralised learning methods. As a result, Federated Learning has the potential to significantly augment diagnostic accuracy, support personalised treatment strategies, and improve clinical decision-making processes. Additionally, the integration of FL into healthcare analytics can enhance applications such as early disease detection, medical image analysis, and remote patient monitoring systems. The chapter also highlights the importance of efficient workflow mechanisms within Federated Learning frameworks, which enable seamless collaboration among healthcare institutions. Techniques such as Federated Averaging (FedAvg) and Federated Stochastic Gradient Descent (FedSGD) play a vital role in coordinating model updates across distributed nodes while maintaining data privacy. These algorithms enable local models to be trained independently at each participating institution and subsequently aggregated to produce a global model with enhanced performance. Such mechanisms confirm that healthcare providers can benefit from collaborative learning while maintaining compliance with strict regulatory frameworks governing patient data protection.

Furthermore, the study demonstrates that the adoption of Federated Learning can contribute to optimising healthcare delivery systems. By enabling efficient distributed data analysis, healthcare providers can generate faster insights, improve diagnostic procedures, and deliver timely medical interventions. This not only enhances the quality of patient care but also reduces operational costs associated with large-scale data storage and management. In this context, FL can play a crucial role in advancing smart healthcare ecosystems, where artificial intelligence, medical technologies, and data analytics collaborate to support patient-centred care. Despite its promising potential, the implementation of Federated Learning in healthcare presents several challenges. Issues such as data heterogeneity, communication overhead, and the need for interpretable models continue to be significant barriers to large-scale adoption. Healthcare data often varies in format, quality, and distribution across different institutions, which can affect model training and performance. Similarly, the exchange of frequent model updates among multiple nodes may increase communication costs and computational complexity. Additionally, clinical environments require high levels of transparency and interpretability in AI-driven decision-making systems to ensure that healthcare professionals can trust and understand the outputs generated by predictive models.

Addressing these challenges will require continued research and technological development in the field of Federated Learning. Future studies may focus on developing personalised federated learning approaches that can effectively handle non-identically distributed data across institutions. Researchers can also explore scalable federated learning frameworks designed for smaller healthcare facilities that may have limited computational resources and infrastructure. Integrating FL with emerging technologies such as explainable artificial intelligence (XAI), blockchain-based data security, and Internet of Medical Things (IoMT) can further enhance its reliability, transparency, and security in healthcare applications. In conclusion, Federated Learning represents a significant advancement in the development of privacy-preserving artificial intelligence for healthcare systems. Its ability to combine collaborative data analysis with strong privacy protection makes it a promising solution for addressing the growing demands of data-driven healthcare innovation. As smart healthcare systems continue to evolve, ongoing improvements in federated learning frameworks will be essential to ensure equitable, secure, and efficient access to advanced medical technologies across global healthcare ecosystems. Through continued research, interdisciplinary collaboration, and responsible technological adoption, Federated Learning has the potential to reshape the future of intelligent healthcare and contribute to improved patient outcomes worldwide.

REFERENCES

Alasmary, H. (2024). Scalable Digital Health (SDH): An IoT-Based scalable framework for remote patient monitoring. *Sensors (Basel), 24*(4), 1346. DOI: 10.3390/s24041346 PMID: 38400504

Albshaier, L., Almarri, S., & Albuali, A. (2025). Federated Learning for Cloud and Edge Security: A Systematic Review of Challenges and AI opportunities. *Electronics (Basel), 14*(5), 1019. DOI: 10.3390/electronics14051019

Alotaibi, B., Khan, F. A., & Mahmood, S. (2024). Communication Efficiency and Non-Independent and Identically Distributed Data Challenge in Federated Learning: A Systematic Mapping study. *Applied Sciences (Basel, Switzerland), 14*(7), 2720. DOI: 10.3390/app14072720

Alowais, S. A., Alghamdi, S. S., Alsuhebany, N., Alqahtani, T., Alshaya, A. I., Almohareb, S. N., Aldairem, A., Alrashed, M., Saleh, K. B., Badreldin, H. A., Yami, M. S. A., Harbi, S. A., & Albekairy, A. M. (2023). Revolutionizing healthcare: The role of artificial intelligence in clinical practice. *BMC Medical Education, 23*(1), 689. DOI: 10.1186/s12909-023-04698-z PMID: 37740191

Babar, M., Qureshi, B., & Koubaa, A. (2024). Investigating the impact of data heterogeneity on the performance of federated learning algorithm using medical imaging. *PLoS One, 19*(5), e0302539. DOI: 10.1371/journal.pone.0302539 PMID: 38748657

Bajwa, J., Munir, U., Nori, A., & Williams, B. (2021). Artificial intelligence in healthcare: Transforming the practice of medicine. *Future Healthcare Journal, 8*(2), e188–e194. DOI: 10.7861/fhj.2021-0095 PMID: 34286183

Bebortta, S., Tripathy, S. S., Basheer, S., & Chowdhary, C. L. (2023). FedEHR: A Federated Learning Approach towards the Prediction of Heart Diseases in IoT-Based Electronic Health Records. *Diagnostics (Basel), 13*(20), 3166. DOI: 10.3390/diagnostics13203166 PMID: 37891987

Chen, Y., Qin, X., Wang, J., Yu, C., & Gao, W. (2020). FedHealth: A federated transfer learning framework for wearable healthcare. *IEEE Intelligent Systems, 35*(4), 83–93. DOI: 10.1109/MIS.2020.2988604

Chiruvella, V., & Guddati, A. K. (2021). Ethical issues in patient data ownership. *Interactive Journal of Medical Research, 10*(2), e22269. DOI: 10.2196/22269 PMID: 34018968

Dara, S., Kanapala, A., Babu, A. R., Dhamercherala, S., Vidyarthi, A., & Agarwal, R. (2022). Scalable Federated-Learning and Internet-of-Things enabled architecture for Chest Computer Tomography image classification. *Computers & Electrical Engineering, 102*, 108266. DOI: 10.1016/j.compeleceng.2022.108266

Dinh-Le, C., Chuang, R., Chokshi, S., & Mann, D. (2019). Wearable Health Technology and Electronic Health Record Integration: Scoping review and Future Directions. *JMIR mHealth and uHealth, 7*(9), e12861. DOI: 10.2196/12861 PMID: 31512582

Esmaeilzadeh, P. (2023). Evolution of health information sharing between health care organizations: Potential of nonfungible tokens. *Interactive Journal of Medical Research, 12*, e42685. DOI: 10.2196/42685 PMID: 37043269

Fang, C., Dziedzic, A., Zhang, L., Oliva, L., Verma, A., Razak, F., Papernot, N., & Wang, B. (2024). Decentralised, collaborative, and privacy-preserving machine learning for multi-hospital data. *EBioMedicine, 101*, 105006. DOI: 10.1016/j.ebiom.2024.105006 PMID: 38377795

Grataloup, A., Jonas, S., & Meyer, A. (2024). A review of federated learning in renewable energy applications: Potential, challenges, and future directions. *Energy and AI, 17*, 100375. DOI: 10.1016/j.egyai.2024.100375

Gu, X., Sabrina, F., Fan, Z., & Sohail, S. (2023). A review of privacy enhancement methods for federated learning in healthcare systems. *International Journal of Environmental Research and Public Health, 20*(15), 6539. DOI: 10.3390/ijerph20156539 PMID: 37569079

Habehh, H., & Gohel, S. (2021). Machine learning in healthcare. *Current Genomics, 22*(4), 291–300. DOI: 10.2174/1389202922666210705124359 PMID: 35273459

Hassan, S. U., Abdulkadir, S. J., Zahid, M. S. M., & Al-Selwi, S. M. (2024). Local interpretable model-agnostic explanation approach for medical imaging analysis: A systematic literature review. *Computers in Biology and Medicine, 185*, 109569. DOI: 10.1016/j.compbiomed.2024.109569 PMID: 39705792

Islam, M. J., Rahman, A., Kabir, S., Karim, M. R., Acharjee, U. K., Nasir, M. K., Band, S. S., Sookhak, M., & Wu, S. (2021). Blockchain-SDN-Based Energy-Aware and distributed secure architecture for IoT in smart cities. *IEEE Internet of Things Journal, 9*(5), 3850–3864. DOI: 10.1109/JIOT.2021.3100797

Johannssen, A., & Chukhrova, N. (2025). The crucial role of explainable artificial intelligence (XAI) in improving health care management. *Health Care Management Science, 28*(3), 565–570. DOI: 10.1007/s10729-025-09720-y PMID: 41026402

Khan, L. U., Saad, W., Han, Z., Hossain, E., & Hong, C. S. (2021). *Federated learning for Internet of Things: Recent advances, taxonomy, and open challenges*. arXiv. https://doi.org//arXiv.2009.13012DOI: 10.48550

Kim, J., Kim, J., Hur, K., & Choi, E. (2026). Federated learning for heterogeneous electronic health record systems with cost effective participant selection. *Scientific Reports*, *16*(1), 6876. DOI: 10.1038/s41598-026-38299-9 PMID: 41622329

Kjwan, A. H., & Mohammad, O. H. (2024). Enhancing Medical Data Analysis with Federated Learning in the Internet of Medical Things. *International Journal of Research in Science & Engineering*, *43*(43), 38–52. DOI: 10.55529/ijrise.43.38.52

Li, X., Gu, Y., Dvornek, N., Staib, L. H., Ventola, P., & Duncan, J. S. (2020). Multi-site fMRI analysis using privacy-preserving federated learning and domain adaptation: ABIDE results. *Medical Image Analysis*, *65*, 101765. DOI: 10.1016/j.media.2020.101765 PMID: 32679533

Lim, W. Y. B., Luong, N. C., Hoang, D. T., Jiao, Y., Liang, Y.-C., Yang, Q., Niyato, D., & Miao, C. (2020). Federated learning in mobile edge networks: A comprehensive survey. *IEEE Communications Surveys and Tutorials*, *22*(3), 2031–2063. DOI: 10.1109/COMST.2020.2986024

Ma, B., Feng, Y., Chen, G., Li, C., & Xia, Y. (2023). Federated adaptive reweighting for medical image classification. *Pattern Recognition*, *144*, 109880. DOI: 10.1016/j.patcog.2023.109880

McMahan, B., Moore, E., Ramage, D., & Hampson, S. Arcas, B.A.y. (2017). Communication-Efficient Learning of Deep Networks from Decentralized Data. Proceedings of the 20th International Conference on Artificial Intelligence and Statistics, in Proceedings of Machine Learning Research 54:1273-1282 Available from https://proceedings.mlr.press/v54/mcmahan17a.html.

Mishra, A., Saha, S., Mishra, S., & Bagade, P. (2023). A federated learning approach for smart healthcare systems. *CSI Transactions on ICT*, *11*(1), 39–44. DOI: 10.1007/s40012-023-00382-1

Moshawrab, M., Adda, M., Bouzouane, A., Ibrahim, H., & Raad, A. (2023). Reviewing federated machine learning and its use in diseases prediction. *Sensors (Basel)*, *23*(4), 2112. DOI: 10.3390/s23042112 PMID: 36850717

N, P. S., Shelke, N., Saini, D. K. J. B., Pimpalkar, A., Pal, M., & Chirchi, V. (2025). Explainable federated learning for secure and transparent medical diagnosis in IoT-based smart hospitals. In *2025 5th International Conference on Soft Computing for Security Applications (ICSCSA)* (pp. 883–889). IEEE. https://doi.org/DOI: 10.1109/ICSCSA66339.2025.11171173

Noor, A., Chaman, U. M., & Kabir, M. S. (2026). Federated learning in healthcare: A comprehensive survey on privacy, scalability and clinical applications. *ICT Express*. Advance online publication. DOI: 10.1016/j.icte.2026.05.011

Oh, W., & Nadkarni, G. N. (2023). Federated Learning in Health care Using Structured Medical Data. *Advances in Kidney Disease and Health*, *30*(1), 4–16. DOI: 10.1053/j.akdh.2022.11.007 PMID: 36723280

Paul, D., Sanap, G., Shenoy, S., Kalyane, D., Kalia, K., & Tekade, R. K. (2020). Artificial intelligence in drug discovery and development. *Drug Discovery Today*, *26*(1), 80–93. DOI: 10.1016/j.drudis.2020.10.010 PMID: 33099022

Paul, M., Maglaras, L., Ferrag, M. A., & Almomani, I. (2023). Digitization of healthcare sector: A study on privacy and security concerns. *ICT Express*, *9*(4), 571–588. DOI: 10.1016/j.icte.2023.02.007

Pham, Q. V., Dev, K., Maddikunta, P. K. R., Gadekallu, T. R., & Huynh-The, T. (2021). *Fusion of federated learning and industrial Internet of Things: A survey* (arXiv:2101.00798). arXiv. https://arxiv.org/abs/2101.00798

Pustokhina, I. V., Pustokhin, D. A., Gupta, D., Khanna, A., Shankar, K., & Nguyen, G. N. (2020). An effective training scheme for deep neural network in edge computing enabled Internet of Medical Things (IOMT) systems. *IEEE Access : Practical Innovations, Open Solutions*, *8*, 107112–107123. DOI: 10.1109/ACCESS.2020.3000322

Qi, P., Chiaro, D., Guzzo, A., Ianni, M., Fortino, G., & Piccialli, F. (2023). Model aggregation techniques in federated learning: A comprehensive survey. *Future Generation Computer Systems*, *150*, 272–293. DOI: 10.1016/j.future.2023.09.008

Rahman, A., Hossain, M. S., Muhammad, G., Kundu, D., Debnath, T., Rahman, M., Khan, M. S. I., Tiwari, P., & Band, S. S. (2022b). Federated learning-based AI approaches in smart healthcare: Concepts, taxonomies, challenges and open issues. *Cluster Computing*, *26*(4), 2271–2311. DOI: 10.1007/s10586-022-03658-4 PMID: 35996680

Rajagopal, S. M., M, S., & Buyya, R. (2023). FedSDM: Federated learning based smart decision making module for ECG data in IoT integrated Edge–Fog–Cloud computing environments. *Internet of Things : Engineering Cyber Physical Human Systems*, *22*, 100784. DOI: 10.1016/j.iot.2023.100784

Rani, S., Kataria, A., Kumar, S., & Tiwari, P. (2023). Federated learning for secure IoMT-applications in smart healthcare systems: A comprehensive review. *Knowledge-Based Systems*, *274*, 110658. DOI: 10.1016/j.knosys.2023.110658

Reddy, K. D., & Gadekallu, T. R. (2023). A comprehensive survey on federated learning techniques for healthcare informatics. *Computational Intelligence and Neuroscience*, *2023*(1), 8393990. DOI: 10.1155/2023/8393990 PMID: 36909974

Rieke, N., Hancox, J., Li, W., Milletarì, F., Roth, H. R., Albarqouni, S., Bakas, S., Galtier, M. N., Landman, B. A., Maier-Hein, K., Ourselin, S., Sheller, M., Summers, R. M., Trask, A., Xu, D., Baust, M., & Cardoso, M. J. (2020). The future of digital health with federated learning. *NPJ Digital Medicine*, *3*(1), 119. DOI: 10.1038/s41746-020-00323-1 PMID: 33015372

Sandhu, S. S., Gorji, H. T., Tavakolian, P., Tavakolian, K., & Akhbardeh, A. (2023). Medical imaging applications of federated learning. *Diagnostics (Basel)*, *13*(19), 3140. DOI: 10.3390/diagnostics13193140 PMID: 37835883

Santos, M. R., Guedes, A., & Sanchez-Gendriz, I. (2024). SHapley Additive ExPlanations (SHAP) for efficient feature selection in rolling bearing fault diagnosis. *Machine Learning and Knowledge Extraction*, *6*(1), 316–341. DOI: 10.3390/make6010016

Seh, A. H., Zarour, M., Alenezi, M., Sarkar, A. K., Agrawal, A., Kumar, R., & Khan, R. A. (2020). Healthcare data breaches: Insights and implications. *Health Care*, *8*(2), 133. DOI: 10.3390/healthcare8020133 PMID: 32414183

Shaik, T., Tao, X., Higgins, N., Li, L., Gururajan, R., Zhou, X., & Acharya, U. R. (2023). Remote patient monitoring using artificial intelligence: Current state, applications, and challenges. *Wiley Interdisciplinary Reviews. Data Mining and Knowledge Discovery*, *13*(2), e1485. Advance online publication. DOI: 10.1002/widm.1485

Sheller, M. J., Edwards, B., Reina, G. A., Martin, J., Pati, S., Kotrotsou, A., Milchenko, M., Xu, W., Marcus, D., Colen, R. R., & Bakas, S. (2020). Federated learning in medicine: Facilitating multi-institutional collaborations without sharing patient data. *Scientific Reports*, *10*(1), 12598. DOI: 10.1038/s41598-020-69250-1 PMID: 32724046

Sheller, M. J., Reina, G. A., Edwards, B., Martin, J., & Bakas, S. (2019). Multi-institutional deep learning modeling without sharing patient data: A feasibility study on brain tumor segmentation. *Lecture Notes in Computer Science*, *11383*, 92–104. DOI: 10.1007/978-3-030-11723-8_9 PMID: 31231720

Shojaei, P., Vlahu-Gjorgievska, E., & Chow, Y. (2024). Security and Privacy of Technologies in Health Information Systems: A Systematic Literature review. *Computers*, *13*(2), 41. DOI: 10.3390/computers13020041

Teo, Z. L., Jin, L., Liu, N., Li, S., Miao, D., Zhang, X., Ng, W. Y., Tan, T. F., Lee, D. M., Chua, K. J., Heng, J., Liu, Y., Goh, R. S. M., & Ting, D. S. W. (2024). Federated machine learning in healthcare: A systematic review on clinical applications and technical architecture. *Cell Reports Medicine*, *5*(2), 101419. DOI: 10.1016/j.xcrm.2024.101419 PMID: 38340728

Tharini, V. J., & Vijayarani, S. (2019). IoT in healthcare. In *Advances in medical technologies and clinical practice book series* (pp. 1–22). https://doi.org/DOI: 10.4018/978-1-7998-1090-2.ch001

Tian, S., Yang, W., Grange, J. M. L., Wang, P., Huang, W., & Ye, Z. (2019). Smart healthcare: Making medical care more intelligent. *Global Health Journal (Amsterdam, Netherlands)*, *3*(3), 62–65. DOI: 10.1016/j.glohj.2019.07.001

Xu, J., Glicksberg, B. S., Su, C., Walker, P., Bian, J., & Wang, F. (2020). Federated Learning for Healthcare Informatics. *Journal of Healthcare Informatics Research*, *5*(1), 1–19. DOI: 10.1007/s41666-020-00082-4 PMID: 33204939

Yang, D., Xu, Z., Li, W., Myronenko, A., Roth, H. R., Harmon, S., Xu, S., Turkbey, B., Turkbey, E., Wang, X., Zhu, W., Carrafiello, G., Patella, F., Cariati, M., Obinata, H., Mori, H., Tamura, K., An, P., Wood, B. J., & Xu, D. (2021). Federated semi-supervised learning for COVID region segmentation in chest CT using multinational data from China, Italy, Japan. *Medical Image Analysis*, *70*, 101992. DOI: 10.1016/j.media.2021.101992 PMID: 33601166

Yang, Q., Liu, Y., Chen, T., & Tong, Y. (2019). Federated Machine Learning. *ACM Transactions on Intelligent Systems and Technology*, *10*(2), 1–19. DOI: 10.1145/3298981

Zhang, F., Shuai, Z., Kuang, K., Wu, F., Zhuang, Y., & Xiao, J. (2023). Unified fair federated learning for digital healthcare. *Patterns (New York, N.Y.)*, *5*(1), 100907. DOI: 10.1016/j.patter.2023.100907 PMID: 38264718

Chapter 5
LBOAF:
Lady Bug Optimizer-Enabled AI-Driven Framework for Preserving Patient Data

Prasanna Guduru
http://orcid.org/0000-0003-1186-9935
Sri Venkateswara University, India

K. Vijaya Lakshmi
Sri Venkateswara University, India

Swathi Pothala
http://orcid.org/0000-0002-9093-4469
Sri Venkateswara University, India

P. Jyotsna
Sri Venkateswara University, India

Vinuthna Kondipati
Sanofi, USA

N. V. Keerthana
http://orcid.org/0000-0001-8878-2083
Velalar College of Engineering and Technology, India

ABSTRACT

In the field of healthcare, artificial intelligence is increasingly being used in decision support systems, and there is a major concern about the privacy and security of sensitive patient data. This research proposes a robust artificial intelligence-based framework that uses federated learning, differential privacy, homomorphic encryption, blockchain, and Lady Bug Optimization (LBO) for the secure and private analysis of patient data. In the proposed system, the data of the patients is stored locally in the hospital network, and the federated learning mechanism is used for collaborative training of the model. Differential privacy is used to protect sensitive patient data by adding noise during the training of the model. Homomorphic encryption is also used in the proposed system to improve the security of the data. Lady Bug Optimization is used to adaptively tune the parameters of the differential privacy and the parameters of the model to achieve the optimal results. In addition, blockchain is used in the proposed system to monitor the training of the model.

DOI: 10.4018/979-8-2600-3070-7.ch005

1. INTRODUCTION

Artificial Intelligence (AI) has turned into a groundbreaking technology in numerous areas such as healthcare, architecture, energy systems, environmental analysis, and enterprise applications. In particular, in the healthcare sector, AI-based deep learning models are demonstrating great effectiveness in disease diagnosis and clinical decision support. Some examples of breast cancer detection with EfficientNet and U-Net architectures (Abdel-Wahab et al., 2025), sepsis prediction models (Barkas et al., 2025), fetal arrhythmia detection with AI-enabled the cardiotocograph (Bhosale, 2025), and diagnosis of hormonal disorders with machine learning and optimization methods (Dhanka et al., 2025). The studies represent just a few examples of the healthcare industry increasingly depending on data and AI-based models for medical diagnosis and patient care improvement.

However, the use of more and more sensitive patient data also brings up very serious questions of data privacy, security, and ethical usage (Martínez et al., 2023). For example, centralized AI systems are perpetually vulnerable to data breaches, model inversion, and inference attacks, which can be very harmful to patient confidentiality. Similar security issues were also found in AI-enabled Internet of Things (IoT) networks (Nazari et al., 2025) phishing and denial-of-service mitigation systems (Sofiyan, 2021) and AI- powered wireless communication infrastructures (Qin et al., 2024). Thus, the need for effective privacy-aware AI architectures has been highlighted.

Extensive multi-objective optimization methods have been used across a range of fields, including low-carbon building design (Noorzai et al., 2023), adaptive facade systems (Manesh et al., 2025) and performance-driven architectural layouts (Zhou & Xue, 2025). Metaheuristic optimization algorithms, including honey bee algorithms (Ponnusamy et al., 2024) genetic optimization and hybrid ladybug, hawk optimization methods (Shanmugam & Arumugam, 2025)are found to effectively address the often conflicting criteria such as accuracy, energy efficiency, and system robustness. Simultaneously, explainable and trustworthy AI has become a major focus, particularly in systems that are safety-critical and decision-critical. For example, explainable geospatial AI helps to assess climate-induced landslide susceptibility (Yousefi et al., 2025), contrastive multimodal insect recognition (Liu et al., 2025), and intelligent safety systems for assault detection (Sthankiya et al., 2024). All highlight the need for transparency and accountability in AI-based systems. Such demands are most of the time a matter of life and death in healthcare environments where, at least, a lack of transparency in decision-making may lead to loss of trust and non-compliance with regulations.

Decentralized and real-time AI supported by digital twin technologies and interactive AI platforms is another rising trend. For instance, digital twins were used for energy forecasting and business optimization (Boukaf et al., 2024) and LLM-assisted platforms have allowed efficient design optimization workflows (Islam & Khan, 2024). In the same way, real-time crop optimization (Sridhar et al., 2025) And AI pandemic preparedness models stress the importance of having scalable and distributed intelligence. But merely decentralizing will not automatically ensure privacy, as model updates can still reveal sensitive data (Elkhateeb & Anwar, 2025) (Datta & Namasudra, 2024).

Federated and decentralized learning approaches reduce the risk of direct data sharing. However, if privacy mechanisms are unchanged and poorly optimized they are still vulnerable to gradient-based privacy attacks (Arunprasath & Annamalai, 2024) (Rao et al., 2025). Most of the existing systems do not adjust the privacy controls for heterogeneous data sensitivity and system dynamics. Thus, a critical research gap exists in an adaptive, optimization-driven, preserving AI framework (Khan, 2025).

To solve this problem, the present study suggests a Lady Bug Optimizer AI-driven Framework (LBOAF) for safe and privacy-preserving healthcare AI. The framework employs federated learning to train the model in a decentralized manner, differential privacy to protect the inference, homomorphic encryption for the secure aggregation, and LBO for the dynamic adjustment of privacy parameters. The framework, being optimization-driven adaptable the paper demonstrates that the proposed framework can provide data privacy and model performance simultaneously, paving the way to a scalable and trustworthy solution for next-generation AI-driven healthcare analytics.

2. LITERATURE SURVEY

The fast introduction of AI in different areas like healthcare, cybersecurity, and enterprise systems has caused a rise in demand for privacy, maintenance, explainability, and ethical accountability of AI architectures. Features of today's AI technologies. Traditionally, AI systems have mainly been seen as prediction machines. However, they are increasingly required to comply with data protection laws, be transparent, and adhere to regulations, as illustrated recently. Against this background, federated learning, decentralized intelligence, security, driven optimization, and explainable AI are the main research directions. Explainable, privacy, preserving AI and mutual attention have been two concepts that have naturally emerged after AI's influence in high, risk decision, making scenarios. For example, the study linking explainable, automated and privacy-aware AI shows how security and intelligent systems are mainly made up of interpretability and trust (Harrath et al., 2025).These writers have figured out that explainability and privacy are not at odds with each other but that they go together and are particularly important in the areas of healthcare and cybersecurity. Equally, AI ethics-based mental health interventions necessitate data handling that is responsible, transparent, and fair to sustain public trust (Saeidnia et al., 2024).

Federated learning is one of the most common answers to centralized data exposure. A case study of federated learning models at the corporate level shows that decentralized training hardly compromises privacy while enabling collaborative intelligence among different organizations (Hasan, 2025). On the other hand, the authors point out that the models are still prone to gradient leakage and fixed privacy controls, which means that there is a need for privacy mechanisms that can change according to the situation. Regulatory aspects also show that to be General Data Protection Regulation (GDPR) and Health Insurance Portability and Accountability Act (HIPAA) compliant, AI systems must embed privacy from the very beginning of system development, not as an aftereffect (Ashraf & Haile, 2023).

Decentralization and data authenticity issues are solved by blockchain, backed by AI systems, as well. Research on auditable reconciliations in decentralized financial systems reveals that blockchain can offer tamper-proof record-keeping, transparency, and accountability in AI-powered environments (Alaka et al., 2025) (Masood et al., 2024). Similar ideas have been used for smart city environments, where the security system breach detection based on optimization has increased the sturdiness of Internet of Health Things (IoHT) systems (Jayanthi et al., 2025).

Optimization, intelligence, and being driven are essential for enhancing the performance and adaptability of AI. Nature-inspired algorithms, such as the hybrid metaheuristic ladybug and hawk optimization method for Parkinson's disease classification, are highly capable of dealing with complicated, multimodal healthcare data (Hosen et al., 2025). Optimization algorithms have been able to demonstrate through these experiments that they can adjust in real time different aspects that are often in conflict, e.g., accuracy, stability, and computational efficiency. This is the reason why they are combined with privacy, preserving optimization strategies to achieve this balance. (Ansari et al., 2025) and (Periáñez et al., 2024) emphasize that healthcare systems using AI, neuromodulation technology, and going through a digital transformation, see AI more and more as a trusted clinical decision support tool at the system level for optimization.

Existing works are of a significant, loud call for safe and adaptable AI models that would be capable of functioning in a distributed systems setting in healthcare. Also, basic research in computer science and information technology explains how AI, software engineering, and intelligent system design lead to the creation of modular and scalable architectures(Mathew & Krishnan, 2025). The recent advances, like federated learning, differential privacy, homomorphic encryption, and blockchain technologies, have tried to solve the issues mentioned above independently. Federated learning does away with direct data transfer problems but is susceptible to attacks by way of gradient leakage. Differential privacy adds security through statistics but reduces the usability of models when privacy-related hyperparameters are set statically. Homomorphic encryption ensures computations can be performed without decrypting the input data but involves computational costs.

The literature still shows a very important gap: Firstly, a majority of privacy-preserving AI frameworks today mainly depend on fixed privacy parameters and a lack of adaptive optimization mechanisms. Secondly, bringing together the elements of federated learning, optimization algorithms, encryption, and auditability into one single healthcare-oriented architecture has not been extensively done. In fact, the LBOAF proposed in this study is a step further from the previous work, as it presents variable privacy tuning in a decentralized, secure, and law-abiding AI environment.

2.1 Motivation

The motivation of this work derives from the increased dependence on AI- based healthcare systems that need access to very private patient data, while the currently centralized and static privacy-preserving methods are still exposed to data leakage, inference attacks, and non-compliance with regulations. Federated learning, on the one hand, minimizes the sharing of raw data but does not eliminate privacy risks arising from unprotected gradient exposure and a fixed privacy budget. On the other hand, the existing healthcare AI systems are missing the adaptive mechanisms that can dynamically balance data confidentiality, model accuracy, and system efficiency, taking into account varying clinical and regulatory conditions. Hence, the working out of an LBOAF has been geared towards this project. The framework will merge federated learning, differential privacy, secure aggregation, and auditability smartly through LBO, and be capable of providing strong, scalable, and regulation-compliant patient data protection at no expense of AI performance.

2.2 Contribution

- Provide a new LBOAF that intelligently adjusts the trade-off between patient data privacy and model performance in AI-powered healthcare systems.
- Uses federated learning combined with adaptive differential privacy to ensure that no raw data is shared and to reduce gradient-based inference attacks.
- Uses an optimization approach to privacy budget and noise parameter tuning that leads to better results in terms of both accuracy and privacy preservation than static privacy mechanisms.
- Besides, using secure aggregation and auditability mechanisms, the authors improve the trust, transparency, and regulatory compliance of their healthcare AI application.

- Tests the proposed framework under real-world medical data analytics scenarios that are privacy-sensitive and show the framework's efficiency and capability.

3. METHODOLOGY

The LBOAF is essentially a secured, adaptable, and privacy-enhancing AI pipeline for healthcare analytics. Patient data are first of all kept at local healthcare institutions only, where data preprocessing and normalization are done for data quality and consistency. AI models can be developed locally on-site via federated learning, which does not allow the raw patient data to be shared across institutions.

Moreover, the local training process applies differential privacy to model gradients by adding calibrated random noise, so that a typical record will not be identifiable in a subsequent reconstruction or inference attack. Without the LBO algorithm, it is very hard to allow privacy settings to be changed adaptively. Here, the LBO serves as such an adaptive optimization layer that quietly and regularly adjusts critical privacy and training parameters, which also include differential privacy budget, noise scale, learning rate, and update frequency in accordance with feedback from model performance and privacy loss metrics. Besides, the present optimization procedure is concerned with the best possible trade-off of data privacy and predictive accuracy given different data sensitivity and system scenarios. The model updates, both privacy-protected and LBO, optimized, are encrypted with homomorphic encryption and then securely sent to the central aggregation server. Secure aggregation is done on encrypted updates only, so the server or any intermediaries cannot peek at sensitive model data.

A blockchain-based audit mechanism commits model update transactions, optimization decisions, and access logs to an immutable ledger to guarantee transparency, traceability, and compliance with regulations. In the end, the worldwide aggregated model is sent back to the contributing institutions for the next cycle of training and evaluation, while system performance is measured based on accuracy, privacy loss, computational overhead, and scalability criteria. Figure 1 illustrates the integrated architecture combining federated learning, adaptive optimization, privacy preservation, secure aggregation, and auditability for healthcare AI.

Figure 1. Lady Bug Optimization–Based Adaptive Framework (LBOAF) Architecture

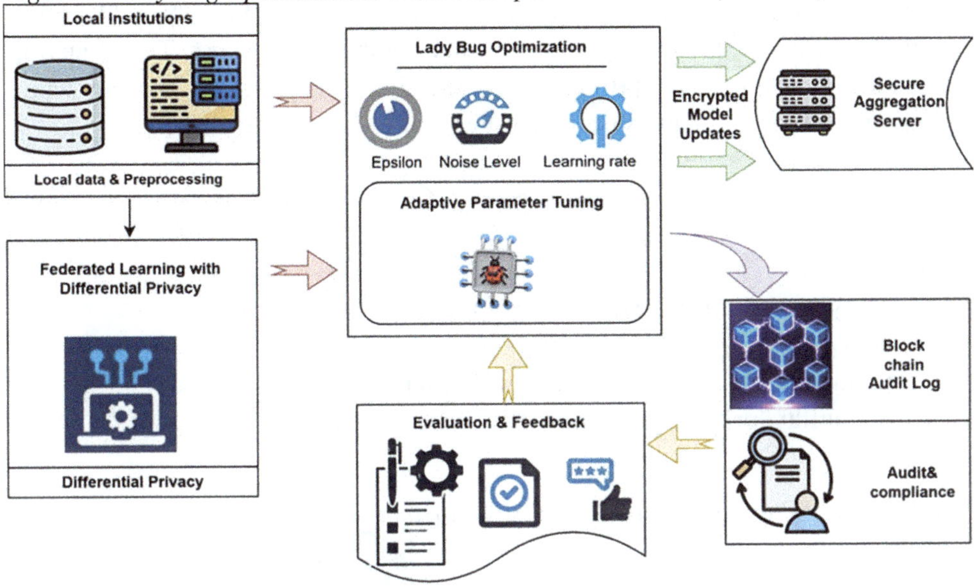

3.1 Lady Bug Optimization Algorithm (LBO)

The LBO Algorithm significantly facilitates adaptive privacy control in the LBOAF in this project. The primary reason for choosing LBO is that it can effectively perform a search over complicated, nonlinear solution spaces and can dynamically reconcile multiple, rather conflicting objectives, such as patient data privacy, model accuracy, and computational efficiency. In the proposed system, LBO is utilized to find the optimum value of some essential federated learning hyperparameters such as differential privacy budget (ε), noise level, learning rate and communication frequency. A ladybug is basically a candidate solution that specifies a certain combination of these parameters. By using iterative exploration and exploitation techniques inspired by ladybug foraging behaviour, the algorithm assesses candidate solutions against the defined fitness function. This fitness function simultaneously measures prediction performance and privacy loss; thus, the system can adaptively determine optimal configurations given different data sensitivity and training scenarios.

During each iteration, parameter sets that perform poorly are discarded and replaced by better-performing ones, while the elite solutions are preserved to ensure the stability of convergence. This adaptive tuning prevents the framework from depending on fixed privacy budgets, which usually result in either too much noise or insufficient privacy protection. Rather, LBO keeps tweaking parameters so that it can achieve a strong balance between secrecy and learning utility. Figure 2 shows how the Lady Bug Optimization algorithm dynamically tunes privacy and learning parameters to balance accuracy, privacy, and computational cost. This equation defines the multi-objective optimization goal of LBO to maximize accuracy while minimizing privacy loss and system overhead, as defined in equation (1).

$$L = \max(\alpha . Accuracy - \beta . PrivacyLoss - \gamma . ComputationalCost) \quad (1)$$

Where,
Accuracy = predictive performance of the global AI model
PrivacyLoss = differential privacy budget ε
ComputationalCost = communication & encryption
α, β, γ = utility, privacy protection, and system efficiency.

Figure 2. Lady Bug Optimization (LBO) Algorithm

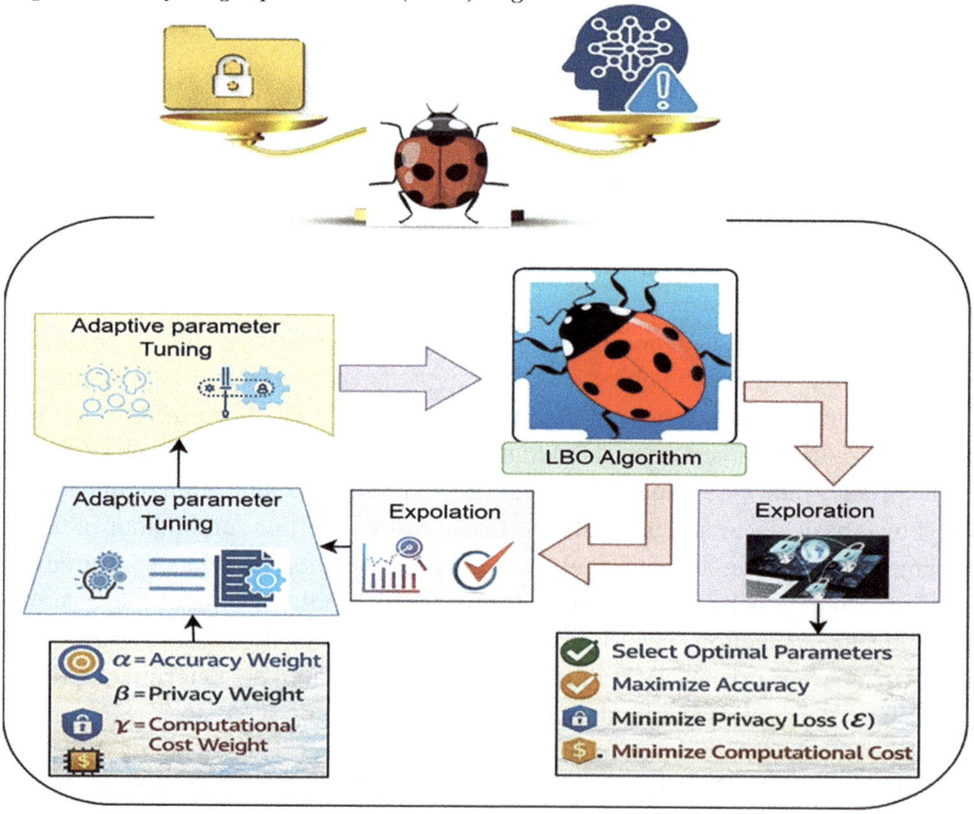

3.2 Federated Learning

Federated Learning forms the core idea of the LBOAF Framework. Federated Learning is basically a decentralized, privacy-protected model training technique. The main reason why Federated Learning is used in this project is to allow cross-institutional learning among the multiple healthcare facilities without downloading or transporting the raw patient data, thus minimising the chances of data breaches and regulatory violations. After secure preprocessing, every healthcare institution (client) participating in Federated Learning locally trains an AI model on its private patient dataset.

During the local training, the data does not go outside the local environment, so obviously, security and confidentiality are ensured. Rather than sharing data, only model parameters or gradients are produced. Moreover, Differential Privacy techniques are applied to these local updates, and to top it all, they are encrypted before sending them across the wire. The encrypted updates are sent to a central aggregation server, where they are securely combined to form a global model. The global model, after it has been updated by combination, is sent back to all the institutions that took part to allow them to keep learning and adjusting. Figure 3 depicts decentralized model training across multiple healthcare institutions without sharing raw patient data. Here, federated learning is deeply combined with LBO, which automatically adjusts the training parameters like learning rate, communication frequency, and privacy budget, thus enhancing convergence speed and ensuring a proper trade-off between privacy and accuracy. This expression aggregates locally trained model parameters into a global model without sharing raw patient data, and is defined as equation (2).

$$F^{a+1} = \sum_{n=1}^{N} \frac{b_n}{B} F_n^{(a)} \qquad (2)$$

Where,

F^{a+1} = Updated global model

$F_n^{(a)}$ = Locally trained model

b_n = Number of data samples

$B = \sum_{n=1}^{N} b_n$ = Total number of samples

N = Total number of federated clients

Figure 3. Federated Learning Algorithm

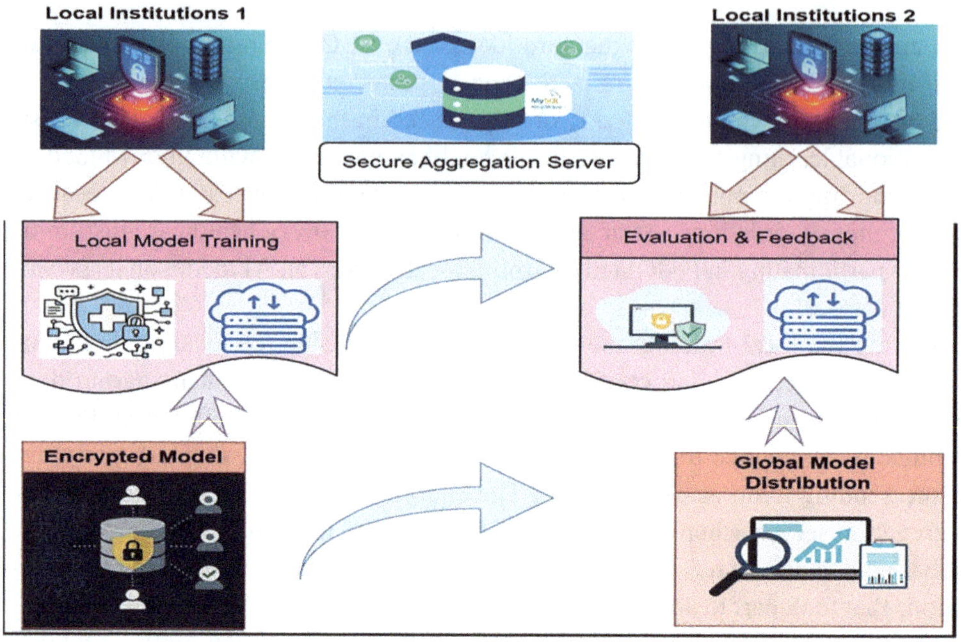

3.3 Differential Privacy Mechanism

The Differential Privacy mechanism is used to secure the sensitive information of patients and thus prevent its leakage in the course of federated learning. Federated learning does not entail the sharing of raw data; however, model updates may still be used to extract private information through gradient inversion or inference attacks. Differential privacy eliminates this problem by making sure that the trained model is hardly affected by any single patient record.

This research employs differential privacy locally at the client side before sending model updates to the aggregation server. At the time of local training, the gradients or model parameters that have been calculated are injected with the calibrated noise, which serves to conceal the individual's data contributions. The privacy level is determined by the privacy budget (ε), where decreasing the value of ε increases the level of privacy. Instead of a fixed privacy budget, the framework that is proposed here uses LBO to continuously adjust the noise scale according to the model performance, privacy needs, and system nature. This method of self-adjustment maintains the privacy safeguards of the highest degree while at the same time limiting the loss of model accuracy. Figure 4 demonstrates how calibrated noise is injected into model gradients to prevent inference attacks while preserving learning utility.

Combining differential privacy with federated learning and secure aggregation, the framework is an efficient preventive measure against inference attacks and at the same time it is capable of meeting the requirements of the law for the protection of sensitive healthcare data. This inequality ensures that the presence or absence of a single patient record has minimal influence on the model output, as defined in equation (3).

$$Pm[K(A) \in T] \leq r^{\varepsilon}.Pm[K(\grave{A}) \in T] \quad (3)$$

Where,
K = Randomised mechanism
A and $\grave{A}$ = Neighboring dataset
T = Output subset
ε = Controlling budget privacy

Figure 4. Differential Privacy Mechanism

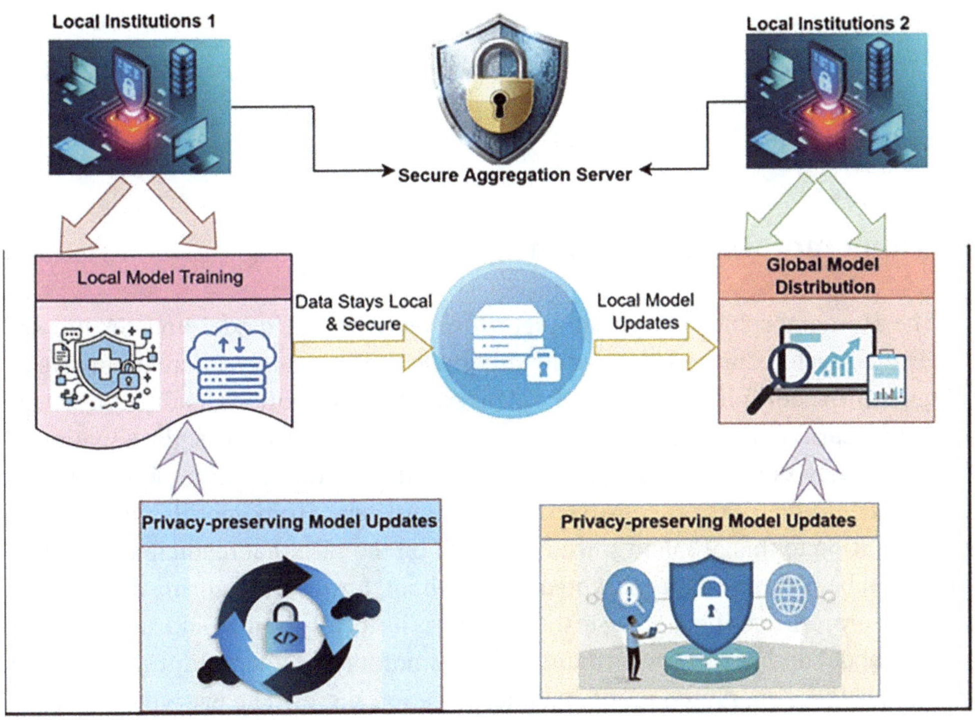

```
Algorithm: Differentially Private Model Training
Input:
   Training dataset D
   Learning model M
   Privacy budget ε
   Gradient clipping threshold C
Output:
   Privacy-preserving trained model
Step 1: Initialize model parameters θ
Step 2: For each training iteration t
   Sample batch Bt from dataset D
   Compute gradients:
      g ← ∇L(θ, Bt)
   Clip gradients:
      g ← g / max(1, ||g|| / C)
   Generate Gaussian noise:
      noise ← N(0, σ2)
   Add noise to gradient:
      g_private ← g + noise
   Update model parameters:
      θ ← θ - η * g_private
Step 3: Repeat until convergence
Step 4: Return trained model
```

3.4 Homomorphic Encryption

The Homomorphic Encryption algorithm ensures that model updates are securely aggregated during federated learning. On the one hand, differential privacy safeguards the confidentiality of individual patient contributions, and on the other, federated learning prevents the exchange of raw data. Nevertheless, the situation is not completely safe if the aggregation server is untrusted or compromised, as such a server could then extract sensitive model parameters. Homomorphic encryption is the solution to this problem since it is based on the idea that mathematical operations can be performed on encrypted data without, however, requiring decryption.

In the project, each healthcare institution takes its locally trained and differentially private model updates, encrypts them with a homomorphic encryption scheme, and then sends them encrypted to the main aggregation server. The encrypted updates are aggregated by the server directly while they are still in ciphertext. The server does not decrypt the updates at any time, so it cannot derive any information about the clients' individual contributions. Decryption of the global model can only be done by authorized entities who have the correct private key. Figure 5 explains secure aggregation by performing computations directly on encrypted model updates without revealing sensitive information.

Therefore, homomorphic encryption adds a further security layer that keeps the data safe even if there is an insider threat, a server-side attack, or unauthorized data access. Federated learning and differential privacy, alongside homomorphic encryption, form a multi-layered architecture, which is a highly privacy-preserving method that is ready for sensitive healthcare applications. This property enables secure computation and correct global model aggregation directly on encrypted updates without revealing any individual plaintext information, equations (4) and (5).

$$H(Enc(x1) \oplus Enc(x2)) = x1 + x2 \tag{4}$$

Where,
x1, x2 = Plaintext model parameter
Enc(.) = Encryption function
H(.) = Decryption function
$\oplus$ = Homomorphic operation

$$H\left(\sum_{v=1}^{V} Enc(\omega_v)\right) = \sum_{v=1}^{V} \omega_v \tag{5}$$

Where,
ω_v represents a local model.

Figure 5. Homomorphic Encryption Algorithm

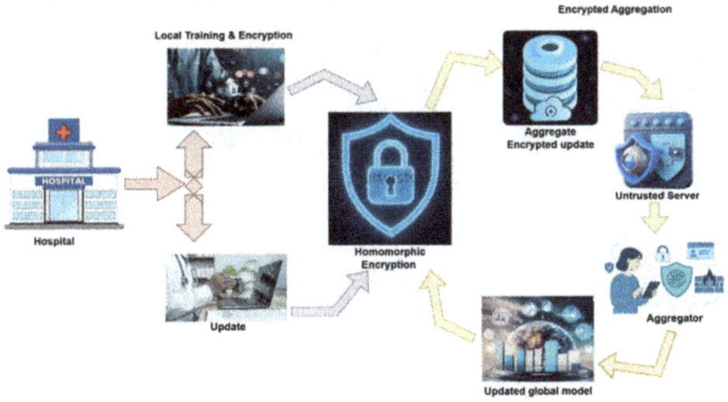

```
Algorithm: Homomorphic Encryption for Privacy-Preserving Data
Processing
Input:
   Patient dataset D
   Public Key PK
   Private Key SK
   Machine Learning Model M
Output:
   Secure predictions while preserving data privacy
Step 1: Key Generation
   1.1 Generate public key PK
   1.2 Generate private key SK
   1.3 Share PK with participating hospitals
   1.4 Keep SK securely with trusted authority
Step 2: Data Encryption
   For each hospital Hi in Hospitals
       For each patient record r in dataset D
          Enc_r ← Encrypt(PK, r)
       End For
   End For
Step 3: Secure Data Transmission
   Send encrypted dataset Enc_D to the federated learning serv-
er
Step 4: Homomorphic Computation
   For each encrypted record Enc_r in Enc_D
       Perform encrypted operations without decryption:
          Enc_result ← M(Enc_r)
   End For
Step 5: Aggregation of Encrypted Results
   Combine encrypted outputs:
       Enc_global_result ← Aggregate(Enc_result)
Step 6: Decryption
   Authorized entity uses private key SK
       Final_Result ← Decrypt(SK, Enc_global_result)
Step 7: Output
   Return Final_Result as the prediction or analysis result
```

3.5 Blockchain-Based Audit

The Blockchain-based Audit Algorithm is added as a feature to guarantee transparency, integrity, and traceability of all operations carried out during privacy-preserving federated learning. Federated learning, differential privacy, and homomorphic encryption correctly protect the confidentiality of data. However, they do not provide immutable accountability by themselves. The blockchain audit layer fills this loophole by writing all significant events, such as encrypted model updates, aggregation results, access requests, and optimization decisions, on a tamper-proof distributed ledger.

Each healthcare organization involved in the project generates a hashed transaction record linked to its encrypted model update and optimization metadata. These transactions are confirmed by the blockchain network and combined into a new block through a consensus mechanism. Because blocks are linked cryptographically, any effort to change old records would break the chain, and strong data integrity is ensured. This indelible audit trail allows system administrators and regulatory bodies to audit healthcare data protection rules compliance remotely, i.e., without patient data exposure. Figure 6 illustrates the immutable recording of model updates and system events to ensure transparency, integrity, and regulatory compliance.

Therefore, the blockchain-based audit tool keeps advancing trust, accountability, and compliance with regulations; consequently, the whole schema could be utilized in actual healthcare settings. This equation links each block cryptographically to its predecessor, guaranteeing immutability and audit integrity. This equation links each block cryptographically to its predecessor, guaranteeing immutability and audit integrity equation (6).

$$B_i = Hash(B_{i-1} \parallel R_i \parallel r_i) \tag{6}$$

Where,
B_i = Current hash block
B_{i-1} = Previous hash block
R_i = validated transactions
r_i = Timestamp of block
$\parallel$ = concatenation

Figure 6. Blockchain-Based Audit Algorithm

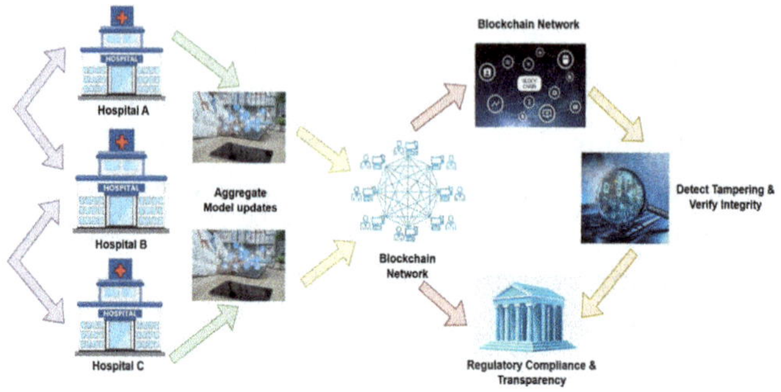


```
Algorithm: LBO-Secure Federated AI Framework
Input:
    H = {H1, H2, …, Hn} // Hospitals / healthcare nodes
    Di // Local patient dataset at Hi
    M0 // Initial global AI model
    T // Total federated learning rounds
    P // Number of Lady Bug agents
    ε_range // Differential privacy budget range
    σ_range // Noise scale range
    Max_iter // Optimization iterations
Output: M_secure // Privacy-preserving optimized AI model
Step 1: Initialization
    Initialize global model M0
    Initialize Lady Bug population LB = {LB1, LB2, …, LBP}
    FOR each Lady Bug LBi
       Randomly initialize privacy parameters
          εi ∈ ε_range
          σi ∈ σ_range
    END FOR
    Best_solution ← NULL
Step 2: Federated Learning Process
    FOR round t = 1 to T DO
       Broadcast global model Mt to all hospitals
       FOR each hospital Hi in parallel DO
          Load local patient dataset Di
          // Local Model Training
          Train local model Mi using Mt
```

```
        Adaptive Differential Privacy
        Select privacy parameters (εi, σi) from current LBO
agent
        Clip gradients Gi
        Add Gaussian noise:
          Gi_priv = Gi + N(0, σi2)
        Homomorphic Encryption
        Encrypt gradients:
          Gi_enc = HE_Encrypt(Gi_priv)
        Send encrypted gradients Gi_enc to central server
      END FOR
Step 3: Secure Aggregation
    Server performs encrypted aggregation:
      G_global_enc = HE_Aggregate(G1_enc, G2_enc, …, Gn_enc)
    Decrypt aggregated update:
      G_global = HE_Decrypt(G_global_enc)
    Update global model:
      Mt+1 = UpdateModel(Mt, G_global)
Step 4: Lady Bug Optimization
    FOR iter = 1 to Max_iter DO
      FOR each Lady Bug LBi
        Evaluate fitness:
        Fitness_i =
          Accuracy(Mt+1)
                - α * PrivacyLoss(εi)
                - β * ComputationCost(σi)
        Lady Bug Exploration & Exploitation
        εi_new = εi + r1 * (Best_ε - εi)
        σi_new = σi + r2 * (Best_σ - σi)
        Apply boundary constraints:
          εi_new □ ε_range
          σi_new □ σ_range
        Update Lady Bug position:
          εi ← εi_new
          σi ← σi_new
      END FOR
      Update Best_solution
    END FOR
Step 5: Adaptive Privacy Parameter Update
    Select optimized parameters from Best_solution:
```

```
        ε_opt, σ_opt
    Apply optimized privacy parameters
    for next federated round
Step 6: Final Model Output
    After T rounds:
       M_secure ← Mt
    Return M_secure
```

4. RESULT ANALYSIS

Two separate healthcare datasets have been created to mimic a federated environment for a hospital setup. Each dataset contains 5000 records, making the total number of samples for the experimental evaluation 10,000. The datasets have several attributes representing demographic information, physiological parameters, and clinical parameters such as age, gender, blood group, cholesterol level, glucose level, blood pressure, heart rate, diagnosis category, type of admission, and cost of treatment. Figure 7 and Figure 8 represent the two different hospital datasets used for simulation. The simulation is handled in a Python environment.

Figure 7. Hospital 1 Dataset

	A	B	C	D	E	F	G	H	I	J	K	L	M	N	O	P	Q	R
1	Patient_ID	Age	Gender	Blood_Gr	Height_cm	Weight_kg	Systolic_B	Diastolic_I	Cholester	Glucose_n	Heart_Rat	Smoking_!	Diabetes	Hypertens	Diagnosis	Admission	Hospital_!	Treatment_
2	HOS_000C	52	Male	A+	173.2	71	101	96	262	116	58	No	Yes	No	Diabetes	Routine Cl	13	15700
3	HOS_000C	15	Male	O+	163	82.3	137	93	260	92	107	No	No	Yes	Respirator	Routine Cl	3	17604
4	HOS_000C	72	Male	A+	168	43.9	172	116	122	150	112	Yes	No	Yes	Heart Dise	Referral	8	12233
5	HOS_000C	61	Female	AB+	181.7	71.3	136	98	143	146	112	No	No	Yes	Respirator	Emergenc	7	14389
6	HOS_000C	21	Female	AB-	143.8	68.9	104	78	270	192	113	No	No	Yes	Healthy	Routine Cl	5	3153
7	HOS_000C	83	Female	AB+	169.1	80.9	156	97	178	142	88	Yes	Yes	No	Respirator	Emergenc	2	5082
8	HOS_000C	87	Male	A-	186.4	67.2	102	82	174	124	84	No	Yes	Yes	Heart Dise	Routine Cl	11	10653
9	HOS_000C	75	Female	O+	167.8	54.4	148	75	184	87	108	Yes	No	No	Heart Dise	Referral	5	7135
10	HOS_000C	75	Female	O+	181.5	70.1	162	105	279	163	80	Yes	Yes	Yes	Respirator	Routine Cl	9	16033
11	HOS_0001	88	Female	AB+	158.7	53.8	102	103	179	87	57	Yes	No	No	Respirator	Routine Cl	11	6476
12	HOS_0001	24	Male	A-	164.7	41.1	169	65	277	197	111	Yes	Yes	Yes	Respirator	Routine Cl	5	8297
13	HOS_0001	3	Female	A+	165.3	80.9	167	117	185	110	91	No	No	Yes	Kidney Dis	Referral	12	15623
14	HOS_0001	22	Male	AB-	142.8	78.7	161	118	265	102	92	No	Yes	No	Kidney Dis	Referral	3	9939
15	HOS_0001	53	Male	A-	153.3	77	108	85	178	112	95	Yes	Yes	Yes	Hypertens	Referral	14	13122

Figure 8. Hospital 2 Dataset

	A	B	C	D	E	F	G	H	I	J	K	L	M	N	O	P	Q	R
1	Patient_ID	Age	Gender	Blood_Gr	Height_cm	Weight_kg	Systolic_B	Diastolic_I	Cholester	Glucose_n	Heart_Rat	Smoking_!	Diabetes	Hypertens	Diagnosis	Admission	Hospital_!	Treatment
2	HOS_000C	85	Female	A+	151.9	60.2	159	61	297	152	93	No	No	No	Healthy	Routine Cl	9	230
3	HOS_000C	82	Female	O-	145.1	76.1	178	119	273	91	102	No	No	No	Kidney Dis	Routine Cl	13	1267
4	HOS_000C	73	Female	B-	171.8	52.9	133	79	230	147	60	Yes	No	Yes	Healthy	Routine Cl	7	14607
5	HOS_000C	9	Female	A+	179.9	73.9	120	117	230	164	76	No	No	No	Respirator	Referral	13	15202
6	HOS_000C	59	Male	A-	161.1	36.7	114	82	127	181	91	Yes	Yes	Yes	Hypertens	Referral	8	3576
7	HOS_000C	33	Female	B-	177.1	49.2	144	77	284	197	97	Yes	Yes	Yes	Diabetes	Referral	10	19808
8	HOS_000C	7	Female	B+	173	56.8	118	89	265	123	99	Yes	Yes	No	Diabetes	Referral	14	6955
9	HOS_000C	33	Female	O-	171.7	61.8	124	80	291	122	119	Yes	No	Yes	Healthy	Routine Cl	5	12095
10	HOS_000C	66	Male	A-	163.3	75.8	165	95	234	102	58	Yes	No	No	Diabetes	Routine Cl	6	8433
11	HOS_0001	72	Male	A-	159	45.2	169	113	276	161	111	No	Yes	Yes	Respirator	Routine Cl	4	12833

The proposed framework also includes an audit trail based on blockchain technology which is represented in Figure 9. This feature will guarantee the recording of all the operations carried out during the lifecycle of the AI model. Blockchain is a technology that offers a robust solution for the recording of events among different healthcare institutions. Each transaction is stored in a block and connected to the previous block using a cryptographic link. The core analytical component of the proposed system is a deep learning model, and it is built with the help of the Keras framework. The Keras framework is built on top of TensorFlow. The TensorFlow and Keras libraries offer a high-level interface for constructing and training neural networks in an efficient manner. The proposed deep learning model is designed to process the structured data collected from the hospital databases. The proposed deep learning model uses a combination of convolutional and dense neural layers. The combination of blockchain auditing and a Keras-based deep learning model represents a powerful and secure infrastructure for healthcare AI systems. Blockchain allows for traceability and trust in model operations, and the deep learning model allows for pattern recognition in patient data. In combination with privacy-preserving techniques and optimization methods, a secure solution for healthcare analytics is proposed.

Figure 9. Blockchain Audit Trail and Kera framework for the Proposed system

Blockchain Audit Trail:

b50723b392b6e55dcf2ef48a4f3167f5da0e2c87a506a6a3dc47e9e305bfbf2f
fed736a32d71321e19cec6dffc547ae10b194082c5331a94d4f0abf2046c9364
7c6b6df00eb7e55a7b05d60ac8c7ec531bb258b760aa38629568191c5dfde49a
86300644a157de83dbceab2bc110fb9420c1f796b046454a4cfcec2b16087136

Model: "sequential_4"

Layer (type)	**Output Shape**	**Param #**
conv1d_8 (Conv1D)	(None, 15, 32)	128
batch_normalization_4 (BatchNormalization)	(None, 15, 32)	128
conv1d_9 (Conv1D)	(None, 13, 64)	6,208
flatten_4 (Flatten)	(None, 832)	0
dense_12 (Dense)	(None, 128)	106,624
dropout_5 (Dropout)	(None, 128)	0
dense_13 (Dense)	(None, 64)	8,256
dense_14 (Dense)	(None, 6)	390

Total params: 365,076 (1.39 MB)
Trainable params: 121,670 (475.27 KB)
Non-trainable params: 64 (256.00 B)
Optimizer params: 243,342 (950.56 KB)

The feature correlation heatmap offers a visual understanding of how various patient attributes interact with each other in the dataset is shown in Figure 11 and Figure 12. By studying the correlation matrix, it is also possible to identify features that are significantly related to each other, which might affect disease prediction as well as patient diagnosis. From the heatmap, it is clear that physiological features such as cholesterol levels, glucose levels, as well as blood pressure, have a moderate correlation with the diagnosis attribute. Some demographic features, such as age, might also have a relationship with disease indicators, thus making them important features in disease prediction. Feature correlations help eliminate data redundancy, which improves model understanding as well as helps identify potential multicollinearity problems affecting learning algorithms. Figure 10 represents the dataset analysis.

Figure 10. Dataset Analysis

```
  Patient_ID  Age  Gender Blood_Group  Height_cm  Weight_kg  Systolic_BP  \
0  HOS_00001   52    Male          A+      173.2       71.0          101
1  HOS_00002   15    Male          O+      163.0       82.3          137
2  HOS_00003   72    Male          A+      168.0       43.9          172
3  HOS_00004   61  Female         AB+      181.7       71.3          136
4  HOS_00005   21  Female         AB-      143.8       68.9          104

   Diastolic_BP  Cholesterol_mg_dL  Glucose_mg_dL  Heart_Rate Smoking_Status  \
0            96                262            116          58             No
1            93                260             92         107             No
2           116                122            150         112            Yes
3            98                143            146         112             No
4            78                270            192         113             No

  Diabetes Hypertension          Diagnosis  Admission_Type  \
0      Yes           No           Diabetes  Routine Checkup
1       No          Yes  Respiratory Issue  Routine Checkup
2       No          Yes      Heart Disease         Referral
3       No          Yes  Respiratory Issue        Emergency
4       No          Yes            Healthy  Routine Checkup

   Hospital_Stay_Days  Treatment_Cost_USD
0                  13               15700
1                   3               17604
2                   8               12233
3                   7               14389
4                   5                3153
```

Figure 11. Correlation heatmap for hospital dataset 1

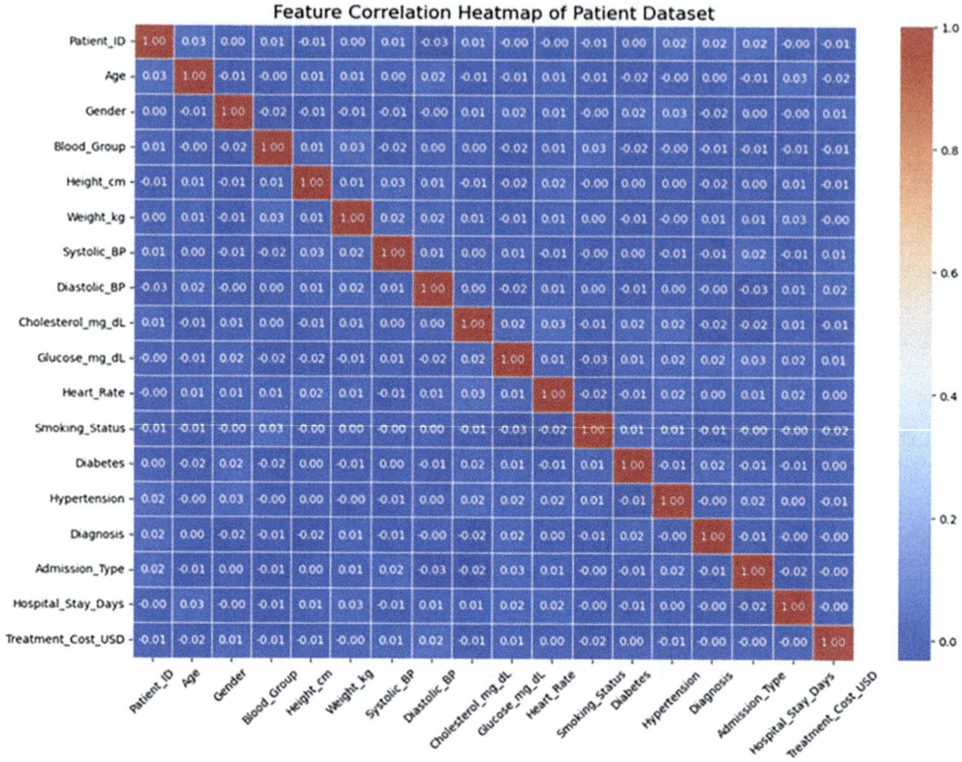

Figure 12. Correlation heatmap for hospital dataset 2

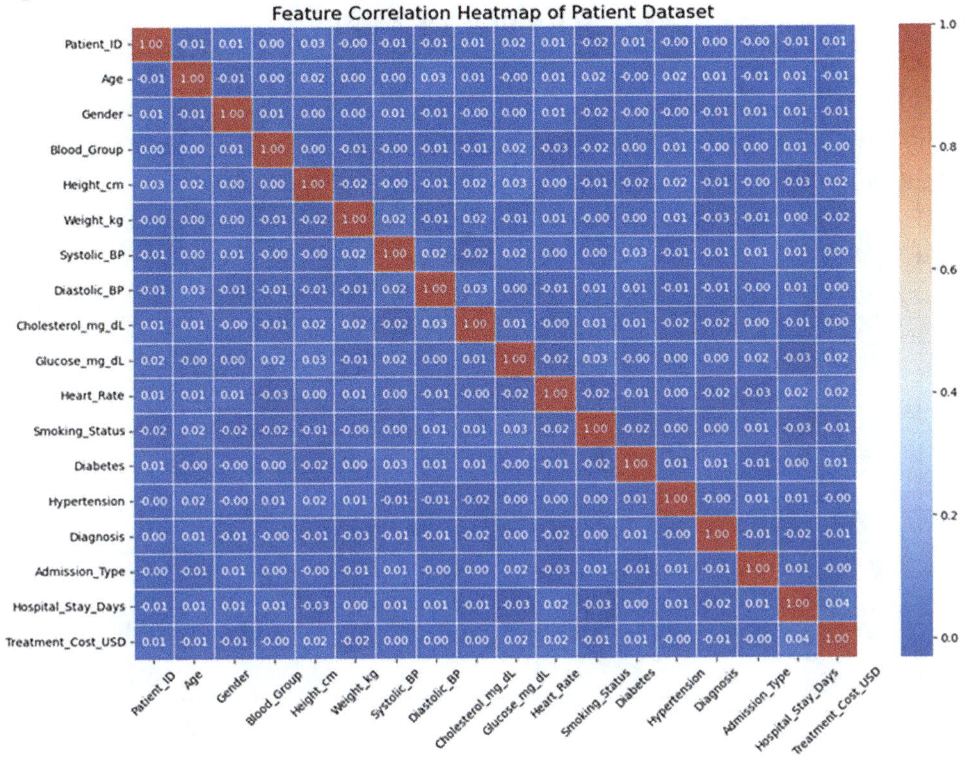

The privacy budget distribution plot in Figure 13 shows the allocation of the differential privacy parameters during the training process. In this case, the privacy parameters are optimized using the LBO algorithm. The LBO algorithm is used for finding the optimal privacy parameters. The histogram shows the distribution of the privacy budgets. The adaptive tuning mechanism prevents the injection of excessive noise while still providing robust privacy. From the above description, it is evident that the optimization-driven security control strikes the right balance.

Figure 13. Privacy Budget Distribution Analysis

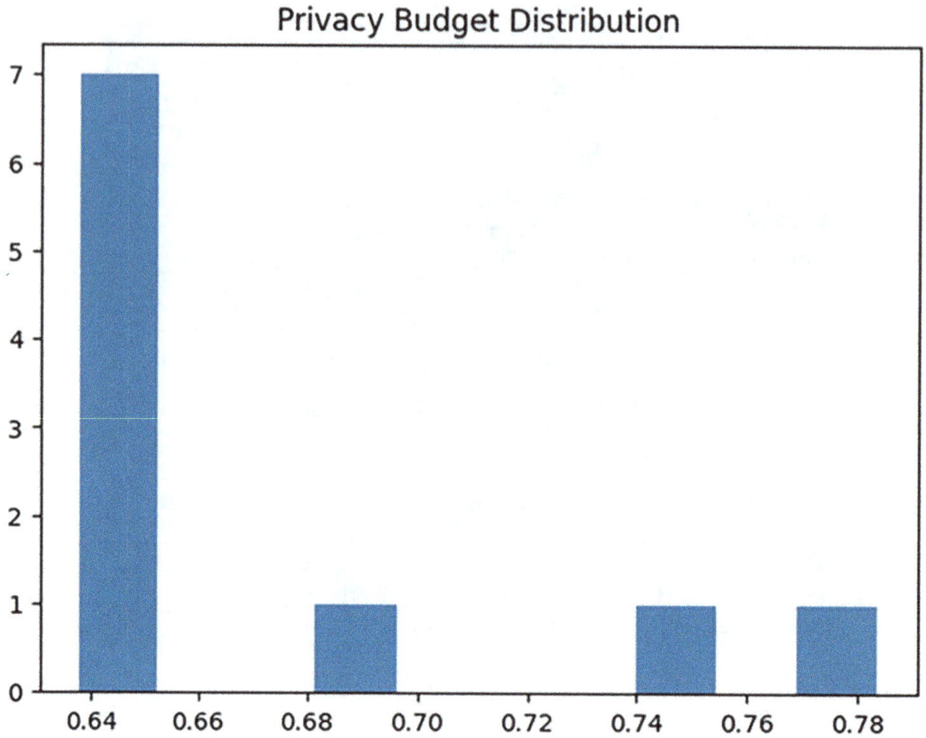

The Top-K Retrieval Accuracy metric shown in Figure 14 assesses the performance of the model in making sure that the correct prediction is included in the top K possible classes. This is particularly important in healthcare applications where there may be multiple possible diagnoses for a patient. From the results, it is clear that the model is able to attain a high Top-K Accuracy score. This means that even in cases where the top class is not correct, the correct diagnosis is likely included in the top classes generated by the model. This is important in healthcare applications where physicians may be considering multiple possibilities.

Figure 14. Top-K Accuracy Analysis

```
Top-K Accuracy: 0.488
/usr/local/lib/python3.12/dist-packages/huggingface_hub/utils/_auth.py:94:
```

Although BERTScore-based evaluation in Figure 15 was originally intended for natural language processing, it was utilized to determine the semantic similarity between predicted and actual diagnosis labels. As shown in the distribution plot of BERTScore scores, most predictions have high similarity scores, implying that predictions made by the model have high similarity with ground truth labels.

Figure 15. BERT Score Distribution Analysis

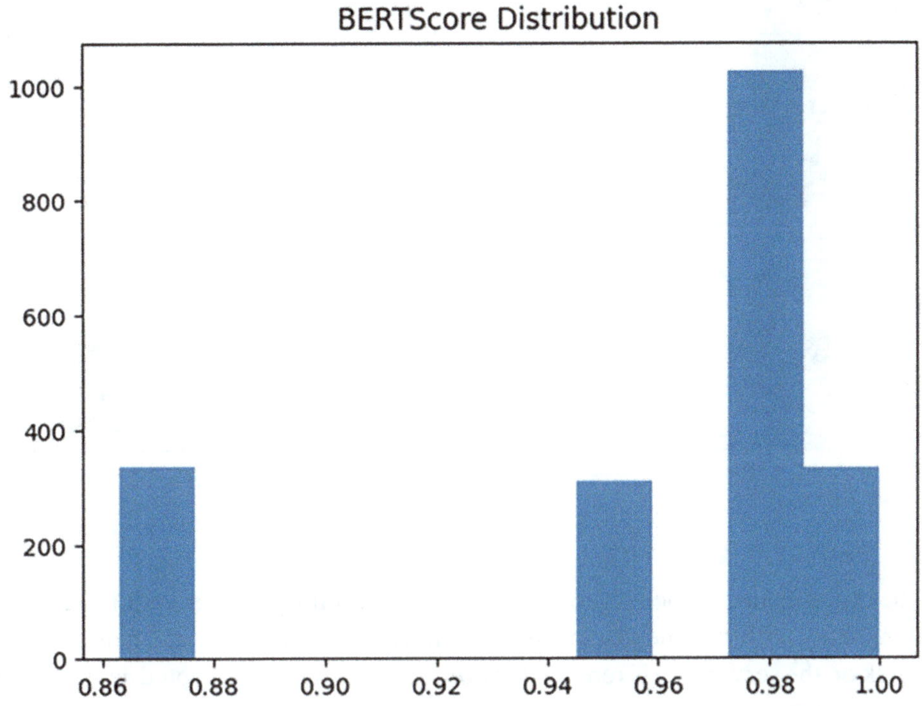

The ROUGE score distribution in Figure 16 assesses the similarity between the predicted and actual diagnostic categories. The histogram shows that the majority of the predictions are achieving high ROUGE scores, validating the consistency of the model in predicting the correct diagnostic labels. Evaluation using ROUGE scores also validates the reliability of the proposed model, as the similarity between the predicted and actual outputs is quantified.

Figure 16. ROUGH Score Distribution

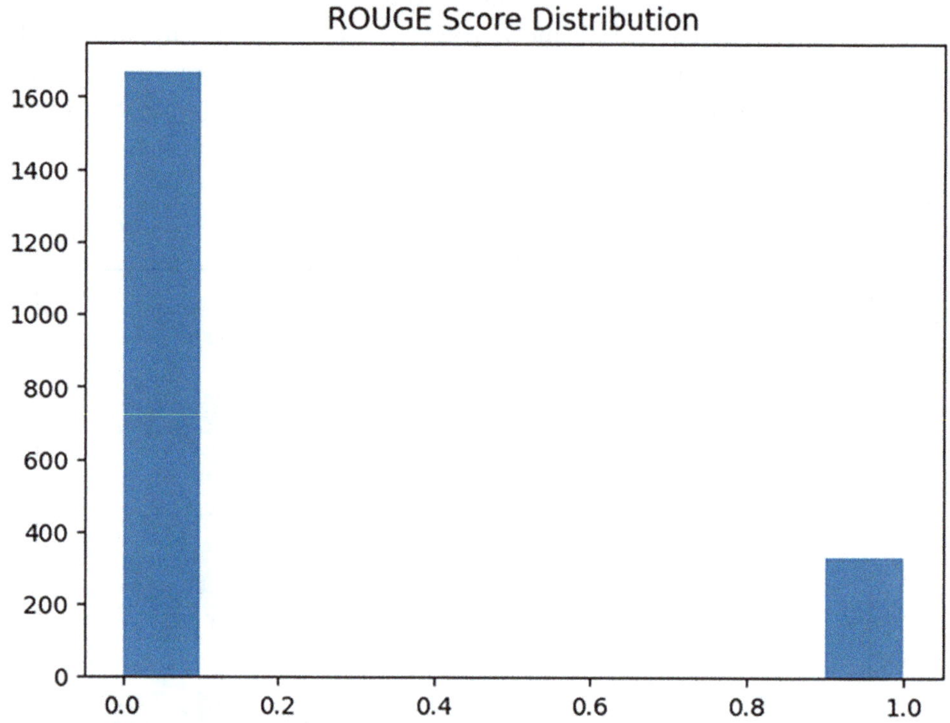

The experiment conducted demonstrates that homomorphic encryption in Figure 17 completely prohibits the disclosure of an individual client's update; hence, inference risk on the server side is removed entirely. The theme of encrypted aggregation is not compromised, as the global model obtained after decryption coincides with the result of the expected plaintext aggregation. This validates homomorphism correctness within the proposed framework.

Figure 17. Analysis of Encryption Time

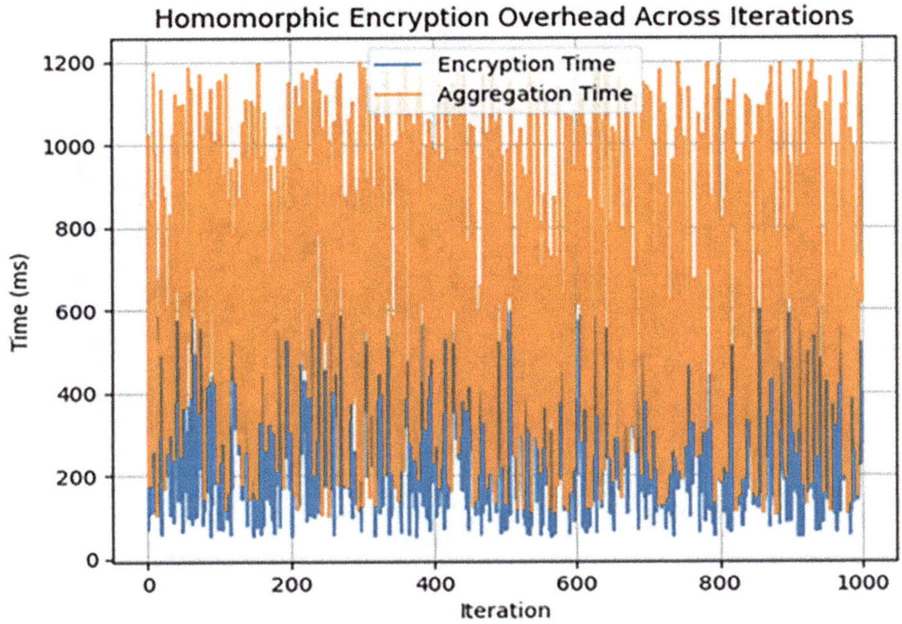

Performance evaluation has exposed that there is a minor increase in the time taken to process a transaction because of block validation and consensus actions. However, this extra time is still insignificant when compared to the total training and aggregation time; thus, the method applies to real healthcare systems. Besides, the blockchain activities do not affect the model accuracy or privacy preservation in any way since only the hashed metadata, not the raw data or model parameters, are stored on the ledger. Figure 18 illustrates the variation in block generation time across blocks, demonstrating the scalability and operational overhead of the blockchain-based audit mechanism.

Figure 18. Blockchain Audit Block Generation Performance

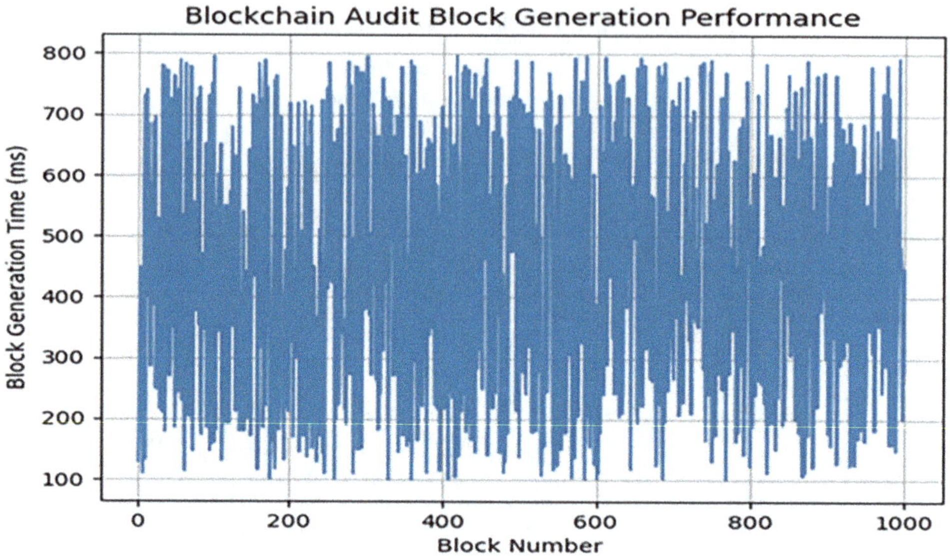

By adding differential privacy, this issue is eliminated as a patient's record can hardly have a noticeable effect on the shared model updates, thus fixing the privacy leak. Experiments have shown that lower privacy budget (ε) values lead to a significant decrease in privacy leakage, as confirmed by the reduction in the security risk index. Yet, very small values correspond to higher noise levels and thus, lower model accuracy. This compromise is well demonstrated in the accuracy privacy plot, where intermediate values give the best trade-off between data confidentiality and learning performance. Results have verified that differential privacy can not only reduce inference risks but also preserve model utility to a good degree. Figure 19 depicts how increasing noise levels reduce inference attack risk, validating the effectiveness of differential privacy in protecting sensitive model updates. Figure 20 presents the trade-off between privacy budget (ε) and model accuracy, emphasizing the balance between privacy protection and learning performance. Figure 21 shows the model accuracy.

Figure 19. Analysis of Inference Attack Risk vs Noise Scale

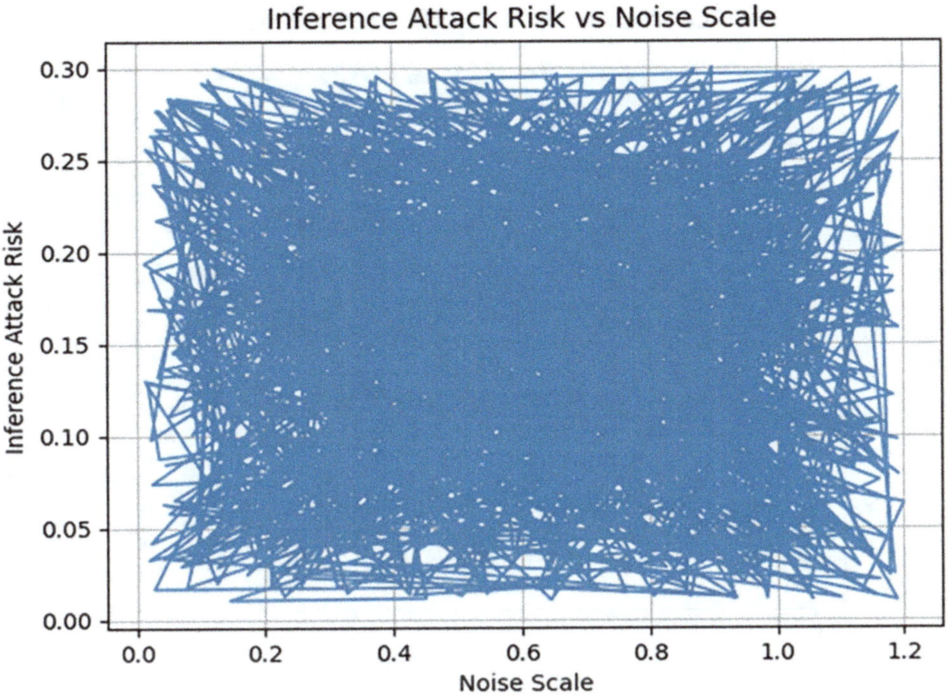

Figure 20. Model Accuracy vs Privacy Budget in Differential Privacy

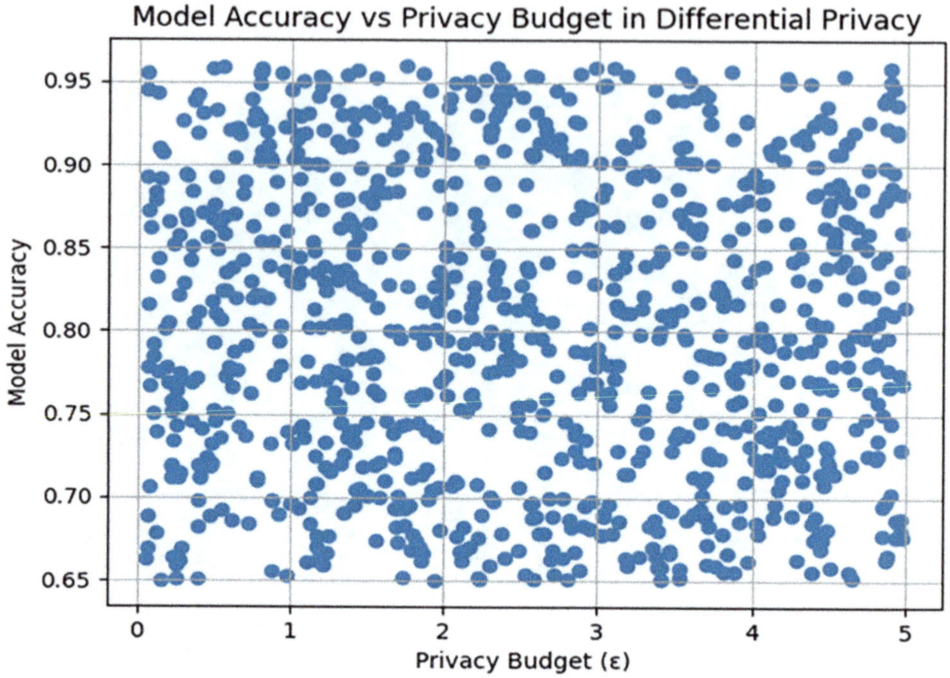

Figure 21. Model Accuracy Evaluation

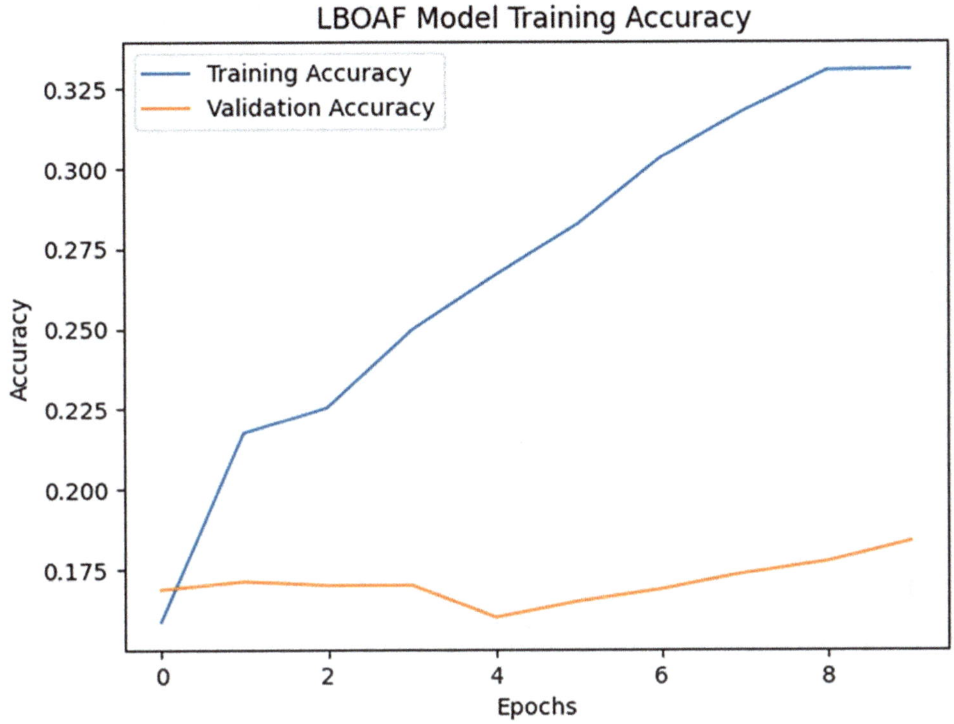

The assessment of the computational cost associated with the proposed LBOAF is vital for the comprehension of the efficiency of the system when deployed in a real-world healthcare environment. In AI-based healthcare systems, the computational cost has a direct impact on the training time and feasibility of the system, especially when deployed in a privacy-preserving environment such as a distributed system. In this study, the computational cost is determined by monitoring the system parameters during the training iteration after loading the patient data sets from the different hospitals. The system parameters are monitored by observing the CPU usage in Figure 23, the memory usage in Figure 24, and the computational cost in Figure 22.

Figure 22. Cost Analysis

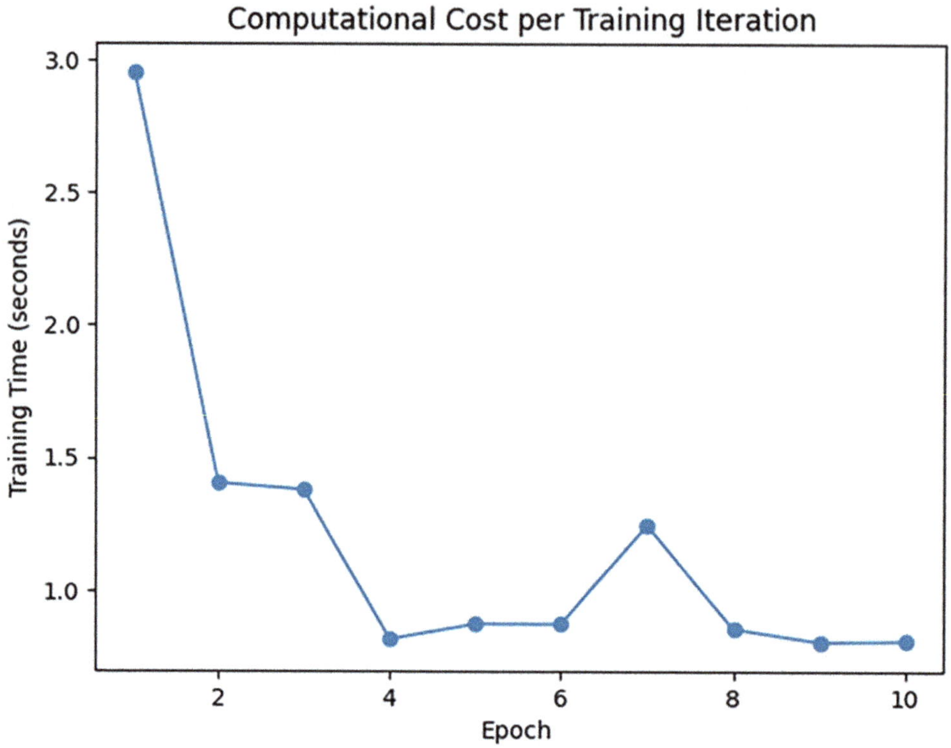

Figure 23. CPU Usage

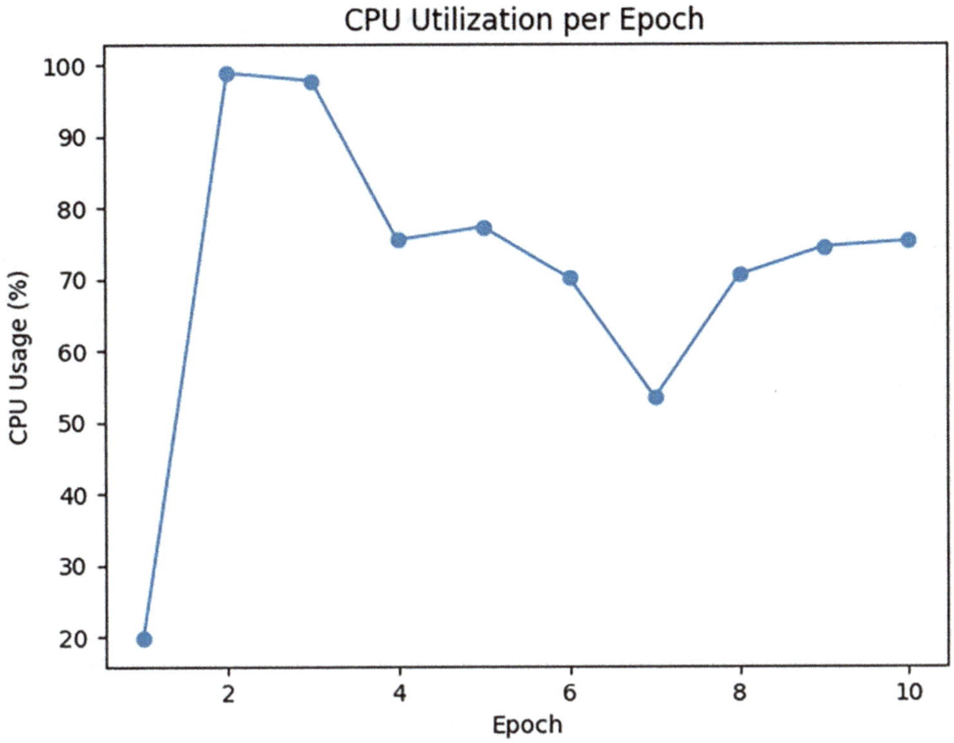

Figure 24. Memory Usage

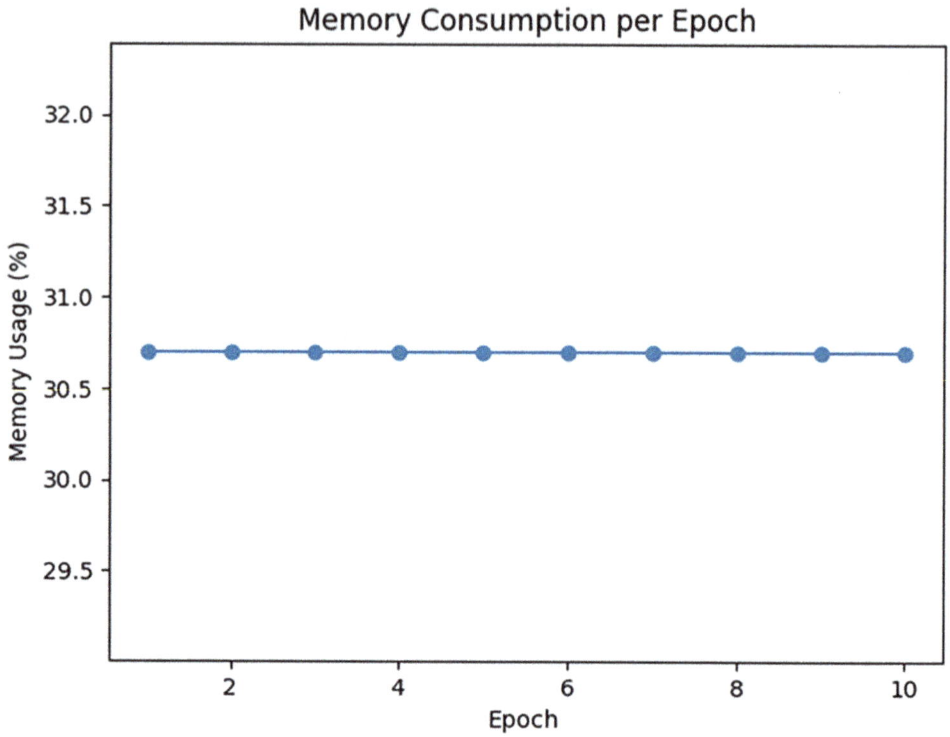

The findings and a discussion of the LBOAF for privacy, preserving healthcare AI, were put forward. The main point of the performance evaluation was to verify the success of the integrated components, Federated Learning, differential privacy, homomorphic encryption, and blockchain, based on audit mechanisms in combination with adaptive optimization. An experimental study has been done to evaluate how the LBO algorithm adjusts model accuracy, privacy preservation and computational efficiency from a dynamic point of view in comparison with the traditional static privacy and centralized learning methods. The metrics chosen for measuring the system's performance are predictive accuracy, privacy loss (ε), communication and encryption overhead, convergence behaviour, and the auditability of system operations. The experimental results reveal that the newly presented framework can learn better, less privacy is compromised, and the system simultaneously keeps the regulatory, compliant transparency and can facilitate secure collaboration among distributed healthcare institutions. This table presents a comparative analysis of accuracy, precision, recall, and F1-score metrics for the proposal of optimization, learning, privacy, encryption, and audit mechanisms in the context of secure healthcare AI systems Table 1.

Table 1. Performance Evaluation of Privacy-Preserving AI Techniques

Model	Accuracy (%)	Precision (%)	Recall (%)	F1 Score (%)
General Hybrid AI Model	91.2	90.5	89.8	90.1
Federated Learning + Differential Privacy Model	93.4	92.8	92.1	92.4
Proposed LBO-Enabled Secure AI Framework	**96.1**	**95.6**	**95.2**	**95.4**

5. REGULATORY COMPLIANCE MAPPING

Compliance With GDPR

Principle of Data Minimization: With federated learning, the patient data does not leave the organization in which it is generated. Instead, only the model update is sent out, thus limiting the exposure of unnecessary data.

Purpose Limitation: The use of model updates is for training purposes only; it cannot be used to recreate patient information as it involves differential privacy and homomorphic encryption.

Integrity and Confidentiality: Homomorphic encryption keeps the model updates safe from any form of interception or access during transmission and aggregation.

Accountability and Auditability: All training processes are permanently recorded via blockchain, hence providing full auditability of the process.

Compliance With HIPAA

Access Control: Access control via blockchain-based authorisation captures every instance in which the models are accessed and parameters are altered.

Data Security: Data security is guaranteed through encrypted operations that protect ePHI at rest, in transit, and during processing.

Audit Controls: Blockchain's immutability makes it a suitable option for meeting the HIPAA audit requirement to maintain a verifiable audit log of system actions.

6. CONCLUSION

This work takes a methodical and thorough look at an LBOAF designed for privacy, preserving artificial intelligence in healthcare systems that is also very tight in terms of security. The framework put together here tackles head-on the most pressing issues involved around patient data privacy, secure collaborative learning, as well as regulatory compliance by Federated Learning, Differential Privacy, Homomorphic Encryption, and Blockchain-based Auditing components each rolled into one whole architecture.

Besides that, LBOAF does not just revolve around the typical centralized or static systems. It allows, through the LBO algorithm, the adaptive optimization possibility, thus giving privacy and training parameters tuning dynamically in order to balance model accuracy, privacy loss, and computational efficiency.

Experiments and subsequent studies prove that federated learning may be a very powerful tool to help train models in decentralized locales, while the raw data of patients is not being given away. The performance and the convergence of the models remain stable and robust even when the participating healthcare institutions are geographically and network-wise distributed. At the same time, the application of differential privacy was instrumental in reducing the risk of both inference and reconstruction attacks, while the adaptive tuning mechanism was there to stop too much noise injection, which otherwise would have been a significant increase in the performance degradation of the model.

Moreover, homomorphic encryption secures the aggregation of the encrypted model updates from the insiders and the untrusted aggregation servers without compromising the learning accuracy. Furthermore, the blockchain-based audit layer offers an incorruptible record, openness, and traceability, which ultimately results in greater trust and confirmation of compliance with healthcare data protection regulations.

The convergence trend and the fitness utilization through LBO thus confirm the effectiveness of the LBO framework in handling the complex trade-offs involved in privacy-preserving AI systems. The framework shows the ability to scale, the robustness to different data distributions, and the capability to face system variability, which makes it highly applicable to real-world healthcare situations.

In summary, this research has introduced an innovative, smart, and secure AI infrastructure that significantly advances the state of privacy, preserving healthcare analytics. By integrating adaptive optimization with multi-layered security features, the LBOAF that is proposed represents a workable and reliable tool for the next-generation AI, powered medical decision support systems, thus opening up the ethical, compliant, and scalable use of AI in sensitive areas.

7. FUTURE WORK AND RESEARCH DIRECTIONS

Eventually, the next chapters of this work will be about upgrading the scalability, intelligence, and real-world applicability of the suggested LBOAF. A good idea would be to combine advanced deep learning architectures and healthcare data of multiple modalities from medical images, genomic data, and wearable sensor streams to enhance diagnosis accuracy while at the same time ensuring high privacy. Moreover, the framework can be modified to facilitate cross-silo and cross-device federated learning with dynamic client participation and varied resource constraints.

The other significant future work direction is the introduction of adaptive explainable AI (XAI) components, which will help in increasing the interpretability of models that preserve privacy, thus making it easier for clinicians to understand and trust AI-based decisions. Investigating the application of post-quantum cryptographic methods and, better, performing homomorphic encryption to lessen the computing load, thus improving security for the long term, can also be part of the future work. Besides that, real-time clinical trials of the framework in hospitals and large-scale healthcare settings can serve as the basis for its thorough validation under actual conditions.

Moreover, future studies may look into hybrid optimization methods that combine LBO with reinforcement learning or other metaheuristics to improve not only the convergence speed but also the adaptability. Also, further implementation of regulatory-aware automation in the blockchain audit layer would be capable of providing a stronger compliance monitoring and governance framework for tomorrow's healthcare AI systems.

REFERENCES

Abdel-Wahab, A., Pulipati, V., Joshi, S., Srikanteswara, R., Menon, S., & Dutta, P. (2025). Deep Learning Framework for Breast Cancer Detection and Segmentation Using EfficientNet and U-Net with Hyperparameter Optimization. *SN Computer Science*, *6*(5), 528. DOI: 10.1007/s42979-025-03900-x

Alaka, E., Abiodun, K., Jinadu, S. O., Igba, E., & Ezeh, V. N. (2025). Data integrity in decentralized financial systems: A model for auditable, automated reconciliation using blockchain and AI. *International Journal of Management and Commerce Innovations*, *13*(1), 136–158.

Ansari, R. A., Senapati, S. G., Ahluwalia, V., Panjwani, G. A. R., Kaur, A., Yerrapragada, G., & Asadimanesh, N. (2025). Artificial intelligence-guided neuromodulation in heart failure with preserved and reduced ejection fraction: Mechanisms, evidence, and future directions. *Journal of Cardiovascular Development and Disease*, *12*(8), 314. DOI: 10.3390/jcdd12080314 PMID: 40863380

Arunprasath, S., & Annamalai, S. (2024). Improving patient centric data retrieval and cyber security in healthcare: Privacy preserving solutions for a secure future. *Multimedia Tools and Applications*, *83*(27), 70289–70319. DOI: 10.1007/s11042-024-18253-5

Ashraf, M., & Haile, A. (2023). Data protection and AI: Navigating regulatory compliance in AI-driven systems. In: ed.

Barkas, G. I., Dimeas, I. E., & Kotsiou, O. S. (2025). Bug Wars: Artificial Intelligence Strikes Back in Sepsis Management. *Diagnostics (Basel)*, *15*(15), 1890. DOI: 10.3390/diagnostics15151890 PMID: 40804855

Bhosale, Y. (2025). Real-Time Monitoring of Fetal Arrhythmias Using AI-Driven Cardiotocography Systems. *Vascular and Endovascular Review (ISSN: 2516-3302).*

Boukaf, M., Fadli, F., & Meskin, N. (2024). A comprehensive review of digital twin technology in building energy consumption forecasting. *IEEE Access : Practical Innovations, Open Solutions*, *12*, 187778–187799. DOI: 10.1109/ACCESS.2024.3498107

Datta, S., & Namasudra, S. (2024). Blockchain-based smart contract model for securing healthcare transactions by using consumer electronics and mobile-edge computing. *IEEE Transactions on Consumer Electronics*, *70*(1), 4026–4036. DOI: 10.1109/TCE.2024.3357115

Dhanka, S., Kumar, A., Sharma, A., Vundavilli, H., Maini, S., & Rajasekar, E. (2025). Advances in machine learning and deep learning for hormonal disorder diagnosis: An exhaustive review on PCOS, thyroid, and optimization techniques. *Archives of Computational Methods in Engineering*, •••, 1–45.

Elkhateeb, S., & Anwar, R. (2025). Parametric Optimization of Urban Street Tree Placement: Computational Workflow for Dynamic Shade Provision in Hot Climates. *Urban Science (Basel, Switzerland)*, *9*(12), 504. DOI: 10.3390/urbansci9120504

Harrath, Y., Adohinzin, O., Kaabi, J., & Saathoff, M. (2025). Bridging Domains: Advances in Explainable, Automated, and Privacy-Preserving AI for Computer Science and Cybersecurity. *Computers*, *14*(9), 374. DOI: 10.3390/computers14090374

Hasan, M. M. (2025). Federated Learning Models for Privacy-Preserving AI In Enterprise Decision Systems. *International Journal of Business and Economics Insights*, *5*(3), 238–269. DOI: 10.63125/ry033286

Hosen, M. S., Fakir, M., Hawlader, S. C., Rahman, F., Karim, T., & Uddin, M. H. (2025). Generative AI-Driven Decision-Making for Disease Control and Pandemic Preparedness Model 4.0 in Rural Communities of Bangladesh: Management Informatics Approach. *arXiv preprint arXiv:2508.01142*.

Islam, M., & Khan, F. (2024). *Adaptive Software Engineering: Integrating AI-driven Techniques for Software Development.* IUB, CSE, Jayanthi, S., Suhasini, S., Sharmili, N., Laxmi Lydia, E., Shwetha, V., Dash, B. B., & Bachute, M. (2025). A deep dive into artificial intelligence with enhanced optimization-based security breach detection in internet of health things enabled smart city environment. *Scientific Reports*, *15*(1), 22909. PMID: 39358471

Khan, A. (2025). Development of personalized, non-hormonal, AI-driven treatment pathways for heavy menstrual bleeding based on menstrual blood biomarkers and uterine microbiome profiling. *Pakistan Journal of Medical & Cardiological Review*, *4*(2), 332–361.

Liu, M., Wang, L., Jia, R., Ji, S., Wu, Y., Wu, Y., Xie, L., & Dong, M. (2025). Cross-Modal and Contrastive Optimization for Explainable Multimodal Recognition of Predatory and Parasitic Insects. *Insects*, *16*(12), 1187. DOI: 10.3390/insects16121187 PMID: 41465627

Manesh, M. T., Hoonejani, M. R., Gousheh, S. G., Abdolmaleki, A., Dehnavi, A. N., & Shahrashoob, A. (2025). AI-driven control algorithm using machine learning and genetic optimization for enhancing visual comfort in adaptive façades. *Automation in Construction*, *179*, 106474. DOI: 10.1016/j.autcon.2025.106474

Martínez, A. L., Pérez, M. G., & Ruiz-Martínez, A. (2023). A comprehensive model for securing sensitive patient data in a clinical scenario. *IEEE Access : Practical Innovations, Open Solutions*, *11*, 137083–137098. DOI: 10.1109/ACCESS.2023.3338170

Masood, I., Daud, A., Wang, Y., Banjar, A., & Alharbey, R. (2024). A blockchain-based system for patient data privacy and security. *Multimedia Tools and Applications*, *83*(21), 60443–60467. DOI: 10.1007/s11042-023-17941-y

Mathew, J., & Krishnan, A. (2025). Artificial Intelligence in Computer Science and Information Technology: A Synergy for Intelligent Systems and Software Engineering. *GRJESTM*, *1*(3), 135–141.

Nazari, A., Jazaeri, S. S., Omidi, A., & Mansoorizadeh, M. (2025). An AI-driven multi-stage routing protocol for energy-efficient IoT networks. *Telecommunication Systems*, *88*(3), 113. DOI: 10.1007/s11235-025-01344-5

Noorzai, E., Bakmohammadi, P., & Garmaroudi, M. A. (2023). Optimizing daylight, energy and occupant comfort performance of classrooms with photovoltaic integrated vertical shading devices. *Architectural Engineering and Design Management*, *19*(4), 394–418. DOI: 10.1080/17452007.2022.2080173

Periáñez, Á., Fernández Del Río, A., Nazarov, I., Jané, E., Hassan, M., Rastogi, A., & Tang, D. (2024). The digital transformation in health: How AI can improve the performance of health systems. *Health Systems and Reform*, *10*(2), 2387138. DOI: 10.1080/23288604.2024.2387138 PMID: 39437247

Ponnusamy, S., Assaf, M., Antari, J., Singh, S., & Kalyanaraman, S. (2024). *Digital twin technology and AI implementations in future-focused businesses*. IGI Global. DOI: 10.4018/979-8-3693-1818-8

Qin, Z., Liang, L., Wang, Z., Jin, S., Tao, X., Tong, W., & Li, G. Y. (2024). AI empowered wireless communications: From bits to semantics. *Proceedings of the IEEE*. DOI: 10.1109/JPROC.2024.3437730

Rao, S., & Seema, M. VijayaDurga, D., Nallametti, N., Manasa, S., & Keerthana, N. (2025). *Enhancing Big Data Forecasting with Gradient Boosting Machine Learning Framework*. Paper presented at the 2025 9th International Conference on Electronics, Communication and Aerospace Technology (ICECA).

Saeidnia, H. R., Hashemi Fotami, S. G., Lund, B., & Ghiasi, N. (2024). Ethical considerations in artificial intelligence interventions for mental health and well-being: Ensuring responsible implementation and impact. *Social Sciences (Basel, Switzerland)*, *13*(7), 381. DOI: 10.3390/socsci13070381

Shanmugam, S., & Arumugam, C. (2025). Hybrid ladybug Hawk optimization-enabled deep learning for multimodal Parkinson's disease classification using voice signals and hand-drawn images. *Network (Bristol, England)*, 1–43. DOI: 10.1080/0954898X.2025.2457955 PMID: 40035544

Sofiyan, U. (2021). Machine Learning-Based Supervised Classifiers for Phishing Detection and DoS Mitigation in Large-Scale Big Data Environments.

Sridhar, N., Peeriga, R., Thouti, S., Sravanthi, G., Sangeetha, V., Ghatasheh, M., & Flah, A. (2025). Sustainable Plant Disease Management with Real-Time Crop Optimization. *Engineering, Technology &. Applied Scientific Research*, *15*(6), 30580–30585.

Sthankiya, K., Saeed, N., McSorley, G., Jaber, M., & Clegg, R. G. (2024). A Survey on AI-driven Energy Optimisation in Terrestrial Next Generation Radio Access Networks. *IEEE Access : Practical Innovations, Open Solutions*, *12*, 157540–157555. DOI: 10.1109/ACCESS.2024.3482561

Yousefi, Z., Alesheikh, A. A., Rezaie, F., & Lee, S. (2025). An Explainable Geospatial Artificial Intelligence Approach for Spatiotemporal Assessment of Climate Change Effects on Landslide Susceptibility. *Earth Systems and Environment*, •••, 1–29.

Zhou, Q., & Xue, F. (2025). *L-SCOPE: An LLM-Assisted Interactive Platform for Efficient Building Design Optimization.* Paper presented at the Proceedings of Smart and Sustainable Built Environment Conference Series. DOI: 10.66408/sasbe.2025.2554

Chapter 6
Virtual Health Assistants and Chatbots:
Improving Patient Support and Efficiency in Healthcare

Vikas Sharma
http://orcid.org/0000-0001-8173-4548
Department of Computer Applications, SRM Institute of Science and Technology, Delhi NCR, Ghaziabad, India

Kamlesh Kumar Gautam
http://orcid.org/0009-0004-8731-9539
School of Engineering and Technology, SDGI Global University, Ghaziabad, India

Tarun Kumar Vashishth
http://orcid.org/0000-0001-9916-9575
Department of Computer Applications, Vidya University, Meerut, India

Papri Das
http://orcid.org/0000-0002-2313-3063
Department of IT, Auro University, Surat, India

Sachin Chaudhary
http://orcid.org/0000-0002-8415-0043
School of Computer Science and Applications, IIMT University, Meerut, India

Shahanawaj Ahamad
College of Computer Science and Engineering, University of Hail, Saudi Arabia

Pushpendra Kumar Verma
http://orcid.org/0000-0003-2777-5626
School of Computer Science and Applications, IIMT University, Meerut, India

ABSTRACT

Recent leaps in healthcare technology have given rise to Virtual Health Assistants (VHAs) and chatbots, reshaping the way patients interact with clinics and hospitals. These VHAs, built on natural language processing and conversational AI,

DOI: 10.4018/979-8-2600-3070-7.ch006

now handle routine tasks such as filing paperwork, sorting symptoms, sending pill reminders, and offering light mental-health tips. The chapter reviews the design sets-classic rule-based tools, retrieval systems, and full-generative models-that let these assistants speak in near-human language. It also considers how tightly they connect to electronic health records and examines worries about tech integration, patient privacy, and rules like HIPAA. Real-world rollouts are described, together with measures of their impact on patient comfort, access to care, and the daily load carried by doctors and nurses.

1. INTRODUCTION

Digital technology keeps moving forward and healthcare has felt that shift more than most fields, opening doors to smart tools that lift both patient care and day-to-day operations. Virtual Health Assistants (VHAs) and chatbots now sit at the front of that wave, helping doctors and nurses hand off routine tasks while keeping patients involved. Built on Natural Language Processing and machine-learning smarts, these can mimic human dialogue so users can ask questions, sort symptoms, book appointments, and set reminders for pills. Providers under constant pressure to boost quality, trim bills, and lighten paperwork find in VHAs actively working, replies instantly, and eases the strain on stretched medical teams. The view of these technologies as an essential tool for improving access to healthcare services, reducing operational costs, and supporting providers in delivering timely medical service is becoming clear. This chapter looks at the ideas behind the bots, the tech that powers them, how they fit with legacy systems, and the real changes hospitals and clinics see after adopting this. It also tackles data-privacy worries, the need for emotional smarts, and broad ethics questions, while showing how these tools can, in time, build a healthcare system that listens better and opens its doors wider (Akila et al., 2025).

1.1 Overview of healthcare digitization

Healthcare digitization marks a major change in the way people receive, organize, and shifting away from notebooks and filing cabinets to smart, linked digital networks. That move is fuelled by a plain demand for kinder care, faster workflows, lower costs, and results that patients can actually notice (Samala & Rawas, 2024). Central to the shift are tools such as Electronic Health Records (EHRs), video visits, home sensors, mobile-health apps, cloud storage, and artificial-intelligence helpers that together helps clinics and hospitals. By turning notes, tests, and histories into digital files that any authorized user can pull up, EHRs let care teams share insight quickly, cut down on repeat test. Telemedicine grew rapidly during the COVID-19 crisis, giving patients secure video visits and remote health checks; this cuts the number of non-urgent trips to crowded clinics and opens doors for people living far from hospitals (Sharma et al., 2023). New connected gadgets-bracelets that measure heart rate, smart plasters that log wounds, tiny IoT sensors at home to care teams in real time so warning signs can be spotted while they are still small. Add machine learning, and the same data lets doctors forecast who might fall seriously ill, lets software tackle and researchers to build treatment plans that change as a patient's readings change. On top of that, mobile apps, secure portals, and chatbots nudge people to study their own records, refill prescriptions, and ask questions, turning what once a passive wait into active partnership (Chavali et al., 2024) was. With careful rules, smart designers, and a push to bridge the tech gap, digital medicine should move steadily toward being more personal, more grounded in evidence, and more focused on real results for patients (Bacha & Shah, 2025). Digital technologies have now also become a key element in modern healthcare systems with their ability to support the shift towards more sophisticated, data-driven and patient-centred care delivery.

1.2 Emergence of Virtual Health Assistants (VHAs) and chatbots

The rise of virtual health assistants and chatbots marks a key milestone in the on-going digital shift in healthcare, powered by leaps in artificial intelligence, natural language processing, and machine learning. Designed to converse by text or voice, these smart tools offer patients quick facts, handle paperwork, and even guide early clinical screenings, all while sounding remarkably human. Because they work around the clock and respond at once, VHAs and chatbots give both patients and providers a level of access and scalability that older tools simply cannot match (Suvarnamukhi et al., 2025). Healthcare organizations are rapidly implementing conversational AI systems in order to better serve customers and improve communication with patients. Early versions were little more than menu-driven robots that could book a follow-up or confirm a test time yet demand for instant help pushed developers to dream bigger. Now, thanks to stronger algorithms, the newest assistants grasp layered questions, remember a user's history, adjust to mood swings, and may flag signs of distress before a human notice. Whether tucked inside a hospital portal, loaded on a phone, or built into a smart speaker, they guide users through symptom checks, refill reminders, therapy check-ins, fitness tips, and everyday management of long-term conditions. As healthcare staff become harder to find and patients expect faster help, hospitals, clinics, insurers, and telehealth apps are turning to virtual health assistants (VHAs) more than ever. Because these tools lighten therapist's daily tasks, boost patient happiness, and give steady answers, they are widely seen as an easy way to widen access and streamline operations (Batista, 2025). On top of that, VHAs can gather and study patient clues in the moment, giving care teams fresh insights for quicker, personal decisions. With the tech still growing, many experts believe VHAs and similar chatbots will soon sit at the heart of smart health systems, stitching together cutting-edge tools and the people they serve. Figure 1 illustrates how a chatbot can help patients, particularly those who are illiterate, better understand their health and take appropriate actions. A visual guide for using chatbots in healthcare illustrates how conversational AI makes it easier for patients to understand and engage with their health by making it easier to get the information and answers they need.

Figure 1. Chatbot Architecture for Illiterate Patients for Self-Care

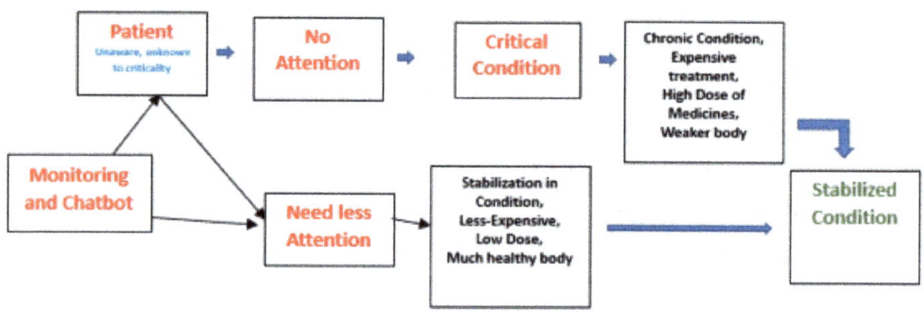

2. FOUNDATIONS OF VIRTUAL HEALTH ASSISTANTS AND CHATBOTS

It is important to understand the technology behind virtual health assistants (VHAs) in order to properly evaluate their capabilities and limitations as well as their applications in a variety of healthcare settings. VHAs and healthcare chatbots sit on a mix of core technologies that let them mimic human talk and give real help inside doctor offices and clinics. Natural Language Processing (NLP), Artificial Intelligence (AI), Machine Learning (ML), and other knowledge engines work together so the system can read, grasp, and reply to questions in ways that make sense for each user. At heart, these tools try to take over routine conversations-whether clinical or admin-by building digital helpers that talk, listen, and settle basic inquiries without pulling a staff member away from patient care.

2.1 Definitions and classifications

VHAs and health chatbots are AI-driven programs that carry on conversation and deliver medical services through text or voice, acting like a virtual receptionist or first-line advisor. They stand between patients and providers, handing out tips, appointment details, and symptom guidance on demand. Though the names overlap, VHAs usually pack extra power, blending text, voice, and pictures, hooking directly to Electronic Health Records (EHRs), and holding onto richer context so follow-up answers stay on target.

Classifications of VHAs and Chatbots in healthcare can be broadly categorized based on their architecture, interaction style, and use case:

1. Based on System Architecture:
   - **Retrieval-Based Chatbots:** Retrieval-Based Chatbots pull a response using machine-learning ranking, matching each user question to the best answer from a set. They feel smoother than rules yet still stumble when the pattern is new.
   - **Generative Chatbots:** Built using advanced NLP models such as transformer architectures (e.g., GPT), these bots can generate novel responses, allowing more dynamic and context-aware interactions.
2. Based on Communication Modality:
   - **Text-Based Assistants:** Interact through written language via apps, websites, or SMS.
   - **Voice-Based Assistants:** Utilize speech recognition and synthesis to interact with users through smart speakers or phone calls.
   - **Multimodal VHAs:** Combine text, voice, and visual cues (such as avatars or video) for a richer user experience.
3. Based on Functional Scope:
   - **Administrative Chatbots:** Handle non-clinical tasks like appointment booking, reminders, billing inquiries, and insurance verification.
   - **Clinical Support Chatbots:** Provide symptom checking, medication guidance, post-discharge care, and chronic disease monitoring (Anandavally, 2024).
   - **Mental Health and Wellness Bots:** Offer emotional support, stress management, mindfulness coaching, and preliminary mental health assessments.

Understanding these categories lets a health organization pick the right virtual health assistant or chatbot for its goals, audience, and tech setup. As the tools mature, the boundaries between types keep fading, leading to smarter, and more flexible digital care systems. Using these classifications, healthcare organizations can assess the best chatbot architecture for the services needed due to the complexity and number of services offered.

2.2 Consumer Health Chatbots vs Clinical Decision Support Systems

Health chatbots that offer a service to consumers by sharing general information about wellness and offering guidance for lifestyle modification, as well as mentally assist individuals, remind them about appointments, and offer educational information regarding health. The focus of consumer health chatbots is on improving patient engagement and increasing access to health information, rather than providing a direct medical diagnosis or recommend specific treatments. Clinical virtual health assistants are more sophisticated tools developed specifically for use by healthcare systems. These systems are intended to assist healthcare professionals with clinical support tasks that include but are not limited to: symptom triage and clinical documentation. Because of the potential impact of clinical virtual health assistants on clinical decision-making, they are subject to additional regulations, validation processes, and clinical accountability. Thus, it is critical to differentiate clinical virtual health assistants from consumer health chatbots, as the acceptable levels of risk, evaluation methodologies and legal obligations differ significantly between both of these categories of virtual health assistants.

2.3 Evolution of conversational AI in healthcare

Health care chatbots have travelled a long road since their clunky, rules-only beginnings; today they act like smart, talkative helpers who can mimic a real back-and-forth with patients. Early versions were little more than decision trees-canned questions, rigid scripts, and a limited bag of tricks for posting hours, answering the same FAQs, or shuttling visitors around a website. Because these bots had no sense of context and never strayed off their map, they served only predictable, repeatable tasks. Real progress kicked in when Natural Language Processing and Machine Learning were added, allowing the programs to grasp what people typed or said instead of just matching keywords. Often labelled retrieval-based, these second-generation bots generated a wider answer pool and tweaked replies to fit each user's intent (Zulzilah & Isa, 2024). Because they seemingly learned from past chats, smiles rose and so did the things they handled: symptom checks, pill nudges, appointment bookings, and more. Today's virtual agents run on deep-learning powerhouses- transformer models like BERT, GPT, and versions fine-tuned just for medicine. Recent chat-style models grasp the context of a talk, follow the thread across multiple turns, and reply on the spot in surprisingly polished language. That leap forward has given rise to Virtual Health Assistants (VHAs) that do more than answer questions; they mimic caring, recall what a patient said last time, and dish out advice tailored to each person's needs. When these bots plug into Electronic Health Records, voice-to-text engines, mood-sensing software, and multilingual engines, they grow even smarter and more welcoming. Because of that, hospitals are now using them for mental health check-ins, daily disease coaching, early screening, and post-surgery nudges, cutting clinicians workloads and getting patients to engage more (Nivedhitha et al., 2024). Due to improvements in deep learning algorithms, combined with access to large amounts of healthcare data, there has been rapid development of conversational AI used in healthcare settings. Therefore, most VHAs are capable of supporting a variety of healthcare services ranging from patient education and remote monitoring to basic health assessments.

2.4 Key capabilities and limitations of VHAs

VHAs still stumble, they sometimes misinterpret jargon, drop important context, or struggle with edge cases, which can leave patients and providers frustrated. Their growing presence in care shows promise, yet these quirks remind us that, for now, a human partner still holds the final word.

Key Capabilities of VHAs:

1. **24/7 Patient Support:** VHAs provide continuous access to healthcare information and services, making them valuable tools for addressing non-emergency queries outside of clinic hours, thereby improving healthcare accessibility.
2. **Symptom Triage and Self-Assessment:** Many VHAs are trained to ask a series of questions and assess symptoms to help patients understand the urgency of their condition, directing them toward appropriate care options.
3. **Administrative Assistance:** VHAs streamline administrative tasks such as appointment booking, reminders, insurance inquiries, and medical record retrieval, reducing the burden on healthcare staff.
4. **Medication Reminders and Treatment Adherence:** VHAs can deliver personalized alerts for medication schedules, follow-up appointments, and health monitoring routines, which improves adherence and patient outcomes.
5. **Mental Health and Emotional Support:** Some advanced VHAs provide basic mental health screening, emotional support, and self-help tools for stress, anxiety, and depression, promoting mental well-being.
6. **Multilingual and Accessible Communication:** Equipped with natural language processing and speech recognition technologies, VHAs can support multiple

languages and interaction modes (text, voice, chat), making healthcare more inclusive.

7. **Integration with Electronic Health Records (EHRs):** By interfacing with EHR systems, VHAs can retrieve or update patient information, allowing for personalized and context-aware responses.

Limitations of VHAs:

1. **Limited Clinical Judgment:** VHAs lack the deep clinical reasoning and diagnostic abilities of human healthcare professionals. While they can triage symptoms, they cannot replace expert medical advice or perform physical examinations (Laymouna et al., 2024).
2. **Dependence on Predefined Data and Models:** Most virtual health assistants work with fixed training sets and pre-built models, so they wobble when faced with odd questions, rare symptoms, or situations that need local know-how.
3. **Inability to Handle Complex or Emotional Conversations:** Some systems spot simple mood signals, yet they do not feel real empathy and often stumble during tense or subtle talks that demand human touch.
4. **Privacy and Security Concerns:** Because these tools handle sensitive patient records, any leak could harm lives, so strict safeguards and compliance with rules like HIPAA or GDPR are a must.
5. **Technological Accessibility and Digital Literacy:** VHAs assume people own smartphones and know how to swipe; that expectation can lock out frail seniors or neighbours in resource-poor clinics.
6. **Language and Cultural Limitations:** Even with dozens of tongues onboard, slang, local dialect, or folk beliefs about health may drift past the bot, leaving advice that feels off-key.

3. CONVERSATIONAL DESIGN FRAMEWORKS

How well a healthcare chatbot or virtual health assistant performs boils down to how thoughtfully its conversations are designed. When every exchange is laid out carefully, talking to the bot feels smooth, natural, and directly tied to what the user actually needs. That layout covers the logic, pathways, and knowledge that let the tool grasp a question and reply with something useful. Because health care demands precision, empathy, and clear language, designers also have to protect users' safety and match clinical tone. Broadly speaking, three main styles guide this work: rule-based dialogues, retrieval-based systems, and generative models. Each type comes with its own strengths and weaknesses, so developers choose one based on task complexity, desired interaction depth, and available technology.

3.1 Rule-Based Systems

Rule-based systems sit at the head of the class when it comes to the conversation engines behind many virtual health assistants and chatbots. They run on a playlist of set scripts, yes-or-no branches, and tidy if-this-then-that rules that keep the dialogue on a tight path. Every piece of user text gets lined up with a pre-chosen reply, so the chat flows like clockwork. In hospitals and clinics, these bots take on orderly jobs: booking a slot, nudging someone to take medicine, answering the usual FAQs, or gathering intake details. That neatness brings real upsides. Building, testing, and rolling out such a bot does not drain time or budget, and the replies stay predictable-a big win when patient safety is on the line. Because they do not lean on huge training files, smaller practices with slim digital wallets can still give one a try. Yet all that order comes with a downside. The bot clams up when a patient types something outside the script, uses slang, or packs several questions into one message. When that happens, the talk stalls, and the user is left wondering what went wrong. Even so, rule-based virtual health assistants still shine when users stick to a short list of clear tasks, quietly keeping safety, compliance, and dependability on track within well-marked limits.

3.2 Retrieval-Based Models

Retrieval-based models push the design of virtual health assistants and chatbots a step further. Instead of fixed decision trees, they lean on machine-learning tools to pick the best reply from a set that was written in advance. The system analyses the users question with natural-language processing, matches it against a stored question-and-answer bank, and pulls the option that fits the intent and context most closely. In healthcare, this approach lets a VHA guide patients through a wider mix of inquiries while sounding more fluid and human. Retrieval-based chatbots routinely handle symptom checks, simple health questions, wellness tips, and guided decision support-so long as the system can lean on a predefined but context-sensitive script. Behind the scenes, features like intent spotting, entity tagging, and dialogue state tracking let them keep the chat rolling across multiple turns, giving users a noticeably livelier experience. The catch is that these systems are enslaved by their answer library; if a query drifts too far from the stored templates, they either recycle an awkward match or fall silent because nothing fresh can be invented. Keeping that library up-to-date and clinically sound requires tireless editing, a job that only gets harder as research and guidelines shift almost daily. Still, the effort pays off;

the result blends firm control with a chat-like flow, making the bot ideal for routine medical chats where precision, consistency, and patient safety come first.

3.3 Generative Models

Generative models now sit at the front of conversational design for virtual health assistants (VHAs) and chatbots because they bend to real dialogue far better than older methods. Rule-based setups stick to set scripts and retrieval bots pull answers from a pre-packed library, yet a generative system craft each reply on the spot using deep learning tricks from sequence-to-sequence work and transformer giants like GPT, BERT, or specialty cousins built for medical talk. Fed on vast piles of text, these models catch context, stitch together smooth back-and-forth over multiple turns, and handle nearly any user query with surprisingly few hard stops. Inside health care that freedom lets generative VHAs sound natural, keep on topic, and match the words they choose to each patient's skill level with language. They prove useful during mental-health check-ins, tricky symptom chats, personal wellness advice, or plain info about treatments-all tasks that thrive on open, empathetic give-and-take. The models can walk a user through jargon, switch to plain terms, and even pick up hints of worry or urgency in the wording. Still, their strength brings real hurdles for medical use. A continuing worry is that generative tools may still spit out wrong, confusing, or even harmful advice whenever clinical topics come up. To guard against that, developers must tighten the models with careful tuning, human review, and direct links to trusted medical references so answers stay factual, consistent, and ethically sound. On top of that, training these systems costs huge computing power, requires vast sets of labelled examples, and needs strong safeguards to protect patient data and meet rules (Husnain, 2025).

4. INTEGRATION WITH HEALTHCARE ECOSYSTEMS

For virtual health assistants (VHAs) and similar chatbots to deliver real, lasting value, they must plug smoothly into the larger healthcare network (Vashishth et al., 2024). When that happens, the smart helpers stop being stand-alone toys and become threads woven into everyday clinical tasks, data systems, and communication lines. Properly anchored in a facility, a VHA can act as a helpful bridge linking patients, providers, and back-office processes, cutting delays, trimming mistakes, and raising the overall standard of care.

4.1 Electronic Health Records (EHRs) Integration

Pairing VHAs with EHRs sits at the heart of offering care that feels personal, runs smoothly, and adjusts to each patient's situation. Behind the scenes, EHRs act as all-in-one digital files, holding everything from past illnesses and allergies to current prescriptions, shot records, lab tests, and ongoing care plans. Figure 2 depicts a chatbot, a patient's Electronic Health Record (EHR) automatically gets updated, enabling personalized care and improved health monitoring.

Figure 2. Automated Chatbot System for Real-time Healthcare Services

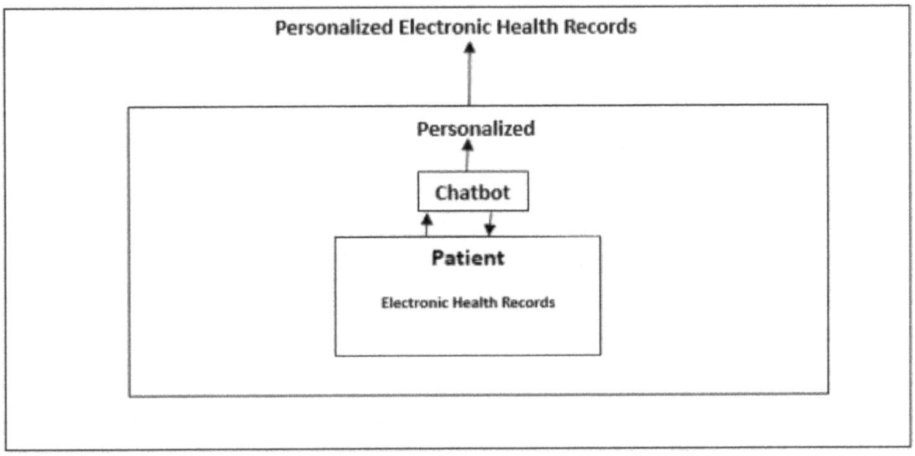

When a virtual health assistant links up with a hospital's electronic record system, it can pull clinical facts in real time and use that knowledge to give each patient more personal help and smarter answers. For example, the virtual assistant can shoot a quick text reminding a patient about Wednesdays check-in, prod them to grab more blood-pressure pills since last month's bottle is running low, or keep an eye on daily sugar logs for someone with diabetes. It can also whisper real-time tips, warning on-screen of drug overlaps after scanning the whole med list or sending step-by-step do-this-dos after knee surgery. Because of that close link, the physician's office spends less time buried in forms; notes slide into the chart, lab results are filed, and usual queries get answered on autopilot. The doctor's decisions therefore rest on a complete picture that appears at a tap, slashing wait times and lowering the odds that an exhausted staffer misses a vital clue. Still, wiring the assistant to the electronic record can be bumpy; mismatched software tongues, patchy data rules, and tight privacy rules can stall progress. Every EHR company guards its own files with different codes and standards, so the bot has to learn many dialects instead of relying on a single, neat template. Any time a person or program glimpses sensitive health records, the rules swing into action. Access has to line up with HIPAA or GDPR: that means encrypting data in transit, confirming who logs in, and keeping careful audit trails. Even with those guardrails, linking virtual health assistants to EHRs is a clear step forward for digital medicine. Suddenly, static numbers and notes turn into insights the care team can use right away; that shift opens the door to timely interventions, clearer communication, and a health system that responds faster to patients' needs (Reddy et al., 2025).

4.2 Health IT System Compatibility

For Virtual Health Assistants (VHAs) and chatbots to take root and grow in today's hospitals and clinics, their back-end technology has to fit smoothly with the tools people already use. Every VHA design should assume it will share space with Electronic Health Records, hospital information systems, clinical decision helpers, pharmacy portals, lab apps, and even wearables that send vital signs straight to the care team. If the virtual helper sits outside that ecosystem because no link was built, it ends up talking to nobody and patients and staff shrug it off. To prevent that, developers lean on industry data languages like HL7, FHIR, and DICOM for images so the VHA can read charts, snap labs, or check a prescription without delays. When these standards are in place, records move in real time, alerts pop up where they should, and the assistant stops being a lonely gadget. Imagine a smart virtual health assistant (VHA) that pulls a patient's latest test results straight from the lab-server, pops up with on-the-spot tips, and even grabs a telemedicine slot the moment the doctor clears a block on her calendar (Vashishth et al., 2025). Beyond that, the same helper slips smoothly into a hospital's website, a cell phone app, a waiting-room kiosk, or even the smartwatch a patient wears to yoga. That degree of stretch lets health systems serve people and staff alike through the same clear, easily remembered channel no matter where or how they log in. Of course, the VHA also needs to play nice with whatever backbone the facility uses-whether everything sits in the cloud, hides behind its own servers, or splits duties across both setups (Chauhan et al., 2024). Getting all those pieces to fit together, however, is anything but simple and costs more than most teams care to admit. Project leaders must sketch out every interface, stick to industry specs, partner closely with tech vendors, and run tiring rounds of real-world tests. Skip any step, and the result is broken links, duplicate entries, wasted time, and, in the worst cases, care gaps that may put a patient at risk. Get it right, though, and the VHA stops being just another app; it becomes a smart, talking node in a single digital-health network, boosting service quality, tightening data trust, and letting all the systems speak the same language.

4.3 Legal and Ethical Compliance

Staying on the right side of the law and maintaining strong ethics is vital when Virtual Health Assistants (VHAs) and chatbots move into hospitals, clinics, and homes. Because these smart helpers now store sensitive health facts and sometimes sway treatment choices, every line of code and conversation needs to follow the rules written by lawmakers and the higher standards set by care providers. Plainly put, good compliance protects a patient's dignity, keeps private data safe, and slowly builds the public trust that new technology desperately needs. At the heart of most legal talk is privacy, and rules like the U.S. Health Insurance Portability and Accountability Act (HIPAA) or Europe's General Data Protection Regulation (GDPR) spell out what that looks like. VHAs therefore have to guard the confidentiality, accuracy, and overall safety of personal health information (PHI). Doing so usually means adding strong encryption, easy-to-use yet solid login checks, and tight access gates so hackers or curious staff cannot peek at or steal data. On top of that, smart assistants must lay out simple consent steps, explaining what data gets collected, why, and who else will ever see it. From an ethical standpoint, virtual health assistants (VHAs) should Respect each patient's choices, stay clear about how they work, and steer away from hidden bias. Providers owe patients a plain heads-up when they log on or call in: the voice on the line is code, not a flesh-and-blood clinician. That basic honesty pairs with the harder job of teaching the software on wide, messy, current data so it skips over, not copies, the gaps already in care. When a symptom is fuzzy, a crisis weighs on the mind, or a moral twist comes up, the virtual health aide should quietly toss the ball to a real nurse or doctor instead of patching together half a reply. Both builders and health systems then need to run routine probes, stress drills, and bias sweeps to keep the helpers inside ethical and legal fences. Such gut checks spot hidden harm, wrong tips, or compliance cracks long before patients are hurt or the hospital faces a lawsuit.

5. USE CASES AND IMPLEMENTATIONS

Once treated as lab curiosities, these same digital helpers have elbowed their way into everyday life, reshaping care in hospitals, clinics, and the smartphone in a pocket. Because they scale almost with a flick, providers shove them into dozens of chores, from booking appointments and tackling billing snarls to guiding cough checkers or serving late-night chat therapy. In all those roles, real-world studies sing the same tune: virtual assistants smooth the patient trip while lightening staff load and lowering the odds of burnout.

5.1 Administrative Support

Virtual Health Assistants (VHAs) and friendly chatbots now fit right into health care wherever the paperwork pile starts leaning. Chores such as booking appointments, answering billing questions, checking insurance, signing up new patients, and shuffling forms drain time and staff energy in busy clinics and hospitals. When these smart helpers grab hold of the grunt tasks, the human workload shrinks, and the entire system runs a little smoother. With automated scheduling and gentle reminder texts, patients can book, shift, or cancel a visit by simply speaking or typing-rather than waiting on hold for a receptionist. That small upgrade eases life for patients, cuts the no-show rate, and opens up slots for others who need care. VHAs also guide people through pre-registration, collecting addresses, medical history, and insurance details so the front desk works quicker and the caregivers enter the room better informed (Hindelang et al., 2024). Billing and insurance queries are yet another corner where chatbots shine. They handle routine asks about co-pays, deductibles, or claim status, and even steer patients through the final payment, freeing staff to focus on more complex issues. This cuts down on mix-ups, boosts patient happiness, and gives front-office staff more time to tackle tricky jobs. When linked to Electronic Health Records, VHAs can also help clinicians by noting encounter details, spinning out reports, and updating charts on the fly. Less time spent on forms means providers devote more energy to caring for patients. So, by handling the repetitive stuff, these assistants lift a huge weight off administration, sharpen the quality of data, slash costs, and offer a smoother, friendlier experience to everyone who walks into a clinic or logs on to a portal. As hospitals and clinics move further into digital territory, VHA-backed support is quickly becoming one of the cornerstones of modern health IT (Singh et al., 2024).

5.2 Clinical Support

Virtual Health Assistants (VHAs) and chatbots are popping up across clinics and homes, lending a hand to doctors, nurses, and patients at nearly every step of care. Because these AI-driven helpers streamline paperwork, lighten staff workloads, and flag the right info faster than a rush-hour pager, they have become prized allies in crowded hospitals and small practices alike. One of their most talked-about tasks is guiding people through symptom triage and initial check-ups. By chatting with patients in simple, step-by-step exchanges, a VHA logs each ache or worry, rates how urgent it feels, and points to the right next move-whether that is a warm salt-water gargle, a Tuesday appointment, or a dash to the ER (Branda et al., 2025). The result is faster, fairer access to care for patients and a calmer, smarter queue for clinicians. VHAs also stay on the line for long-term conditions, nudging folks to report numbers and signs so nothing sneaks by. They might ping a person living with diabetes to double-check glucose, remind someone with high blood pressure to write down a reading, or ask an asthmatic to note when coughs or wheezes flare up. Linked directly to Electronic Health Records and the patient's wearables, modern virtual health assistants can ping doctors the moment some vital slips off its usual line. In the exam room or on the ward, the same VHA pulls up research-backed tips, links to the latest studies, and flags patient-specific red lights-drug clashes, allergy notes, or other hard no-thanks. That real-time support helps keep orders safer and cuts the odds of costly mix-ups. More sophisticated versions even track after-surgery progress, nudge folks through rehab, and deliver bite-sized lessons so recovery stays on course. On top of that, they walk patients through pill timetables, translate lab jargon, and calmly chat about what comes next, boosting confidence and basic know-how. Still, no gadget is a substitute for a caring clinician; these helpers show up beside the human team, not in its place. When they are tested, tagged for updates, and watched over, VHAs add an extra pair of eyes and ears, turning reactive care into something quicker, more personal, and much harder to ignore.

5.3 Mental Health and Wellness

Virtual health helpers and friendly chatbots now sit quietly yet successfully in mental health care, offering quick, stigma-free support the moment worry knocks. As anxiety, depression, and plain-old stress climb worldwide, people hunt for speedy relief-especially in remote villages or under resourced neighbourhoods where a therapist may be miles away. These purpose-built wellness agents lean on warm conversational A I that strives to sound caring rather than cold machine. They coach slow breaths, log moods, push gentle journaling, and hand over simple CBT tools so users spot harsh thoughts, ease pressure, and stay steady through daily bumps. Well-known companions such as Woebot, Wysa, and Tess-Walk users through step-by-step chats that slowly build self-awareness and inner strength. VHAs now run around the clock, giving anyone overwhelmed by feelings a safe place to ask for help whenever the need strikes-and doing so without a hint of judgment. That kind of always-on access knocks down the usual walls that stop people from reaching out, nudges them toward early care, and gives even the folks wary of a human therapist because of stigma or privacy fears a way to start (Wah, 2025). Yet, although these virtual allies can chip in with mild and moderate struggles, they never take the place of a licensed clinician. The smarter programs watch for red flags-sudden talk of self-harm or deep, unshakable gloom-and then pass the case up the line to a real therapist, a trusted hotline, or even emergency responders when time is short.

6. IMPACT ASSESSMENT

Virtual Health Assistants (VHAs) and light-touch chatbots have spread quickly through hospitals, clinics, and insurance offices, and their reach keeps growing. Clear benefits are already appearing across clinical workflows, business operations, and the day-to-day experience of patients, making it important to measure what they deliver. By automating routine chores, answering questions around the clock, and nudging people to stay engaged with their care, these digital helpers are steadily reshaping the way health services are delivered.

6.1 Patient Experience and Satisfaction

VHAs meet people where they actually are-on phones, web portals, or quick-service kiosks-so access barriers drop fast. Customers now expect help to appear on demand, and round-the-clock service means care teams are no longer the only gatekeepers. When answers arrive in seconds instead of days, day-to-day stress eases and important choices can move forward without extra delays. Virtual assistants also recall a patient's past visits, wishes, and goals, turning a routine encounter into a custom chat each time. By reading a person's own file-history notes, drug lists, and recent messages-chatbots can build replies that fit, sending the right tip, nudge, or lesson exactly when it is needed. This kind of tailored talk makes people feel noticed and valued, lifting their trust and overall happiness with care. VHAs also boost know-how by breaking down jargon, walking users through steps, and offering help in many languages so medical facts stay plain and easy to grasp. When details click, patients can choose wiser paths for their health and worry less about strange procedures. Another win is smoother admin work. Booking a slot, checking test results, or snagging post-visit tips all happen quicker and with far less hopping around thanks to VHA backup, leaving visitors with a calmer, more fluid experience. Still, technology cannot fully stand in for human touch. Virtual chat can feel cold to some or leave them uneasy about machine-made advice. So savvy systems build in quick switches to live staff whenever a person decides they want a real voice on the line.

6.2 Healthcare Accessibility in Remote Areas

Virtual health assistants (VHAs) and simple chatbots are stepping up as handy links between busy city clinics and the people living far off in remote or neglected areas. Where doctors, drug stores, and lab services are few, these smart, low-cost programs keep care flowing and keep budgets from breaking. Thanks to smartphones, cloud storage, and easy voice or text chat, a VHA can slide onto a patients screen no matter whether that phone sits in a mountain hamlet or a coastal slum. Perhaps the biggest draw for far-flung places is that the assistant is there all day and night, ready to answer questions as soon as they pop up. Someone wondering about a cough can check whether it looks serious, find a list of warning signs, set a note to take the right pills, or pick up tips on preventing the next cold, all while staying at home. That kind of speed matters most where hospitals are crowded, roads are washed out, or the nearest clinic is a full day's hike. Besides sharing quick bits of advice, VHAs act like friendly study partners, explaining topics like diabetes, pregnancy, or vaccines in clear local words so everyone understands. That approach lifts health literacy and gives people the confidence to choose what is best for their bodies. For people living with long-term health issues, virtual health assistants keep an eye on care from afar, let both patients and clinics know as soon as an odd sign appears, nip trouble in the bud, and lower the number of late-night trips to the E.R. In bigger public health drives, chatbots take a starring role, sending out bulk alerts and gathering quick answers during vaccine pushes or outbreak notices. They share handy facts, stand up to false headlines, and scoop instant feedback from neighbourhood's miles away from any health center, all without staff having to hit the road. Yet shaky internet, low comfort with gadgets, and communities mixing several languages still slow things down in some spots. Fortunately, rising smartphone ownership and government-backed digital-inclusion plans are slowly chipping away at these gaps (Maher et al., 2024).

6.3 Clinician Workload Reduction

Bringing virtual health assistants and chatbots into a hospital's routine is quickly changing the day-to-day flow for care teams, lifting a pile of small, steady tasks off clinician's backs so they can zero in on tricky cases and hard medical calls. Because providers are already stretched thin by swelling patient volumes, staff shortages, and mountains of paperwork, these smart helpers step in with an easy way to cut daily busywork and sharpen overall efficiency. The biggest win shows up when VHAs grab the dull-but-critical jobs: booking appointments, entering intake data, welcoming new arrivals, and sending gentle follow-up nudges. Since those chores can swallow huge blocks of time, passing them to a chatbot lets doctors, nurses, and specialists snag lost minutes for real face-to-face care. For example, a simple chat window linked to the electronic record can quietly ask about allergies, meds, and family history long before the patient sits in the exam room, and that early prep slashes the paperwork mountain for the clinician. VHAs can also run point with a first-pass symptom check and basic assessment. Through guided questions, the assistant logs vital details, sorts cases by urgency, and flags emergencies, giving the care team a clearer queue before the first phone call or appointment begins. By screening cases before a consultation, virtual health assistants let clinicians zero in on urgent patients and set their calendars smartly. Many also nudge doctors with evidence-based tips, drug clash alerts, and ready-made care plan ideas at the moment they are needed. These on-the-spot reminders lighten mental strain and help make each treatment step more precise and uniform. At the same time, VHAs coach patients, firing off gentle prompts for pills, tests, and healthy habits. Because of this, healthcare team's field fewer last-minute questions or follow-up calls, which eases the burden on clinics and keeps long-term patients on track (Mishra et al., 2024).

6.4 Evaluation Metrics for Virtual Health Assistants

Standardized performance metrics must be used to evaluate virtual health assistants' deployment and ensure they can operate safely and successfully. Specific examples of standardized performance metrics include clinical accuracy for symptom triage (primary care), identify complex cases and refer to a human clinician, percent of responses generated by AI that are incorrect or created out of thin air (or hallucination), patient satisfaction, usability in vulnerable populations, adherence to treatment plan and reduction of clinician workload. Metrics that are focused on safety, such as the risk of providing false reassurances and providing particularly reliable escalation methods, are of particular importance when generative AI systems are implemented in clinical settings. Therefore, establishing valid and reliable evaluation frameworks is paramount to provide VHAs operate successfully within the appropriate safety and performance parameters.

7. VIRTUAL HEALTH ASSISTANTS (VHAS) AND CHATBOTS CHALLENGES IN HEALTHCARE

Even with the obvious perks, bringing VHAs into real-world care paths is far from plug-and-play. Developers and providers alike must wrestle with a mix of technical, legal, ethical, and social hurdles if they want patients to trust the service-and each other-properly. However, there are still many challenges that limit the extent to which virtual health assistants can be widely used in healthcare environments.

1. **Data Privacy and Security Risks:** VHAs deal with the kind of personal information most people share only with their doctor: full medical histories, current symptoms, lists of medications, even notes about anxiety or depression. That means end-to-end encryption, locked storage, and strict adherence to HIPAA, GDPR, or whatever rules apply in a given market. Tie the assistant to web portals, insurance apps, or pharmacy clouds, though, and the attack surface widens fast,

exposing systems to hackers, rogue insiders, or careless API links. When the data leaks, trust-erasing headlines follow, and patients rightly question whether AI tools deserve a place in their care.

2. **Limited Diagnostic Accuracy and Scope:** Even though virtual health assistants (VHAs) keep getting smarter, they still miss the subtle insight that a seasoned doctor brings to hard cases. Most replies come from rules or data pools baked into the tool, so real quirks in a patient's history may get overlooked. That gap opens the door to missed clues or bland advice, and in tense moments-or when the picture is hazy-clinical instinct is what people really need.
3. **Integration Challenges with Existing Health IT Systems:** Linking virtual health assistants smoothly with EHRs, hospital networks, and telehealth tools is still hard to do. Many health systems find it tough to talk to old servers, which dumps data into silos, makes people enter the same info twice, and leaves records looking patchy. To close the gaps, experts need common standards, custom APIs, and usually a big budget for wiring upgrades.
4. **Ethical and Legal Concerns:** Rolling out these assistants raises knotty issues about consent, who pays when something goes wrong, and how clear the AI reasoning really is. If a chatbot hands out poor advice and a patient is hurt, no one knows if the coder, the clinic, or the supervising doctor picks up the blame. On top of that, patients don't always realize they are chatting with software, which can warp consent and chip away at trust.
5. **Lack of Emotional Intelligence and Empathy:** People-centred settings like healthcare run on feeling, and that's where virtual health assistants lag. They can parrot caring phrases from a script, yet they miss most non-verbal signals-shaken hands, worried faces or the silence that speaks volumes. Because of that gap, turning to a bot for news about a terminal diagnosis, a mental health scare or a death in the family frequently feels wrong.
6. **Digital Literacy and Accessibility Barriers:** Any tool is only as good as the person who can use it, and VHAs sit on shaky ground when patients lack tech comfort. Elderly users, people with disabilities, and anyone facing slow internet, poor English or simply the fear of clicking the wrong button can quickly hit a wall. When that happens, the hoped-for bridge to equal care becomes yet another gap, especially in rural clinics or clinics with thin budgets.
7. **Trust and Acceptance Among Users and Providers:** Patients and providers alike tend to eye AI helpers with caution, wondering how reliable, open, or useful they really are. Push-back often arises from worries about job loss, feelings of lost control, or bad memories of clunky apps that let everyone down. To win hearts, the VHA team must spell out what the tool can-and cannot-do and back those claims with solid, real-world proof.

8. FUTURE DIRECTIONS WITH VIRTUAL HEALTH ASSISTANTS (VHAS) AND CHATBOTS IN HEALTHCARE

As Artificial Intelligence continues improving and digital health technology advances at a fast rate, the potential capabilities of VHAs will be improved substantially. Better AI, sharper language skills, and tighter links with existing records will drive the next wave. When the dust settles, these helpers should not only spark stronger patient engagement but also lend a timely hand to clinicians, flag risks early, and keep whole systems running more smoothly.

1. **Emotionally Intelligent and Empathetic AI Systems:** Future virtual health assistants (VHAs) will be tuned to feelings, reading a person's mood through the lilt of their voice, choice of words, and-even when cameras are on-the set of their face. Instead of rehearsed phrases, the VHA will learn to spot worry, tension, or bewilderment and reply with words that match the moment. This skill matters most in mental-health chats, end-of-life talk, or daily coaching for long illnesses, because gentle, human-like concern can lift satisfaction and keep patients on track with care (Zhang et al., 2024).
2. **Seamless Integration with Wearable and IoT Devices:** As the Internet of Things floods more homes, VHAs will hook up with wristbands, patches, and connected fridges that quietly report heart rate, blood pressure, glucose, sleep, and more. Streaming that data live lets the assistant craft advice on the spot and flag trouble before it blooms. For instance, after spotting restless nights, the VHA could nudge safer habits or-even quicker-message the doctor if readings drift into danger, putting early-warning power into everyday hands.
3. **Predictive Analytics for Preventive Care:** By melding machine learning with big-data crunching, future virtual health assistants (VHAs) will shift from reactive helpers to savvy early-warning systems. They will sift through a patient's records, meds, and daily habits, spotting telltale patterns that hint at trouble before symptoms show. Imagine a humble chatbot quietly flags risk for diabetes, low mood, or heart trouble after weighing blood sugar logs, sleep hours, and family notes. Acting on these alerts, doctors can issue referrals, sketch care plans, and cut the need for expensive ER visits, placing VHAs squarely at the helm of community health.
4. **Multilingual and Culturally Sensitive Communication:** Coming VHAs will speak many languages and adjust to local customs, opening healthcare to more people around the world. By learning neighbourhood dialects, folk remedies, and community beliefs about illness, an assistant can give help that feels personal and respectful. This upgrade will matter most in mixed cities and remote

towns, where cultural differences and language gaps keep people from the care they need.

5. **Integration into Telehealth and Virtual Clinics:** Soon, VHAs will sit right inside telehealth apps, playing the part of front-desk staff, patient teachers, and first-round screeners. Before anyone talks to a doctor, the bot can note key details, summarize what hurts, and even offer basic tips. That head starts speeds up virtual visits and lets the clinician spend time on real diagnosis and treatment. In time, these helpers may run entire online clinics for simple check-ins, refill requests, and steady-watch programs for chronic illness (Singh et al., 2025).
6. **Enhanced Clinical Decision Support for Providers:** VHAs will also back doctors and nurses with real-time clinical decision help, not just patient-facing tools. Pulling together the latest guidelines, research, and a patients record, the system flashes easy-to-see tips during each consult. A VHA, for example, might flag a risky drug combo or point out an up-to-date care pathway, lifting diagnostic confidence, boosting outcomes, and cutting mistakes (Vashishth et al., 2024).
7. **Voice-First Healthcare Interfaces:** With the advancement of voice recognition technology, future virtual health assistants (VHAs) will lean almost entirely on voice. Such an upgrade will open the door for seniors, people with low vision, and anyone who finds typing tough. With these voice-first systems, patients will be able to chat naturally, ask about medicines, schedule visits, or get quick medical tips using only spoken words, making the whole care process easier.

9. CONCLUSION

Virtual health assistants and chatbots are quietly reshaping how people access and move through the healthcare system. Thanks to leaps in natural-language processing, conversational AI, and machine-learning patterns, these digital helpers lift much of the routine chatter off clinician's shoulders, guide patients through bookings and basic questions, and stretch care farther into remote or underserved neighbourhoods. When they plug directly into electronic health records, Internet-of-Things sensors, and telehealth software, VHAs pull apart the data silos that slow follow-up and make care feel disconnected. Yet promise comes with worry; privacy, narrow clinical knowledge, ethical grey areas, and the digital divide still bark at designers and lawmakers and demand serious fixes. Tomorrow teams will push for emotionally aware, culturally tuned, and multilingual versions that scan history and context, then gently nudge patients toward prevention or treatment before symptoms swell. While health systems chase better patient focus and broader reach, these friendly bots sit at the wheel, ready to steer a new road toward fairer, smarter, and faster digital care. By advancing technology and creating regulatory policy structures that are appropriate for VHAs, healthcare chatbots could become a key part of the next phase of high-class digital healthcare systems.

REFERENCES

Akila, K., Gopinathan, R., Arunkumar, J., & Malar, B. S. B. (2025). The Role of Artificial Intelligence in Modern Healthcare: Advances, Challenges, and Future Prospects. *The European Journal of Cardiovascular Medicine*, *15*, 615–624.

Anandavally, B. B. (2024). Improving Clinical Support Through Retrieval-Augmented Generation Powered Virtual Health Assistants. *Journal of Computer and Communications*, *12*(11), 86–94. DOI: 10.4236/jcc.2024.1211006

Bacha, A., & Shah, H. H. (2025). AI-Powered Virtual Health Assistants: Transforming Patient Care and Engagement. *Global Insights in Artificial Intelligence and Computing*, *1*(1), 15–30.

Batista, A. S. (2025). The Transforming Clinical Practice: The Role of AI-Powered Medical Assistants in Enhancing Healthcare Efficiency and Decision-Making. Journal of Next-Generation Research 5.0.

Branda, F., Stella, M., Ceccarelli, C., Cabitza, F., Ceccarelli, G., Maruotti, A., Ciccozzi, M., & Scarpa, F. (2025). The Role of AI-Based Chatbots in Public Health Emergencies: A Narrative Review. *Future Internet*, *17*(4), 145. DOI: 10.3390/fi17040145

Chauhan, S., Paliwal, M., Manchanda, N., & Gupta, M. (2024). AI and Machine Learning in Modern Healthcare. In Transforming Gender-Based Healthcare with AI and Machine Learning (pp. 1-13). CRC Press. DOI: 10.1201/9781003473435-1

Chavali, D., Dhiman, V. K., & Katari, S. C. (2024). AI-Powered Virtual Health Assistants: Transforming Patient Engagement through Virtual Nursing. *International Journal of Pharma Sciences*, *2*, 613–624.

Hindelang, M., Sitaru, S., & Zink, A. (2024). Transforming Health Care through Chatbots for Medical History-Taking and Future Directions: Comprehensive Systematic Review. *JMIR Medical Informatics*, *12*(1), e56628. DOI: 10.2196/56628

Husnain, A. (2025). Smarter Healthcare: Harnessing AI for Faster, More Accurate, and Accessible Medicine. *Global Trends in Science and Technology*, *1*(2), 1–22. DOI: 10.70445/gtst.1.2.2025.1-22

Laymouna, M., Ma, Y., Lessard, D., Schuster, T., Engler, K., & Lebouché, B. (2024). Roles, users, benefits, and limitations of chatbots in health care: Rapid review. *Journal of Medical Internet Research*, *26*, e56930. DOI: 10.2196/56930

Maher, C., Singh, B., Wylde, A., & Chastin, S. (2024). Virtual health assistants: A grand challenge in health communications and behavior change. *Frontiers in Digital Health*, *6*, 1418695. DOI: 10.3389/fdgth.2024.1418695

Mishra, S., Chaudhury, P., Tripathy, H. K., Sahoo, K. S., Jhanjhi, N. Z., Hassan Elnour, A. A., & Abdelmaboud, A. (2024). Enhancing health care through medical cognitive virtual agents. *Digital Health*, *10*, 20552076241256732. DOI: 10.1177/20552076241256732

Nivedhitha, D. P., Madhumitha, G., Sri, J. J., Jayashree, S., Surya, J., & Divya, D. M. (2024, April). Conversational AI for healthcare to improve member efficiency. In *2024 International Conference on Science Technology Engineering and Management (ICSTEM)* (pp. 1-6). IEEE. DOI: 10.1109/ICSTEM61137.2024.10561046

Reddy, K. V., Saketh, G., Priyanshu, S. S., Nitesh, M., Hussain, S. K., & Sharma, K. V. (2025). AI-Driven Healthcare Management Platform: Enhancing Accessibility, Efficiency, and Security in Digital Health Systems. Synthesis: A Multidisciplinary Research Journal, 3(1), 1-14.

Samala, A. D., & Rawas, S. (2024). Generative AI as Virtual Healthcare Assistant for Enhancing Patient Care Quality. *International Journal of Online & Biomedical Engineering*, *20*(5), 174–187. DOI: 10.3991/ijoe.v20i05.45937

Sharma, V., Vashishth, T. K., Kumar, B., Sharma, K. K., Vidyant, S., & Chaudhary, S. (2023, December). Health Interpretation of Covid-19 Patients using Artificial Intelligence. In *2023 International Conference on Artificial Intelligence for Innovations in Healthcare Industries (ICAIIHI)* (Vol. 1, pp. 1-5). IEEE Computer Society. DOI: 10.1109/ICAIIHI57871.2023.10488924

Singh, M., Mittal, M., Dewan, P., Kaur, A., Kaur, G., & Gupta, A. (2024, February). From Text to Treatment: An Overview of Artificial Intelligence Chatbots in Healthcare. In 2024 11th International Conference on Computing for Sustainable Global Development (INDIACom) (pp. 690-696). IEEE.

Singh, S., Rathee, T., & Singhal, N. (2025). AI-Enabled Medical Chatbots: Advancements in Patient Query Handling and Automated Healthcare Delivery. *International Journal of Environmental Sciences*, *11*(4s), 796–810. DOI: 10.64252/1n1waz11

Suvarnamukhi, B., Praveena, A., Prakash, C. R. C., & Babu, K. N. (2025). Automated Chatbot for Healthcare Using NLP and ML. *International Journal of Information Technology and Computer Engineering*, *13*(1), 1–10.

Vashishth, T. K., Sharma, V., Kumar, B., Panwar, R., Sharma, K. K., & Chaudhary, S. (2024). AI-Integrated IoT in Healthcare Ecosystem: Opportunities, Challenges, and Future Directions. AI and IoT Technology and Applications for Smart Healthcare Systems, 37-54.

Vashishth, T. K., Sharma, V., Sharma, K. K., Kumar, B., Chaudhary, S., & Agarwal, S. (2025). IoT-Enabled Multimedia Applications in Healthcare, Telemedicine, and Imaging. *Multimedia Technologies in the Internet of Things Environment*, *4*(173), 135–160. DOI: 10.1007/978-981-96-4356-1_7

Vashishth, T. K., Sharma, V., Sharma, K. K., Kumar, B., Kumar, A., & Panwar, R. (2024). Artificial Intelligence (AI)–Powered Chatbots: Providing Instant Support and Personalized Recommendations to Guests 24/7. In Technology and Luxury Hospitality (pp. 211-236). Routledge.

Wah, J. N. K. (2025). Revolutionizing e-health: The transformative role of AI-powered hybrid chatbots in healthcare solutions. *Frontiers in Public Health*, *13*, 1530799. DOI: 10.3389/fpubh.2025.1530799

Zhang, Q., Wong, A. K. C., & Bayuo, J. (2024). The role of Chatbots in enhancing health Care for Older Adults: A scoping review. *Journal of the American Medical Directors Association*, *25*(9), 105108. DOI: 10.1016/j.jamda.2024.105108

Zulzilah, S., & Isa, J. R. (2024). Decoding Patient Interactions with AI-Based Virtual Health Assistants. *CARAKA: Indonesia Journal of Communication*, *5*(2), 180–190. DOI: 10.25008/caraka.v5i2.173

Chapter 7

Security of Image Transmission and Internet of Things Networks for Telemedicine

Neha Jain
http://orcid.org/0009-0009-3822-3780
Poornima University, Jaipur, India

Digvijay Pandey
http://orcid.org/0000-0003-0353-174X
Department of Technical Education, Government of Uttar Pradesh, India

Srijib Shankar Jha
http://orcid.org/0000-0001-7687-7771
SoML, IMS Unison University, India

A. Shaji George
http://orcid.org/0000-0002-8677-3682
Wincom Information Technology, Dubai, UAE

Blessy Thankachan
JECRC University, Jaipur, India

Shivani Kharra
http://orcid.org/0009-0007-2010-9598
Stantec, USA

ABSTRACT

This chapter examines the integration of Internet of Things (IoT) networks and secure image transmission in telemedicine to demonstrate their importance in modern medical treatment. The telemedicine of uses IoT to increase patient monitoring, medical access and healthcare system efficiency. Due to the increased use of medical imaging for accurate diagnosis and secure transmission methods are essential to protect sensitive patient data from unauthorized access and cyber threats. Healthcare IoT network components are described. Data-collection and transmission sensors are

DOI: 10.4018/979-8-2600-3070-7.ch007

included. This approach solves data privacy, bandwidth, and device compatibility issues in Internet of Things-based telemedicine. Secure picture communication is stressed due to data manipulation, eavesdropping and unwanted access. Advanced encryption and blockchain technologies can improve medical imaging data integrity and transparency. These technologies provide reliable solutions for securing patient data and maintaining quality for accurate medical evaluations. To demonstrate how data reduction, prioritizing.

INTRODUCTION

The purpose of this chapter is to study the integration of Internet of Things (IoT) networks and secure picture transmission in telemedicine. The purpose of this study is to emphasize the importance of these two ideas in the provision of modern medical care. Telemedicine makes use of the Internet of Things (IoT) to improve accessibility to medical services, simplify remote patient monitoring and bring about an increase in the effectiveness of healthcare systems. It is very important to have secure ways to communicate so that sensitive patient information does not get into the wrong hands or get exposed to cyber threats. This aspect is especially important in light of the rising reliance on medical imaging for correct diagnosis. In this chapter we will cover the many components that make up Internet of Things (IoT) networks in the healthcare industry. Among these components are sensors and other devices that are capable of data collection and transmission. This approach addresses the challenges encountered in telemedicine that relies on the Internet of Things. These challenges include constraints on bandwidth, difficulties in interoperability between devices and concerns over data privacy. It is important to underline the necessity of secure image transmission because of the common hazards that are posed by data tampering and unauthorized access. There are various methods of encryption that are technologically advanced. In addition to the potential of blockchain technology can improve the data integrity and transparency in the field of medical imaging. Additionally, it is essential to maintain the quality required for accurate medical evaluations. Utilizing these methods ensures the security of patient data while maintaining the necessary quality. The efficient transmission techniques such as data compression, prioritizing and energy saving protocols play a crucial role in maximizing bandwidth usage in Internet of Things networks. So explaining the function of these strategies is necessary (Brenner, B., et al., 2022). Ongoing research and technological evolution fuel this confidence. This confidence is driven by ongoing research and technological evolution, which makes it possible to execute medical interventions quickly and accurately. This approach also safeguards patient privacy and enhances the overall quality of care.

The successful integration of Internet of Things networks will change the delivery of healthcare. These goals will be accomplished by making it possible to undertake medical interventions. Telemedicine refers to the process of providing medical care to patients remotely through the use of various forms of telecommunications technology. This technology allows patients and medical staff to communicate even when they are not in the same place. Telemedicine allows for the delivery of a wide range of services, including consultations, diagnoses, treatments and follow up care, among other aspects of medical care. It is possible to facilitate these services through the use of phone conversations, video conferencing and messaging apps or specialist software designed for medical purposes. The concept of telemedicine was established to overcome the logistical and geographic constraints that sometimes limit access to healthcare particularly in locations that are underserved or rural. As a result of the utilization of telecommunications patients no longer need to travel extensive distances or schedule appointments with their treating physicians and specialists in person. When it comes to the management of mental health consultations, post-surgical follow ups and chronic conditions, such services can be extremely helpful. Technological improvements such as wearables, high-speed internet, smartphones and sensors connected to the Internet of Things (IoT) have contributed to the enormous rise that telemedicine has undergone at the present time. The use of these tools that encourage ongoing care and the early identification of potential health problems makes it feasible for healthcare personnel to monitor the health data of their patients in real time. Wearable technology has the capability to monitor vital signs such as blood pressure, heart rate and glucose levels and then transmit the information to medical specialists for examination. The COVID-19 pandemic accelerated the shift toward the use of telemedicine since it provides a safe and efficient method of providing medical care while simultaneously eliminating the need for face to face interaction and the associated danger of infection. In response to the pandemic the concept of telemedicine has emerged as an indispensable instrument as numerous healthcare systems have expanded their services to accommodate the increased number of patients who are receiving care remotely.

ROLE OF IOT IN HEALTHCARE

The Internet of Things (IoT) is a technology that is playing a disruptive role in the healthcare business by connecting various devices, sensors, and operating systems. This technology makes it feasible to gather, transmit, and analyze data in real time. The Internet of Things (IoT) in the healthcare business makes it possible to deliver better patient care, improve diagnoses, and optimize medical processes. This task is made possible with the assistance of smart devices and advanced communication technology. By utilizing this network of interconnected devices, medical personnel are able to remotely monitor the health of their patients, provide assistance in the management of chronic illnesses, and perform interventions at the appropriate time. One of the most significant aspects of the Internet of Things in the field of healthcare is the ability to remotely monitor patients undergoing treatment. As a result of this data being automatically supplied to medical personnel, they are able to monitor the status of patients without having to physically visit the hospital. Not only does this functionality reduce the amount of work that needs to be done at healthcare institutions, but it also makes it easier to detect anomalies at an earlier stage, which eventually results in better outcomes for patients. The Internet of Things also includes personalized medicine, which plays a vital role. By gathering large volumes of health data from individuals, Internet of Things devices make it possible for medical professionals to personalize therapies based on the distinct patient profiles of their patients. These individuals are capable of providing the necessary information. To be more specific, insulin pumps that are enabled by the Internet of Things (IoT) have the capacity to automatically alter dosage based on real-time blood glucose readings. This ability ensures that patients with diabetes receive therapy that is accurate (El Khaddar, M. A.et al., 2012, May). Internet of Things devices help streamline inventory management and medical asset tracking in healthcare institutions, both of which contribute to the overall efficiency of the facility. Smart sensors have the capability of monitoring the whereabouts of medical equipment, pharmaceuticals, and even staff members. This capability has the potential to enhance the efficiency of hospitals and lower the costs that are involved with their operations. The amount of time that patients have to wait for care is cut down as a result of this, which also guarantees that vital resources are available at the proper moment. According to Moore (1999), the Internet of Things makes it possible to create smart pill dispensers that remind patients to take their prescription at the appropriate time and inform caretakers if a dose is missed. This technology makes medication management more effective.

SECURE IMAGE TRANSMISSION IN TELEMEDICINE

It is necessary to have secure image transmission since telemedicine is becoming increasingly dependent on digital communication for the diagnosis and treatment of patients. It is vital to ensure the security of these transmissions to maintain patient privacy and data integrity. This is because telemedicine involves the sharing of confidential medical pictures over digital platforms such as MRIs, ultrasounds and X-rays. Providing protection against cyberattacks is one of the primary reasons for implementing secure picture transmission. Due to the sensitive personal and medical information that they contain cybercriminals consider healthcare data and medical photographs in particular to be extremely lucrative targets at this time. Assuming these photographs are intercepted while they are being transmitted. They could be used for identity theft, blackmail or even sold on the dark web. There is a guarantee that these photographs will be delivered without any damage thanks to the use of secure communication methods and robust encryption. Enhanced collaboration among healthcare professionals is facilitated by the exchange of images in a secure manner. Telemedicine typically entails discussions between a number of professionals who rely on the quick and accurate transmission of medical pictures in order to make judgments that are well informed regarding the patient condition. The use of secure communication methods.Which ensure the timely delivery of images that are free from tampering or loss and makes it feasible to improve clinical collaboration and make decisions more quickly. When it comes to situations that require immediate attention, these characteristics might be very crucial (Brian Brenner, M. D. et al., 2022). The process of maintaining image quality is an additional consideration. Either the medical images that are utilized for diagnosis must remain uncompressed or undergo minimal change to preserve their diagnostic clarity while they are being transmitted. Secure transmission mechanisms reduce the chance of misinterpretation due to low image quality. This requirement is accomplished by ensuring that high-quality photos are transmitted among healthcare providers. Secure transmission enables the provision of remote healthcare services in underserved or rural areas. It is possible to improve access to high-quality medical care even in distant places, where patients may not have easy access to advanced medical facilities, by transferring medical images from adjacent healthcare facilities to specialists in urban areas in a secure manner. (Pandian, Safeer, et al., 2007) It is possible to encourage a greater utilization of telemedicine services by assuring the security of these transmissions.

TELEMEDICINE IOT NETWORKS

Components of IoT Networks in Healthcare

A system wherein networked devices and sensors exchange data with one another to gather, send, and evaluate health-related data via the internet is known as an IoT (Internet of Things) network in the healthcare industry. Patient care and operational efficiency within healthcare systems are enhanced by these networks capacity for remote control, data sharing, and continuous monitoring of medical equipment. IoT networks are used in the healthcare industry to link sensors, wearables, and diagnostic equipment to a central system. Medical professionals can obtain vital patient information remotely, in real-time, and without physical contact thanks to this networked systems data analytics, real-time monitoring, and remote access features. Applications such as remote monitoring, early health issue detection, and better chronic disease management are made possible by IoT networks in the healthcare industry.

Figure 1. Elements of IoT Networks in Healthcare

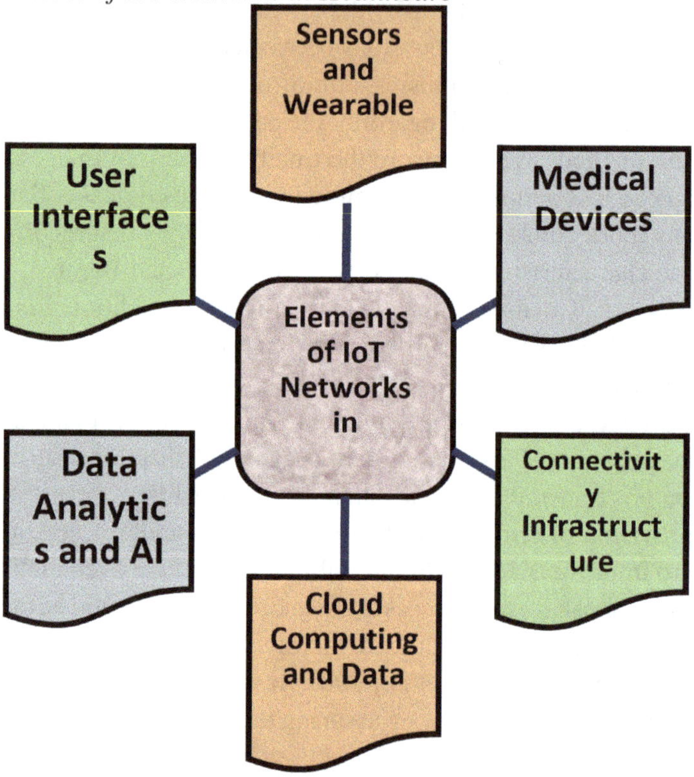

· ***Sensors and Wearable Devices***: Sensors and wearable devices are essential for collecting real-time health data directly from patients. These devices can be worn continuously, facilitating the continuous monitoring of vital signs including heart rate, oxygen saturation, glucose concentration, temperature, and physical activity. Certain advanced sensors can detect specific conditions such as sleep apnea or arrhythmias. These devices enable healthcare providers to monitor patient health trends over time, facilitating early identification of potential issues before they develop into serious conditions. Ongoing monitoring enables proactive care, minimizing hospital visits and permitting patients to receive treatment at home.

· ***Medical Devices***: The Internet of Things (IoT) encompasses an array of medical devices, including insulin pumps, pacemakers, and connected inhalers, which autonomously modify treatment in accordance with the patient's real-time health data. Smart insulin pumps can deliver insulin according to real-time glucose levels, enhancing diabetes management. Likewise, IoT-enabled pacemakers can monitor cardiac rhythms and notify healthcare providers upon detecting irregularities, thereby averting emergencies. These devices can remotely transmit data to healthcare providers, facilitating treatment adjustments without necessitating a patient visit to a clinic or hospital. This instantaneous data exchange can be crucial in scenarios requiring prompt intervention (Devaraj & Ezra, 2011).

· ***Connectivity Infrastructure***: The connectivity infrastructure constitutes the foundation of the IoT network, facilitating uninterrupted communication among devices, healthcare providers, and cloud-based systems. Technologies such as 5G are vital for IoT networks, offering the high-speed, low-latency connections essential for real-time data transmission and remote diagnostics. Dependable connectivity guarantees the prompt delivery of critical data, which is vital for timely interventions, particularly in emergencies. Furthermore, this infrastructure must guarantee secure data transmission to avert breaches, given the highly sensitive nature of healthcare data. The selection of communication protocols (e.g., Wi-Fi, Zigbee, LoRaWAN) is contingent upon variables such as range, data capacity, and security specifications.

· ***Cloud Computing and Data Storage***: The substantial quantity of data produced by IoT devices in healthcare necessitates a scalable and secure cloud infrastructure for storage and processing. Cloud platforms not only store data but also enable sophisticated data analytics, offering insights into patient health trends, forecasting potential health issues, and recommending personalized treatment plans. Cloud computing facilitates remote data access for authorized healthcare professionals, permitting real-time consultations and specialist second opinions. Cloud systems must adhere to stringent data security standards, such as HIPAA, to safeguard patient privacy and guarantee that data is encrypted during transmission and storage.

· ***Data Analytics and AI***: Data analytics, augmented by artificial intelligence (AI), analyzes the raw data obtained from IoT devices to yield actionable insights. AI algorithms can identify patterns and trends in patient data, forecast health decline, and suggest preventive strategies. Predictive analytics can identify patients at risk of chronic conditions such as diabetes or heart disease by analyzing their lifestyle and historical data. Artificial intelligence can also automate administrative functions, such as scheduling follow-up appointments or notifying physicians of anomalies in the data. As additional data is collected,

AI systems evolve and refine, thereby augmenting the precision of diagnoses and treatment strategies over time.

· ***User Interfaces*** **(Mobile Applications/Software):** User interfaces, including mobile applications and specialized healthcare software, serve as the conduit between patients, healthcare providers, and the IoT system. Patients can access their real-time health data, monitor medication compliance, and receive alerts concerning their condition or forthcoming medical appointments via these applications. Healthcare professionals can oversee patient dashboards, retrieve medical records, and react to alerts produced by the IoT system. These interfaces must be intuitive and accessible to facilitate seamless interaction between patients and medical personnel with the system. Mobile applications frequently incorporate communication functionalities that facilitate direct messaging or video calls between patients and physicians for remote consultations (Chakraborty et al., 2013).

The IoT networks in healthcare comprise various components, including sensors, wearable devices, medical imaging apparatus, and cloud-based platforms, as illustrated in Figure 1. These components collaboratively gather, transmit, and analyze patient data in real-time, facilitating remote monitoring, individualized treatment, and enhanced patient outcomes. Device interoperability is crucial for efficient data exchange.

Data Collection and Transfer in Telemedicine IoT

In the context of Internet of Things networks, telemedicine and the collection and transfer of data are crucial processes that provide remote patient monitoring, diagnosis, and the provision of healthcare. The implementation of these protocols ensures that medical professionals have prompt access to reliable health information. Which in turn makes decision-making and patient management more effective. The data collection in Internet of Things networks for telemedicine entails the utilization of a wide range of instruments and sensors to gather information regarding the health of patients. Wearable technology, such as smartwatches and fitness trackers, is able to continuously monitor vital signs, such as the heart rate, blood pressure, glucose levels, and activity levels of the wearer. Additionally, these devices are able to collect data regarding general fitness levels and sleep patterns, providing medical professionals with a comprehensive picture of their patients' health status. In home medical equipment such as blood glucose monitors and smart thermometers will make it simpler to collect certain health measures since they are more convenient to use. Sensors that are incorporated into these devices usually collect readings automatically. This approach lowers the likelihood of errors caused by human intervention and ensures that the data collected is accurate. Many telemedicine platforms include surveys and questionnaires that allow patients to share detailed information about their symptoms, lifestyle and how well they are following their treatment plans. When medical staff use this all-encompassing method of data collection, they will always have an accurate and complete picture of a patient's health. Transfer of Information in Internet of Things-Based Telemedicine Networks: Once we obtain the data. We must ensure its secure transmission to healthcare providers. The Internet of Things networks that are used for telemedicine make use of a wide range of communication protocols and technologies to ensure that the transfer of data is both safe and reliable. The following are some examples of common communication methods: Wi-Fi, Bluetooth, Zigbee (a wireless communication protocol for short-range connectivity) and cellular networks (including 4G and 5G network types). Each one is selected according to several parameters. Such as the compatibility of the devices, the bandwidth needs, and the distance covered. This particular way of sending data relies heavily on encryption. Both Transport Layer Security and Advanced Encryption Standard are examples of encryption protocols that are utilized to safeguard sensitive health information from being accessed by unauthorized parties during the transmission process. Establishing secure routes such as virtual private networks is one way to add an additional layer of protection to sensitive information. The data is routinely moved to databases for healthcare or cloud based systems once it has been transmitted. This allows the data to be processed, saved and analyzed. Because of this centralized storage, medical professionals are able to access patient information from any place. Which enables them to perform real time monitoring and respond quickly to any health concerns that may arise. According to Alenoghena et al. (2022), data analytics tools are able to generate reports, alerts, and insights that are beneficial to treatment planning and patient care. These tools can process the uploaded data.

SECURE IMAGE TRANSMISSION IN TELEMEDICINE

Significance of Medical Image Security

Medical image security is crucial to patient privacy and healthcare system integrity. Medical images like X-rays, MRIs, CT scans, and ultrasounds contain sensitive data that can affect patient care and treatment. Unauthorized access to these images can expose patients health conditions and treatments. HIPAA requires medical image security to protect patient confidentiality and privacy. Healthcare organizations are prime targets for cybercriminals because medical data is valuable. Medical image breaches can cause significant financial losses, legal issues, and brand damage.

Healthcare providers can prevent data breaches and cyberattacks that compromise medical images by using encryption, secure access controls, and regular audits. In addition to financial losses, such breaches can damage patient trust and healthcare institutions' credibility. Accurate diagnosis and treatment depend on medical image integrity. Images that are altered during transmission or storage can cause misinterpretations that harm patient care. Safely transmitting and storing medical images helps healthcare professionals make informed decisions based on unaltered data. In time-sensitive situations where prompt diagnosis can improve patient outcomes, reliability is essential. Healthcare organizations must follow patient data regulations, including medical image handling. Non-compliance can lead to fines, lawsuits, and accreditation loss. Strong medical image security is essential for patient data protection, legal and regulatory compliance, and healthcare providers' credibility and operational integrity. Healthcare data law changes frequently, so organizations must stay informed and compliant. As telemedicine grows, secure medical image transmission is essential. Patients must trust that medical images and other sensitive health data are protected. By protecting medical images, healthcare providers can build trust and increase telemedicine use, improving access to care. Secure telemedicine benefits patients and improves healthcare providers' operational efficiency by reducing data breaches. Healthcare professionals often share medical images for collaboration and second opinions. These images must be secure to build practitioner trust. Secure sharing mechanisms protect data, enabling patient care communication and collaboration without compromise. Multiple specialists can share insights based on secure data, improving patient outcomes and care .

Common Threats: Tampering, Eavesdropping, Unauthorized Access

The protection of medical data, particularly sensitive images, is of utmost importance in the context of telemedicine and Internet of Things networks. This is because there are numerous common threats that threaten the availability, integrity, and confidentiality of healthcare services. "Data tampering," which occurs when unauthorized changes are made to medical images or data related to them while they are being transmitted or stored, is one of the most significant threats. It is possible for even minute changes to medical images to lead to incorrect diagnoses and treatments, which can have potentially life-threatening consequences. Due to the fact that medical imagery plays an essential part in the diagnostic process, it is essential to guarantee the accuracy of this data. Both the detection of unauthorized changes and the maintenance of the information's accuracy are frequently accomplished through the utilization of methods such as digital signatures and sophisticated cryptographic hashing algorithms. The practice of eavesdropping, which involves the act of intercepting data while it is being transmitted, is another significant threat. Unsecured or unencrypted communication channels have the potential to expose sensitive medical images to individuals or groups that are not authorized to view them. Theft of identity, insurance fraud, and even ransomware attacks are all examples of malicious activities that can be carried out by attackers using data that has been intercepted. In order to protect against this danger, it is necessary to implement strong encryption protocols such as Transport Layer Security (TLS) and end-to-end encryption software. The confidentiality of patient information is protected by these security measures, which ensure that even if data is intercepted, it will continue to be inaccessible without the appropriate decryption key. Another significant risk is unauthorized access, which occurs when unauthorised individuals gain access to medical images that have been stored without the appropriate credentials. This has the potential to result in widespread data breaches, which could expose the medical histories of patients, diagnostic images, and other details that are considered sensitive. These kinds of breaches can have severe repercussions for healthcare providers, both financially and legally, and they can also erode the trust that patients have in healthcare institutions. To prevent unauthorized individuals from gaining access to sensitive information, it is essential to implement stringent access controls. Some examples of these controls include multi-factor authentication (MFA), role-based access control (RBAC), and regular auditing of access logs. The critical security challenges that are faced in telemedicine Internet of Things networks are demonstrated by these threats, which include data tampering, eavesdropping, and unauthorized access. When it comes to protecting sensitive medical images and ensuring the privacy and trustworthiness of healthcare services, it is absolutely necessary to implement a combination of techniques that include authentication, monitoring, and encryption (Brenner et al., 2022).

BLOCKCHAIN FOR SECURE IMAGE TRANSMISSION

Blockchain as a Distributed Ledger for Image Security

The blockchain technology provides a novel approach to the protection of medical images by utilizing its decentralized framework to ensure the safety of data. The application of this technology in the field of healthcare guarantees that medical images, once they have been saved, are safeguarded against unauthorized modifications and data manipulation. Since the data is distributed across multiple nodes, each of which contains a copy of the ledger, the decentralized aspect means that rather than relying on a single central authority, the data is distributed across multiple nodes. Considering that this distribution ensures that any attempt to modify the data would require control over the majority of the nodes, tampering is extremely impractical because of this distribution. Blockchain technology offers audit trails that are completely transparent, which enables administrators and healthcare professionals to monitor each and every transaction or access to a medical image. This feature is especially helpful for ensuring accountability and complying with regulatory requirements. By recording each access or update as a time-stamped entry on the blockchain, healthcare providers are able to track the flow of sensitive information and identify any irregularities or unauthorized actions that may have occurred. The consensus mechanisms of blockchain technology improve security. A new transaction, such as the transmission or modification of an image, must be validated by the majority of the network participants before it can be accepted into the blockchain. If it is not validated, the transaction will not be accepted. Due to the fact that the system is based on collective agreement rather than a single point of authority, the risk of data fraud or manipulation is decreased as a result. The incorporation of smart contracts can automate processes such as the granting of access to medical images, thereby ensuring that only authorized parties are able to retrieve or view sensitive information. Blockchain technology provides an additional layer of security in the field of telemedicine, which involves the transmission of images on a regular basis and across multiple networks. This can be accomplished by verifying the origin of the images as well as their authenticity. Together, patients and healthcare providers can have a higher level of confidence that the data that is being shared is accurate and has not been altered, which will ultimately lead to an increase in trust and an improvement in the security framework of telemedicine systems .

Benefits of Blockchain in Data Integrity and Transparency

In the healthcare industry, where protecting sensitive data like medical images is essential, blockchain technology offers major advantages are as shown in the figure 2, in terms of guaranteeing data integrity and transparency. Its ability to maintain data integrity through the use of an immutable, decentralized ledger is one of its main advantages. A medical image or associated patient data added to the blockchain cannot be removed without the network as a whole agreeing to do so. This guarantees the integrity and consistency of medical data, giving medical professionals accurate and dependable information for diagnosis and treatment.

Figure 2. Blockchain Benefits for Data Integrity and Transparency

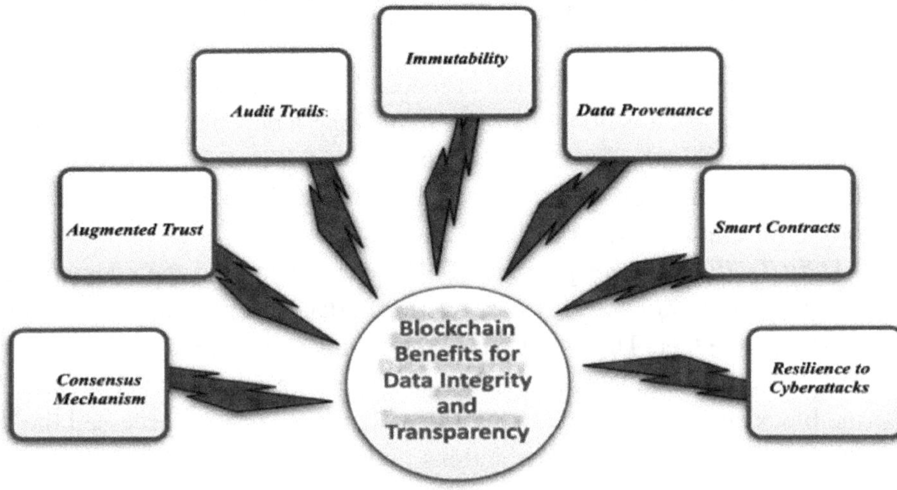

· ***Immutability***: A fundamental characteristic of blockchain is its immutability, guaranteeing that data, once inscribed, cannot be modified or erased. In the realm of healthcare, this signifies that medical records, images, and other patient-related data remain immutable from the instant they are entered into the system. This is crucial as even slight modifications to medical data can significantly impact patient treatment and care. The immutability of blockchain is ensured by cryptographic hashing, which connects each data block to its predecessor. This chain structure guarantees that any modification to a record would compromise the entire chain, rendering it instantly identifiable. This characteristic ensures the integrity of diagnostic data in medical image security, guaranteeing that physicians and healthcare providers utilize accurate and reliable information. Regardless of whether these images are disseminated across various healthcare networks or preserved for extended periods, immutability guarantees that the original data remains unaltered and secure from manipulation. This is particularly vital in legal or compliance contexts, where the veracity of medical records must be established.

· ***Data Provenance***: Blockchain offers a comprehensive record of every data entry, encompassing its creation and all subsequent modifications or accesses. This concept is referred to as data provenance, which is particularly beneficial in the healthcare sector, where monitoring the lifecycle of medical data, including images, is essential. Blockchain enables healthcare providers to ascertain the precise time and individual responsible for capturing, transmitting, or viewing a medical image, thereby guaranteeing that the complete history of the image remains transparent and traceable. This functionality is especially beneficial in multi-specialist contexts where various physicians or technicians require access to and analysis of identical medical data. Blockchain guarantees that every access point is documented, establishing a dependable audit trail. This also inhibits unauthorized modifications or inadvertent alterations by ensuring that every interaction with the data is recorded and can be readily traced to its origin (Everard, K. M. et al., 2022).

· ***Audit Trails*:** The transparency of blockchain facilitates the maintenance of thorough audit trails, as every transaction or data access is documented on the distributed ledger. This feature is essential for maintaining accountability in healthcare. For example, when medical images are disseminated or examined, the blockchain ledger offers an immutable record of who accessed the data, the timing of access, and the actions undertaken. Traceability is crucial for legal compliance, especially concerning regulations like HIPAA in the U.S. and GDPR in Europe, which require stringent supervision of patient data management. Audit trails enhance trust among healthcare providers, patients, and regulators. Blockchain guarantees the provision of clear, traceable records of all actions performed on sensitive medical data, facilitating the prompt identification and resolution of any anomalies or unauthorized access attempts. This additional layer of transparency fosters enhanced accountability among healthcare professionals and guarantees the responsible management of patient data (Muschol et al., 2022).

· ***Augmented Trust*:** Blockchains capacity to furnish a verifiable and transparent ledger of all transactions cultivates trust among all participants in the healthcare system. Patients, healthcare providers, and regulatory authorities can depend on the accuracy, tamper-resistance, and transparent management of data stored in a blockchain. This is particularly crucial in telemedicine, where sensitive information, including medical images, is transmitted across networks. The immutable characteristics of blockchain guarantee that patients can rely on telemedicine platforms to safeguard their confidential information. This trust is augmented by the cryptographic security protocols of blockchain technology. All transactions are encrypted, and access is regulated via cryptographic keys, rendering unauthorized data access nearly impossible. Blockchain enhances the reliability and credibility of telemedicine and other healthcare technologies by promoting a secure and transparent data-sharing environment.

· ***Consensus Mechanism*:** A fundamental principle of blockchain is its consensus mechanism, necessitating the agreement of the majority of network participants on the legitimacy of any new data entry. This guarantees that no individual entity can independently modify or append data without network consent, significantly mitigating the risk of fraudulent actions or unauthorized alterations. This feature is especially advantageous in medical data management, where the precision and veracity of patient records are crucial. In telemedicine, where sensitive data such as medical images is transmitted across various platforms, the consensus mechanism ensures that all transactions involving patient data are accurately validated prior to their acceptance into the blockchain. This adds an extra layer of security and deters malicious entities from injecting false or misleading data into the system, guaranteeing that all parties have access to reliable and verified medical information (Yamin, M. A. Y., & Alyoubi, B. A., 2020)

· ***Smart Contracts*:** Smart contracts are autonomous agreements with the stipulations encoded directly into programming language. In the realm of healthcare, they can facilitate the automation of processes including data sharing and access permissions. A smart contract can autonomously provide access to a medical image for an authorized physician upon the fulfillment of specific prerequisites, such as patient consent or validation of a legitimate request. This automation diminishes the necessity for manual intervention, thereby reducing the likelihood of human error and guaranteeing that only authorized personnel can access sensitive medical images. Smart contracts can augment security by ensuring adherence to data protection regulations, as they can be programmed to record every action involving a patient's medical data, thereby guaranteeing that the entire process is secure, transparent, and accountable.

· ***Resilience to Cyberattacks*:** Blockchains decentralized architecture renders it exceptionally resistant to cyberattacks. Conventional centralized databases are susceptible to attacks, as a breach of the central authority grants the hacker access to all data. Conversely, blockchain disseminates data across numerous nodes, significantly increasing the difficulty for attackers to breach the system. To manipulate blockchain data, a hacker must acquire control of a majority of the nodes, a task that is exceedingly challenging and expensive to accomplish. This resilience is particularly crucial in healthcare, where data breaches can result in significant repercussions. Cyber-attacks on healthcare institutions may lead to the compromise of confidential medical data, financial detriment, and harm to the organization's reputation. Utilizing blockchain for the storage and management of medical images and patient data enables healthcare providers to substantially mitigate the risk of cyberattacks, thereby safeguarding their data against advanced threats (Bembinov & Soenardi, 2023).

IMAGE COMPRESSION AND TRANSMISSION EFFICIENCY

Balancing Compression and Image Quality

Telemedicine requires balancing compression and image quality to transmit medical images over IoT networks for timely diagnosis and treatment. Medical images like CT scans, MRIs, and X-rays are large due to their high resolution, which helps detect subtle anomalies and provide accurate medical assessments. Transferring large files over bandwidth-constrained networks can slow transmission speeds, increase latency, and raise storage costs. Thus, image compression is used to reduce file sizes, but balancing compression and diagnostic image quality is essential. This challenge has been addressed by advanced compression techniques. Some methods use adaptive compression algorithms that analyze image content and apply different compression levels to regions of interest. Image areas with critical diagnostic information are preserved at a higher resolution, while less important regions are compressed to save bandwidth. Medical professionals can still use the images key diagnostic features while reducing file size for faster transmission with selective compression. AI and ML are also improving compression algorithms. AI-based systems can optimize compression without compromising image quality using massive medical image data. These systems intelligently predict which image parts will affect diagnosis and adjust compression parameters. Integrating AI into telemedicine systems allows healthcare providers to maintain medical image integrity while reducing transmission and storage time, improving remote healthcare efficiency. Telemedicine compression and image quality depend on the use case and network infrastructure. Diagnostic images must retain detail for accurate medical decisions, but high-compression methods may be suitable for non-critical data or archiving. As telemedicine grows, sophisticated compression technologies will help deliver high-quality healthcare over IoT networks without compromising quality .

Optimizing Transmission in IoT Networks

Telemedicine requires fast and secure transmission of large amounts of data, including high-resolution medical images, over IoT networks. Sensors, diagnostic equipment, and imaging systems generate and transmit data in healthcare IoT networks. Telemedicine requires efficient medical image transfer through these networks for real-time diagnostics, remote consultations, and continuous monitoring. To optimize transmission efficiency, IoT networks use compression and data prioritization. Over low-bandwidth networks, JPEG 2000 or wavelet-based compression algorithms reduce medical image size without affecting quality, enabling faster data transfer. In IoT networks, 5G and edge computing can boost transmission speed and reduce latency. Instead of using cloud servers, edge computing processes data at the network edge (Laxminarayan & Istepanian, 2000). Faster response times and more efficient data transmission result from reduced main network load. IoT networks can optimize transmission by prioritizing data type, compression, and advanced protocols. Real-time vital signs and emergency images must be transmitted quickly in healthcare. While less urgent data can be transmitted later or compressed, network algorithms can prioritize this critical information and deliver it to healthcare providers quickly. This data prioritisation efficiently handles time-sensitive data in congested or low-bandwidth networks. IoT devices, especially remote patient monitors, must also use less energy for efficient transmission. To maintain data flow and battery life, wearable health sensors must be energy-efficient. IoT systems use energy-saving protocols like data aggregation and selective transmission to send only relevant or abnormal data in real time and less routine or unchanged data. This improves data transmission and device lifespans by reducing network and device strain. Security must be strong without compromising performance for IoT transmission. Medical images and sensitive patient data are secured using lightweight encryption to avoid slowing data transfer. Telemedicine must protect patient privacy and data while balancing security and transmission speed (Pattichis et al., 2002).

CONCLUSION

The integration of various IoT networks with telemedicine improves healthcare delivery and availability. Internet of Things technology collects, shares and secures medical picture data. Secure picture transmission is essential because it affects patient outcomes and care immediately. Protecting sensitive medical data requires robust encryption, blockchain technology for data integrity and effective transmission strategies. The secure image transmission in telemedicine may advance in the future. As artificial intelligence and 5G connectivity increase and more secure data transfer will improve telemedicine for patients and providers. These technologies will improve medical image transmission speed and security against new cyber threats. Continuous research and development in real-time data processing and compression will provide medical image transmission without quality loss. IoT networks influence healthcare transformation. They simplify remote patient monitoring, specialist care and urgent decision making. Telemedicine will require safe and reliable technologies to ensure healthcare accessibility and efficacy. Telemedicine future depends on the successful integration of these technologies. Which will enable a more responsive and integrated healthcare system that prioritises patient safety and quality.

REFERENCES

Alenoghena, C. O., Onumanyi, A. J., Ohize, H. O., Adejo, A. O., Oligbi, M., Ali, S. I., & Okoh, S. A. (2022). eHealth: A survey of architectures, developments in mHealth, security concerns and solutions. *International Journal of Environmental Research and Public Health, 19*(20), 13071. DOI: 10.3390/ijerph192013071 PMID: 36293656

Bembinov, M., & Soenardi, N. (2023). An assessment of client and clinician satisfaction in veterinary teleconsultation compared to in-person consultations. *Vet. Evid, 7*, 1–17. PMID: 42006178

Brian Brenner, M. D., Scott Brancolini, M. D., Yashar Eshraghi, M. D., Maged Guirguis, M. D., Shravani Durbhakula, M. D., David Provenzano, M. D., & Kevin Vorenkamp, M. D. (2022). Telemedicine implementation in pain medicine: A survey evaluation of pain medicine practices in spring 2020. *Pain Physician, 25*, 387–390. PMID: 35901479

Chakraborty, C., Gupta, B., & Ghosh, S. K. (2013). A review on telemedicine-based WBAN framework for patient monitoring. *Telemedicine Journal and e-Health, 19*(8), 619–626. DOI: 10.1089/tmj.2012.0215 PMID: 23841489

Devaraj, S. J., & Ezra, K. (2011, April). Current trends and future challenges in wireless telemedicine system. In 2011 3rd International Conference on Electronics Computer Technology (Vol. 4, pp. 417-421). IEEE. DOI: 10.1109/ICECTECH.2011.5941933

Everard, K. M., Schiel, K. A., Xu, E., & Kulshreshtha, A. (2022). Use of telemedicine in the family medicine clerkship: A CERA study. *PRiMER: Peer-Reviewed Reports in Medical Education Research, 6*, 25. DOI: 10.22454/PRiMER.2022.105712 PMID: 36119909

Laxminarayan, S., & Istepanian, R. S. (2000). UNWIRED E-MED: The next generation of wireless and internet telemedicine systems. *IEEE Transactions on Information Technology in Biomedicine, 4*(3), 189–193. DOI: 10.1109/TITB.2000.5956074 PMID: 11026588

Moore, M. (1999). The evolution of telemedicine. *Future Generation Computer Systems, 15*(2), 245–254. DOI: 10.1016/S0167-739X(98)00067-3

Muschol, J., Heinrich, M., Heiss, C., Knapp, G., Repp, H., Schneider, H., Thormann, U., Uhlar, J., Unzeitig, K., & Gissel, C. (2022). Assessing telemedicine efficiency in follow-up care with video consultations for patients in orthopedic and trauma surgery in Germany: Randomized controlled trial. *Journal of Medical Internet Research, 24*(7), e36996. DOI: 10.2196/36996 PMID: 35896015

Pandian, P. S., Safeer, K. P., Shakunthala, D. T. I., Gopal, P., & Padaki, V. C. (2007). Store and Forward Applications in Telemedicine for Wireless IP Based Networks. *J. Networks*, *2*(6), 58–65. DOI: 10.4304/jnw.2.6.58-65

Pattichis, C. S., Kyriacou, E., Voskarides, S., Pattichis, M. S., Istepanian, R., & Schizas, C. N. (2002). Wireless telemedicine systems: An overview. *IEEE Antennas & Propagation Magazine*, *44*(2), 143–153. DOI: 10.1109/MAP.2002.1003651

Yamin, M. A. Y., & Alyoubi, B. A. (2020). Adoption of telemedicine applications among Saudi citizens during COVID-19 pandemic: An alternative health delivery system. *Journal of Infection and Public Health*, *13*(12), 1845–1855. DOI: 10.1016/j.jiph.2020.10.017 PMID: 33172819

Chapter 8
Advanced AI Techniques for Intrusion Detection and Privacy Preservation in Autonomous Ecosystems

Vikas Sharma
http://orcid.org/0000-0001-8173-4548
Department of Computer Applications, SRM Institute of Science and Technology, Delhi NCR, Ghaziabad, India

Tarun Kumar Vashishth
http://orcid.org/0000-0001-9916-9575
School of Computer Science and Applications, IIMT University, Meerut, India

Shashiraj Teotia
http://orcid.org/0000-0002-0849-3642
Department of Computer Application, Swami Vivekanand Subharti University, Meerut, India

Devendra Singh
Department of Mechanical Engineering, Ajay Kumar Garg Engineering College, Ghaziabad, India

Sonal Shah
Department of IT, Auro University, Surat, India

Sachin Chaudhary
http://orcid.org/0000-0002-8415-0043
School of Computer Science and Applications, IIMT University, Meerut, India

Pushpendra Kumar Verma
http://orcid.org/0000-0003-2777-5626
School of Computer Science and Applications, IIMT University, Meerut, India

DOI: 10.4018/979-8-2600-3070-7.ch008

ABSTRACT

Autonomous systems' growing use across various industries, including transportation, healthcare, and smart city development, has created a serious concern about cyber security. This chapter will provide a brief overview of some of the ways to secure autonomous systems through AI-based intrusion detection systems (IDS) and privacy-preserving mechanisms. In particular, it will identify the use of machine learning to detect anomalies and secure federated learning and blockchain technology to provide integrity of data in autonomous systems. It also provides an overview of how adversarially attacking AI models can be used to reduce cyber risk. Once security frameworks using AI are established, autonomous systems will be able to detect threats and quickly respond, while also preserving user privacy. Finally, this chapter will address regulatory issues regarding autonomous technology and potential future research issues related to the security of autonomous systems.

1. INTRODUCTION

Automation and Artificial Intelligence (AI) are rapidly changing our concept of Autonomous Systems (i.e., systems that perform tasks without human intervention). These changes are happening across many sectors such as Transportation, Health Care, Smart City and Industrial Automation. The majority of Autonomous Systems rely on multiple connected devices and a central computer system that uses AI for information on decisions to allow them to run independently of any human. Artificial Intelligence (AI) based Intrusion Detection Systems (IDS) use Deep Learning to discover abnormal activities with real-time data by analysing very large data volumes and the patterns in that data and identifying unknown threats. Besides, Privacy-Preserving Mechanisms will facilitate the emergence of Federated Learning, allowing the training of AI Models on Autonomous Systems to occur without disclosing any confidential information. The first two points illustrate how decentralised models like Federated Learning can improve the security of the data while at the same time maintain an efficient and effective mechanism for detecting threats using AI. One area where Autonomous Systems face significant challenges is from Cyber Adversaries who have targeted AI systems by way of adversarial attacks. These attacks are designed to cause misclassification or incorrect behaviours of autonomous systems by attacking the inputs into AI Decision-Making Systems (Mollashaik, 2025). Cybersecurity practitioners will need comprehensive defence strategies to prepare their systems and infrastructures for such attacks, and these strategies will include adversarial training, differential privacy and anomaly detection algorithms. The current regulatory environments will need to continue evolving in order to address the new and emerging AI autonomous risks created by these autonomous systems and autonomous technology. Machine Learning anomaly detection methods, secure federated learning models, and blockchain technologies will provide the highest degree of cybersecurity assurance for autonomous systems. The ability to continuously and automatically identify and respond to new and emerging cyber threats, while simultaneously providing user privacy protection, provides a great deal of value to autonomous systems with AI Security Frameworks (AI Security Frameworks), (Cheng et al., 2025).

1.1 Overview of Autonomous Systems in the Various Sectoral Domains

The proliferation of autonomous systems, particularly those employing AI, ML and advanced sensors, is creating new and better solutions to some of the existing problems across various sectoral domains. For example, autonomous vehicles will create a much safer method of transportation and reduce highway congestion through the use of multiple advanced decision maker capabilities and advanced navigation capabilities. Although we refer specifically to driverless vehicles throughout this work, AI perception, planning and control adds many different types of transportation choices for the driver. Alternative forms of transportation may include automated delivery drones, ride serving companies, and automated public transit. Autonomous systems are being used more often in healthcare to assist with surgery, automate diagnoses and monitor patients remotely (Vashishth et al., 2024). Drones and robots also aid disaster relief and environmental management by providing real-time data for better decision making. In manufacturing, autonomous robots and predictive maintenance technologies utilizing AI streamline the manufacturing process thereby reducing overall production costs while producing greater quantities of commodities. In agriculture, drones and AI driven equipment will help improve crop monitoring, irrigation and harvesting. Such advancements will promote sustainable agriculture and protect the environment. As a result of rapid advancements with autonomous systems, new cybersecurity and data privacy concerns have emerged as a result of the connectivity of nearly all autonomous systems over a network infrastructure. Autonomous systems send an enormous amount of data in real-time to be analysed by AI and make real-time decisions; thus, allowing for an increased probability of being attacked through a cyberattack; that adversaries could penetrate into the network; and or that unauthorized parties would gain access to data. In order to preserve the confidence and dependability of autonomous technology, security standards need to be established, AI-based intrusion detection devices need to be developed, and technology solutions that protect individual privacy need to be designed for all autonomous systems (Dhinakaran et al., 2024).

1.2 Increasing Threats to Cybersecurity in Autonomous Technologies

With the rise of advanced technological advancement in automation across many industries (transportation, healthcare, smart cities, and industrial), cyber threats to autonomous technologies will also rise in both sophistication and frequency. The combination of autonomous systems being interconnected with each other, having a requirement for real-time processing of data, and the use of Artificial Intelligence (AI) to make decisions creates an increased chance for cybercriminals to target autonomous systems due to the new attack surface created. By being interconnected with each other, as well as having a requirement for processing data in real-time, cybercriminals have a multitude of opportunities to exploit vulnerabilities in autonomous systems or conduct various types of cyberattacks. Examples of cyberattacks conducted against autonomous systems include data breaches, denials of service (DDoS), and adversarial attacks against AI (intentionally misleading the AI). Attacks against autonomous systems could interfere with operations, hinder their functionality, compromise public safety, and pose a substantial threat to both public safety and personal privacy. Adversarial attack(s) against AI is likely to be one of the more serious concerns associated with cyberattacks currently and in the future for the autonomous technology industry. Through adversarial attacks, cybercriminals can deliberately input carefully crafted information into AI, causing the AI to misclassify, circumvent physical security (human safeguards), and fail to work as intended under various conditions. Cybercriminals that gain unauthorized access to medical robots, smart surveillance systems, and/or industrial automation systems create ethical and legal questions concerning the access to and use of confidential patient records maintained by those systems. Due to the distributed architectures of Autonomous Systems and the way they need to be able to operate in near real-time, securing Autonomous Systems is unique and considerably different than most other types of systems, so traditional cyber protection techniques may not be sufficient for every Autonomous System. New approaches to Cybersecurity are emerging to help alleviate some of the complexity of securing Autonomous Systems (Andreoni et al., 2024).

1.3 Chapter Contribution and Scope

This work consists of a structured analysis and comparison of the use of artificial intelligence (AI) in cybersecurity and privacy-preserving mechanisms for autonomy. Whereas most previous related research has been limited to a single area (e.g., Intrusion Detection, Privacy Preservation, or Adversarial Robustness), this work provides a unified discussion of the full range of security challenges related to autonomous systems through the integration of these previously separate research areas. As part of the current work, the relationship among AI-driven intrusion detection systems, privacy-preserving learning approaches, blockchain-based trust mechanisms, adversarial defense mechanisms and their relationships to one another will be discussed. strengths, limitations, deployment challenges and applicability of these various approaches will also be assessed for the autonomous domains of transportation, healthcare, smart cities and industrial automation. The overall goal is to provide researchers and practitioners with a comprehensive picture of the current state of the various approaches, while also identifying key areas of research gap and future directions.

2. CYBERSECURITY CHALLENGES IN AUTONOMOUS SYSTEMS

Across multiple industries, there is growing reliance on autonomous systems that have introduced cybersecurity challenges of complex nature that can compromise or jeopardize the reliability, safety, and integrity of the systems. Autonomous systems interface with the physical world in dynamic, complex, and interconnected environments. Because of that there is a vast array of cyber threats these systems face, including but not limited to unauthorized access, adversarial attacks on AI, compromises to data, and network vulnerabilities. Of the greatest challenges of Autonomous Systems, is to secure the way these systems make real-time decisions. Real-time decision making is based on overwhelming amounts of data created from sensor information, images, and Communication Networks. Should the integrity of any data source be compromised, this could result in erroneous decisions and could, in turn, result in catastrophic failure, such as accidents in autonomous vehicle, diagnostic errors, in AI medical diagnostics, or cyber security breaches, within smart city infrastructure. An important challenge of Autonomous Systems, is weaknesses of AI Models used within Autonomous Systems, which may be exploited through adversarial attacks, whereby cybercriminals exploit weaknesses with input data and trick AI algorithms into misclassifying objects, misinterpreting threats, or behaving erratically. This is an especially critical issue for safety critical systems, such as those used in self-driving cars and autonomous drones, where split-second decisions are required to protect human safety (Vyas et al., 2024).

2.1 Cyber Threat Landscape for Autonomous Systems

Cyber Threat purposes through new technological developments in the area of autonomous systems, which are becoming an increasingly popular and adopted technology in all types of critical sectors including: transportation, healthcare, smart cities, and industrial automation. The use of artificial intelligence, machine learning, sensor networks, and cloud-based services means that autonomous systems are faced with a growing number of potentially damaging cyber-security threats from criminals targeting autonomous systems networks (ASNs) and their AI-based decision-making capabilities and exploiting any vulnerabilities they may find in such networks. Adversarial attacks using AI to perform adversarial AI attacks on other autonomous technologies are one of the largest threats to the security of autonomous technologies today. An adversarial attack, is when malicious actor uses an adversarial machine or an adversarial algorithm to alter the information that the AI in the autonomous systems uses as input data so to deceive or misinform the AI. Autonomous vehicles are susceptible to cyber-attacks that have the potential to seriously injure their drivers. One commonly used method that the types of attacker's use is to modify the symbols and words on traffic signs, so that the AI model in the autonomous vehicle cannot properly interpret and classify the symbols on the signs, therefore the autonomous vehicle will misinterpret what is a stop sign or how fast to go to obey the posted speed limit. A loss of control because there is an altercation of one of the aforementioned examples will result in serious negative consequences including potential for an accident/incident. The intention of attackers to perform a cyber-attack against the medical AI systems is the same.

Figure 1. Autonomous System Architecture with AI Models

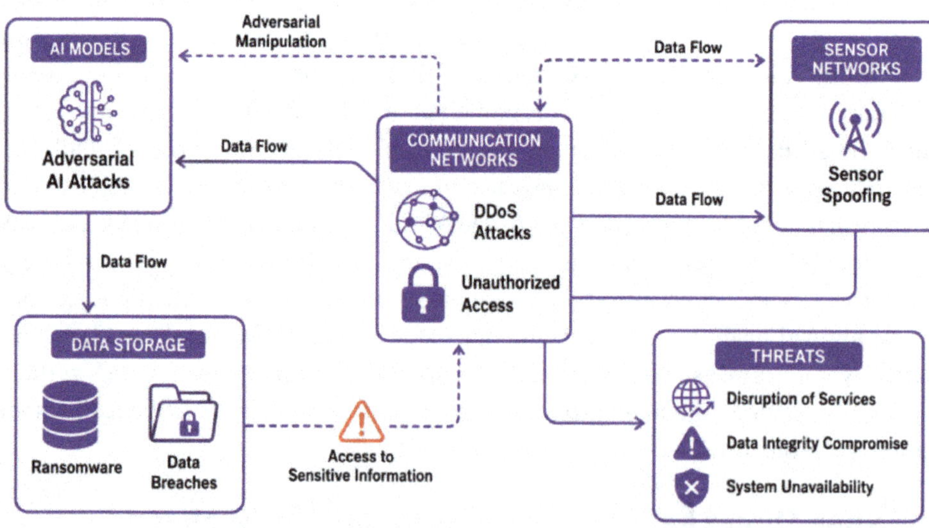

Figure 1 shows a multi-layer architecture of Autonomous Systems and illustrates how the emergence of security vulnerabilities across the various components making up an Autonomous System (i.e., Sensing, Communicating, Processing and Making a Decision). It should also be noted that to effectively manage cybersecurity in an autonomous system, cybersecurity must be addressed across the entire operational stack. It is not sufficient to only address cybersecurity on an individual component basis. Autonomous systems operate over multiple layers of interconnectivity: sensors and IoT devices make up the perception layer; edge or fog layer does real-time processing of data; cloud layer holds data for extensive analytics (or AI model training) across many edges; and application layer executes decisions based upon information received. Each of the four layers adds its specific vulnerabilities (for example, sensor layers can be easily spoofed; edge layers must account for latency-sensitive detection of intrusions; cloud layers introduce risk by way of data breaches and model poisoning). Security solutions reside across both the network and edge layers (ID; privacy-focused methods), while federated learning connects edge and cloud for secure updates to privacy-preserving models and blockchain for ensuring transmission data integrity. The response to an attack occurs by way of data being sent from the sensor and to an edge processing unit, where it undergoes initial analysis, then subsequently validated or aggregated at the cloud level of the system and ultimately executed at the layer (application layer) where the decision was made to perform some action. A thorough knowledge of this architecture is necessary for allowing practitioners to take theoretical concepts and translate them into deployable and operational security frameworks.

The attacks of DDoS and ransomware pose increasing layers of complexity and challenges to the cybersecurity of autonomous systems. They disrupt the operation of autonomous networks by filling them with surplus traffic and preventing access to critical systems, e.g., if there were a DDoS attack on the smart cities system, this would interfere with the operation of traffic management systems leading to excessive congestion and accidents. Ransomware attacks against autonomous healthcare systems could render healthcare professionals unable to access medical equipment and patient records until the ransom was paid. These types of attacks can have devastating financial and operational consequences. There currently exist frameworks and protocols for protecting against such attacks and the potential for cyber-physical attacks from sensor spoofing, which also represents an extreme risk to the safety and integrity of Autonomous Systems, (Nasir et al.,2024) which rely on a number of sensor technologies including LiDAR, radar, and GPS to navigate and make decisions. Due to the interconnected and ever-changing nature of autonomous systems, they are extremely attractive to cybercriminals, nation-state actors, and malicious insiders. The present methods of securing these types of intelligent and automated systems by relying on strict rules and static methods of defence are insufficient to protect these types of systems. (Moustafa et al. 2023). Autonomous Systems implementing Proactive Security Solutions can, therefore, continue to mitigate and respond to Cybersecurity threats in Real Time (to help maintain their S/RC in a growingly Digital World) (Alqubaysi et al. 2025).

Regarding transportation systems, adversarial attacks, and GPS spoofing are two prevalent threats, with established types of defenses available like AI-based intrusion detection systems, as well as new types such as adversarially robust learning models. On the other hand, potential attacks on sensitive health-related patient data would likely involve either loss from theft or unauthorized access, and existing means of defense, such as encryption and access control measures, are readily available, while research is underway into new means of protection, including current developments in federated learning and privacy preserving analytics. With regard to smart city infrastructure, distributed denial-of-service and IOT botnet are primary sources of threats; network-level intrusion detection systems have become common tools for use, while blockchain-based coordination mechanisms and decentralized means of defense remain in development.

2.1.1 System-Level Security Architecture and Operational Integration

Autonomous systems function using layers of interrelated information, including perception, edge computing and cloud systems. Security technologies such as IDS (intrusion detection system), federated learning, blockchain, homomorphic encryption, and differential privacy are suggested but not well defined in how they function in the overall system architecture. At the perception layer (e.g., environmental data using sensors, cameras, LiDAR, radar, GPS devices, and IoT components), this layer is at a significant risk of an attack by spoofing, signal manipulation, sensor tampering or false data injection. Security controls include sensor authentication, secure firmware for sensors, redundant mechanisms, and anomaly detection methods. The Edge Computing Layer is responsible for processing data so that decisions can be made in real time through low latency means. Therefore, it is common for AI-based IDS to be implemented in this layer since immediate detection of threats is necessary for autonomous operations. Edge level security will monitor the characteristics of communication flows, identify abnormal behavior, and initiate immediate mitigation actions as required. The cloud layer has a responsibility for analyzing data on a larger scale, long-term storage, and AI model training. Federated learning allows multiple edge devices to collaboratively improve AI model capabilities without transmitting raw data to a centralized repository. Privacy-preserving technologies such as differential privacy and homomorphic encryption protect sensitive information in the model training and data processing phases. Blockchain technology operates across storage and communication layers providing an immutable audit trail for transactions, transaction verification, and a secure exchange of information. Blockchain can enhance trust between distributed autonomous agents, however they may introduce scalability and latency limitations in real-time environments. Security-related decisions are passed through all architectural layers of the system during a cyber-attack.

Table 1. Domain-Specific Threats and Security Defenses in Autonomous Systems

Domain	Dominant Threats	Mature Defenses	Emerging Defenses
Autonomous Transportation	GPS spoofing, adversarial attacks, V2V attacks	Encryption, authentication, IDS	Adversarially robust AI, federated IDS
Healthcare Systems	Data breaches, ransomware, unauthorized access	Access control, encryption	Privacy-preserving analytics, secure federated learning
Smart Cities	DDoS attacks, IoT botnets, surveillance manipulation	Network IDS, traffic monitoring	Blockchain-based trust management
Industrial Automation	Insider threats, ransomware, operational disruption	Network segmentation, anomaly detection	Zero-trust architectures, automated response systems
Agricultural Systems	Sensor spoofing, data manipulation	Secure communication protocols	AI-driven predictive threat detection

Table 1 demonstrates that there is a vast array of cybersecurity threats that can be encountered in various autonomous system domains. Therefore, security strategies must be developed according to the specific operational environment. The comparison also illustrates that mature cyber defenses are widely deployed using methods such as encryption, authentication, and intrusion detection systems while newer methods including federated learning, blockchain-based trust management, zero trust architectures, and artificial intelligence-driven threat detection are quickly becoming methodologies to be considered for countering emerging security threats.

2.2 Privacy Concerns in AI-Enabled Autonomous Systems

With an ever-increasing number of AI empowered (Autonomous) Systems being created and utilised, the quantity of sensitive information (data) produced by these systems continues to grow. In addition to personal, biometric, and physical location data collected, stored and analysed by Autonomous Systems in Health Care, Transport, Smart Cities etc.; rapidly growing Privacy concerns regarding the use of such sensitive information will also need addressing.

1. **Data Collection and Surveillance Risks:** The greatest challenge for society is to strike a proper balance between leveraging the advantages of the data collection from AI enabled autonomous systems and protecting users' privacy and rights to control their own personal information (Sharma and Bairwa 2025).
2. **Unauthorized Access and Data Breaches:** The most damaging form of data breach involves an AI healthcare system being breached and exposing sensitive personal patient information, enabling identity thieves to steal their identities and commit financial fraud.
3. **Lack of User Consent and Data Ownership:** Due to the nature of autonomous technologies, the collection and processing of their data is done in real-time. Given how difficult it is, in most cases, to obtain explicit consent for processing real time data in AI-enabled Autonomous Technologies, ethical and legal issues arise.
4. **Privacy Risks in Federated Learning and AI Training:** Federated learning provides organizations with a means of enhancing the capabilities of AI models without requiring the organization to centralize their datasets into a single location. As the use of federated learning becomes more common for developing autonomous systems, organizations will need to weigh the benefits of this privacy-preserving method of training against the potential threats posed by malicious actors who may participate in their federated learning networks. Once a malicious user can access a Federated Learning system, they may try to recover any information contained in the individual's model updates from the federated learning system.

The protection of user privacy must be considered by organizations in order to build and maintain trust in the use of AI-enabled autonomous systems. Organizations will also have to take proactive measures to protect against any potential malicious attacks that may occur as the use of AI-enabled autonomous systems continues to grow.

3. AI-BASED INTRUSION DETECTION FOR AUTONOMOUS SYSTEMS

Due to their static methods of detecting threats, traditional methods of detecting intrusion threats (IDS) cannot keep pace with the rapid changes in autonomous systems threats. As a result, AI-based intrusion detection systems (AI-IDS) have been proposed to address this shortcoming. By leveraging machine learning (ML) and deep learning (DL), AI-IDS can quickly identify, analyse, and mitigate cyber threats in real-time. AI-IDS utilise both supervised and unsupervised learning approaches, allowing them to detect all types of attacks, including those already identified and those still unknown (Laghari et al., 2025).

3.1 Fundamentals of Intrusion Detection Systems (IDS) in Autonomous Systems

Autonomous systems rely on an Intrusion Detection System (IDS) to protect them from cyber threats and are therefore important components in the protection of autonomous systems. Due to the complex nature of these systems (involving many interconnected sensors, networks, and AI systems), they are prone to attack by sophisticated cyber threats. Some examples of cyber threats are malware, denial of service (DoS) attacks, data breaches, and unauthorized access attempts, all of which can greatly affect the operation, reliability, and safety of autonomous systems. To mitigate the potential risks of cybersecurity violations against the organizations utilizing autonomous technology, IDS continually monitors network traffic (system traffic) and application activities by users while seeking to ensure compliance with security policies. In addition to improving the operational resilience of autonomous systems through the timely identification and response to cybersecurity violations, NABM helps position organizations mitigating cyber threats that may impact autonomous technologies by providing organizations with the ability to quickly isolate, contain, and remediate potential security breaches. Cybersecurity threats in the autonomous space are dynamic and present unique challenges within the context of a self-driving car, as cyber attackers can take advantage of flaws in the vehicle's V2V communication protocols to create false sensor readings resulting in erroneous navigation decisions. Smart healthcare technology is also susceptible to cyber threats. Cybercriminals will also attempt to gain unauthorized access to patient medical information or disrupt the normal operation of IoT-enabled medical devices. To help combat these types of threats, IDS employs sophisticated techniques to detect and neutralize cyber threats prior to their infliction of harm on the system, including signature-based detection, anomaly detection, and behavioural analysis. When correctly installed, an IDS will help differentiate between standard system operations and unusual activity so that reduce the number of false positives (Muneer & al., 2024). By analyzing extensive amounts of data, intelligent security systems can find patterns and irregularities that indicate cyber-attacks, which are then utilized to proactively defend against them.

Figure 2. Intrusion Detection Systems (IDS) in Autonomous Systems

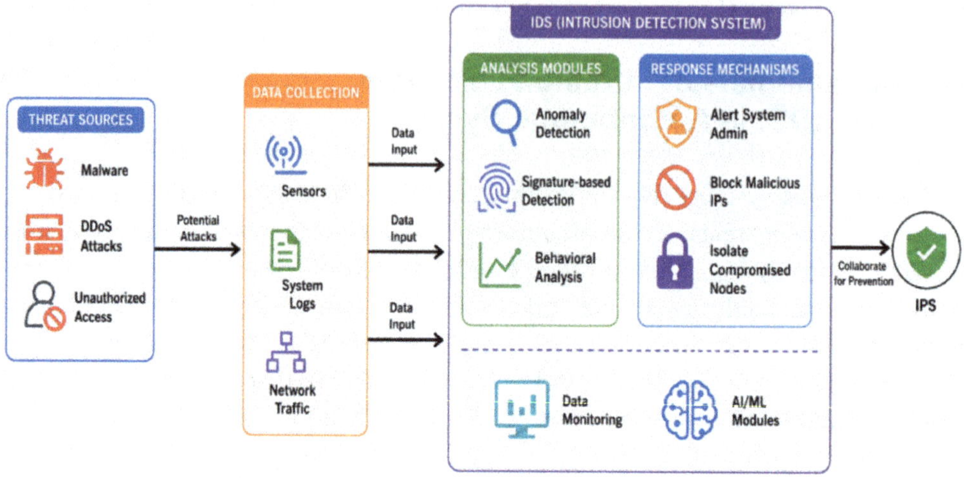

Figure 2 depicts a variety of algorithms employed by AI-enabled intrusion detection systems as they assess network traffic, sensor data, and system logs to identify anomalous behaviours that can then be used for real-time detection of threats. It also illustrates the utilization of machine learning algorithms to further support adaptive threat detection and identification.

3.1.1 Types of Intrusion Detection Systems (IDS) in Autonomous Systems

An IDS's primary purpose is to collect key information on autonomous systems and the way that autonomous systems operate within an increasingly vulnerable world. The significant characteristics of traditional IDSs are NIDSS (network intrusion detection systems) and HIDS (host intrusion detection systems). NIDSS provides monitoring capabilities across an entire network and alerts administrators to potential unauthorised activity on the network.

1. **Network-Based Intrusion Detection Systems (NIDS):** A Network Intrusion Detection System (NIDS) monitors a network by detecting evidence of malicious software (malware), unauthorized use of computer systems, and other such events through examining packets that pass over the network for signs of unauthorized interference with the network and the data contained therein by would-be hackers or other nefarious entities. NIDS installations can be placed at various locations throughout a network, including gateways, routers, or specific segments within the network itself. All traffic flowing between every

device associated with the network will also be monitored by a NIDS without requiring users to intervene. NIDS can identify unusual traffic patterns that may represent potential threats to a network, such as denial-of-service (DoS) attacks, man-in-the-middle (MITM) attacks, and malware infections.

2. **Host-Based Intrusion Detection Systems (HIDS):** HIDS are fixed to standalone machines (hosts) that are set up to monitor the activities of every endpoint connected to the network. HIDS monitor activities by observing application and operating system logs, application activities, and behaviour exhibited by endpoints. Because HIDS monitoring activities focus on the host operating system and application(s), HIDS provide a much clearer picture of activity that occurs at this level than do network-based IDSs. As such, HIDS are able to identify many more types of activity that may take place on a host operating system such as unauthorised logins, changes to files, excessive numbers of system calls. Since HIDS continuously monitor the host and associated logs, they consume a large amount of processing power (Vashishth et al., 2026).

3.2 Machine Learning and Deep Learning for Anomaly Detection

In particular, IDSs trained via supervised learning techniques, such as decision trees, support vector machines (SVMs), and random forests, use labelled datasets of benign and malicious activity to train the IDS. These IDSs learn from previous attacks and have the ability to identify the same types of threats in real-time. The major drawback of using supervised learning to train IDS is that it requires large, well-annotated datasets and, therefore, it does not perform well against new cyber-attack types. An alternative to supervised learning is to use unsupervised learning and deep learning. Examples of unsupervised learning methods include clustering (e.g., k-means clustering and DBSCAN) and autoencoders; both types of unsupervised learning use system behaviour to build a profile of normal behaviour. If an anomaly occurs in system behaviour, it is flagged as a potential threat, regardless of whether or not it has previously been identified. With respect to anomaly detection, CNNs and RNNs increase anomaly detection ability through their capability to automatically extract features from traffic and logs. CNNs and RNNs excel at detecting advanced, complex attack patterns, including stealthy and polymorphic malware. The combined learning of LSTM and GAN-based IDS will eventually provide more reliable and useful models for the detection and mitigation of future adversarial threats, thus improving the adaptability of IDS systems to real-world environments. When additional capabilities are combined with Federated Learning (FL), both LSTM and GAN-based IDS will benefit from the enhanced notification of abnormal behaviour and reduce the amount of time required for analysis. FL will allow for the creation of shared IDS training models amongst multiple autonomous systems without exchanging raw data, thereby preserving individual data privacy while also enhancing the overall threat intelligence for the IDS as a whole. This will be particularly beneficial for smart cities and autonomous vehicles whose networks require high levels of data privacy to secure their networks from both internal and external threats (Zhang et al., 2025).

3.2.1 Comparative Analysis of AI-Based IDS Approaches

Each of the various approaches to intrusion detection based on AI has distinct strengths and weaknesses. For example, supervised learning approaches including Support Vector Machines, Random Forest, and Decision Tree algorithms are capable of high rates of accurate detection when trained on well-labelled data; however, their performance will typically decline when dealing with not yet encountered attack patterns. Un-supervised learning approaches, such as clustering algorithms and autoencoders, allow for the discovery of new types of threats without any input data in the form of labels, thereby making them adaptable, although they tend to have higher false-positive rates as compared to supervised methods. By comparison, deep learning algorithms including Convolutional Neural Networks (CNNs), Recurrent Neural Networks (RNNs), Long Short-Term Memory (LSTM), and Generative Adversarial Networks (GANs) offer advanced features and capabilities for identifying complex types of attacks; however, these types of models typically require significant resources and large amounts of training data in order to operate effectively. Federated learning-based intrusion detection systems can create a greater level of privacy by allowing multiple systems to learn collaboratively without exchanging raw data. While these systems are often more resilient to many types of attacks than those that use traditional methods of intrusion detection, they are still susceptible to model poisoning attacks and overhead due to communication requirements.

Table 2. Comparative Analysis of AI-Based IDS Approaches

AI-Based IDS Approach	Advantages	Limitations
Supervised Learning (SVM, Random Forest, Decision Trees)	High detection accuracy for known attacks; efficient classification	Requires large labelled datasets; limited ability to detect unknown threats
Unsupervised Learning (Clustering, Autoencoders)	Can identify previously unseen attacks without labelled data	Higher false-positive rates and reduced interpretability
Deep Learning (CNN, RNN, LSTM, GAN)	Learns complex attack patterns and high-dimensional features	Computationally intensive and requires substantial training data
Federated Learning-Based IDS	Preserves privacy by keeping data local; supports collaborative learning	Vulnerable to model poisoning attacks and communication overhead

In Table 2, several major AI intrusion detection technologies (IDTs) used for the identification of intrusions in autonomous systems are presented. Each technology is compared for its benefits as well as its downsides. From this comparison, it can be seen that there is no "best" single IDT, therefore the proper choice will depend on factors like data availability, computational resources, privacy needs, and operational context.

3.3 Real-Time Threat Detection and Response Mechanisms

To protect autonomous systems from fast-moving cyber threats, organizations must use real-time threat detection and response processes. Autonomous technologies must function in rapidly changing environments and, as such, timely detection of security threats along with the ability to rapidly respond can help reduce the risk of extensive impact (e.g., disruption to services, compromise of sensitive information, and injury to people). Unlike traditional security methods, which are based on fixed rules, new autonomous technologies can use artificial intelligence (AI) based adaptive security frameworks to detect, investigate, and counteract cyber threats in real-time. Through continuous network traffic monitoring, sensor data gathering, and system log analysis, organizations can quickly recognize malicious behaviour and conduct investigations to eliminate it. Machine Learning (ML) and Deep Learning (DL) based Advanced Intrusion Detection Systems (IDS) monitor system activity to identify both known cyber threats (e.g., malware) and unknown cyber threats (e.g., new attack techniques) (Moulahi et al., 2023). Signature-based IDS can identify previously known threats, but they may not be equipped to identify new threats. To address this limitation, organisations are turning to anomaly detection-based detection methods utilizing unsupervised machine learning techniques (clustering, autoencoders, and GANs) to identify anomalous system behaviour.

Though AI-detection systems for intrusion detection have made great strides since their inception, there are still challenges associated with validation, benchmarking, and operational viability keeping these systems from being implemented in practice. Many new models for this application are developed, validated, and evaluated on small and/or synthetic datasets which do not reflect the actual variability of real-world attacks. Another important issue is the lack of a standard benchmarking framework to allow for cross-system comparisons of model performance. Validation for systems used in safety-critical autonomous contexts will also require testing for more than just an accuracy metric, including testing for reliability, robustness against adversarial input conditions, and real-time response capability. Operational feasibility of advanced AI models at deployment locations where they will be used (edge computing) will also be affected by deployment constraints such as computation requirements/overhead, latency limitations, and energy consumption. Future research in this field will need to address all of these issues through the use of appropriate testing methods, standardized assessment datasets, and optimization strategies that support deployment to confirm that the model will be practically feasible as well as theoretically feasible upon completion.

3.4 Validation, Benchmarking, and Deployment Challenges

Although there have been some advances in the assessment of AI-based intrusion detection systems, validation methods and benchmarks to help provide the basis for an assessment are still not readily available, and are still being developed. In addition, much of the literature regarding AI-based IDSs do not adequately address the different types of datasets that are likely needed to assess AI-based IDS performance, nor has there been a thorough study regarding the main types of performance metrics that can be compared between different studies or evaluated as the same across all studies. One major issue is the lack of an industry-standard methodology for determining datasets and performance metrics for evaluating systems; therefore, most studies are based on different datasets, attack instances, and performance metrics. In addition to accuracy, other characteristics of autonomous systems that could affect the performance of the system include latency, durability, scalability, resistance to adversarial attacks, energy usage, and computational overhead. In safety-critical environments (e.g., autonomous vehicles, healthcare robots, industrial process controls, etc.), additional measures of reliability must be used to assess these systems, including runtime monitoring, fail-safe operational modes, ongoing model validation, and post-deployment evaluation of performance.

4. PRIVACY-PRESERVING MECHANISMS IN AUTONOMOUS SYSTEMS

As autonomous systems grow in use across multiple industries, such as in transportation, healthcare, smart cities, and industrial automation, it is important to secure the data associated with them, both for the sake of the user and for the integrity of the systems themselves.

4.1 Secure Federated Learning for Data Privacy

Federated Learning (FL) is a method of developing machine learning models, that takes advantage of decentralization of computing power when training an AI model. The idea for federated learning originated from many different user domains where there was a concern for the confidentiality of user data, especially in regard to healthcare and transportation applications. Traditionally, in order to create and train an AI model, there must be a central location where the training data is stored. With federated learning, instead of having all the data sent to a single location, users can locally train their own data and then send updates to a single group or organization that will use those updates. FL has significantly decreased the risk of both data breaches and unauthorized access to users' private information because of this. The application of federated learning in health care is when medical devices are employed to collect patient health information, which is then compiled with other medical devices across all medical devices at one centralized location. By aggregating and training multiple datasets, the health care sector can improve upon AI-based models to diagnose diseases and remain compliant with privacy rules and regulations like GDPR and HIPAA. Federated learning also enables autonomous vehicles to learn from the way that the vehicle operates in different types of driving situations, while still preserving sensitive private driving information or the location of the vehicle and its occupants. Secure Federated Learning (SFL) is an enhancement of FL and works to address these security concerns by using advanced privacy-preserving algorithms such as homomorphic encryption, differential privacy, and secure multi-party computation (SMPC) (Narayan, 2025).

4.2 Homomorphic Encryption and Differential Privacy

The protection of sensitive data from being lost as a result of the processing and generation of enormous amounts of sensitive data in AI-based autonomous systems presents challenges associated with both data privacy and computation efficiency. The privacy-securing techniques of homomorphic encryption (HE) and differential privacy (DP) are two examples of techniques that can be used to securely process data while also protecting the confidentiality of users' data in an AI-controlled autonomous environment. There are many examples of how these two advanced techniques will help try to eliminate a host of privacy risks within many sectors (e.g., autonomous healthcare, smart transportation, intelligent surveillance systems) in the event of a breach of data or any other kind of violation of electronic private Web communications (Hendaoui et al., 2024). An example of the capability of HE is that computations can be conducted upon the encrypted data without the requirement of encryption being removed from the data in order to perform computations upon the data. So, for example, an individual's sensitive data (i.e., medical records) can remain encrypted during the entire processing of that data, thus reducing the exposure of the individual's sensitive data. Similarly, for smart cities, HE allows for encrypted data collected via surveillance cameras and traffic sensors to be analysed without a person necessarily being able to identify a specific individual. Even though homomorphic encryption offers a high degree of privacy-security, HE is not optimally efficient in terms of computing; therefore, it will need to continue to be optimized so it can effectively serve in a scalable manner in many of today's rapidly-evolving autonomous vehicle applications. DP is an alternative privacy-boosting technique that prevents unauthorized entities from deriving sensitive personal data from a dataset. Through differential privacy, noise is added to datasets or results so that the individual pieces of information can't be pinpointed, allowing the data to provide many useful insights. This is critical for training models in artificial intelligence because there are attackers who will conduct model inversion attacks to recover the original data.

4.3 Blockchain for Data Integrity and Secure Communications

The use of blockchain technology will play a growing role in ensuring the integrity and security of the information flow within autonomous systems. Autonomous systems depend upon real-time data being exchanged; they require multiple sensors connected to one another and are fully automated via artificial intelligence for decision making. A blockchain offers an alternative method of data security through its decentralized, distributed, immutable ledger. Everything that is written in a blockchain is unalterable so that it cannot be changed or deleted. In the case of autonomous vehicles, blockchain technology will store the sensor readings from the vehicle as well as the location information provided by the GPS receiver. Also, blockchain technology will record all vehicle-to-vehicle (V2V) communications, which is vital for the operation of autonomous vehicles, making it nearly impossible for anyone to forge or otherwise manipulate the critical driving data used in making driving decisions. The Use of Smart Contracts allows Trust to Be Automated between Autonomous Systems. Automated Trust-Based Interactions are achieved by Smart Contracts, a type of Self-Executing Agreement Stored in the Blockchain. Smart Contracts are Geared to Enforce Security Protocols, Verify Identity, Facilitate Secure Transactions, and Eliminate the Need for Middleman for Automated Transactions. In the case of Industrial Automation Smart Contracts will be utilized to Control Communication between Machines to reduce Cyber-attack (Padmavathi and Saminathan, 2025)

5. ADVERSARIAL ATTACKS ON AI MODELS AND DEFENSE STRATEGIES

The implementation of adversarial attacks against AI models that are operating within autonomous systems is of escalating concern. Adversaries will find and exploit the vulnerabilities inherent with machine learning algorithms to adversely affect the manner in which an AI Model takes action on its input by way of the way it was created. Typically, an adversarial attack consists of a "crafted input" that is designed for a human to be unable to detect but has a XY-low probability of causing the AI Model output to produce an incorrect reaction by causing the AI to misclassify or misinterpret data.

5.1 Understanding Adversarial Attacks on AI-Based IDS

In cybersecurity, adversarial attacks against AI-based Intrusion Detection Systems (IDS) pose one of the largest threats to our current security architecture. Adversaries will use many different methods to modify the output results of the machine learning algorithms used by an IDS to ensure that they can pass through the IDS undetected or in some cases as a false positive. For instance, evasion attacks against AI-based IDS can be seen where an adversary alters traffic transmitted over the Internet or changes his/her user behavior within the system prior to their submitting their threat to the IDS. As a result, the IDS would view the traffic as being normal, rather than looking for signs of a threat. Another type of adversarial attack is a poisoning attack. This occurs during the initial training of an AI-based IDS wherein the data being used for training is tainted or corrupted, increasing the likelihood of misclassification and limiting the model's ability to recognize true threats. Through model extraction, attackers can exploit the AI detection mechanisms and use this information to build targeted attacks and identify vulnerabilities within the system. Attackers utilize model probing techniques that have been developed to extract an adversarial model from an AI-DIS. As a result, the detection systems ultimately fail to achieve their intended goal. It is essential to develop resilient defenses that can protect the function, integrity, and performance of AI-based intrusion detection systems that operate in autonomous modes. Organizations must have adaptive AI security frameworks, share threat intelligence in real-time, update their IDS models continually, allowing for resiliency and maintaining the ability to detect intrusions within a dynamic environment (Sharma et al., 2025).

5.2 AI-Driven Defense Mechanisms Against Adversarial Attacks

AI-based defense strategies provide essential protection for autonomous systems from adversarial threats. The utilization of these defense strategies will ultimately allow for the effectiveness and integrity of AI-based Intrusion Detection Systems (IDS) and other security measures.

1. **Adversarial Training:** Adversarial training is designed to serve as one type of defense against adversarial attacks on AI-based IDS models. This training procedure creates the potential adversarial examples by adding adversarial modifications to the training data set. This training allows the AI model to identify and respond to similar adversarial challenges in operational use. The primary benefit is that adversarially trained AI models are able to differentiate between authentic and adversarial input and thus, are better able to protect against adversarial attacks.
2. **Defensive Distillation:** Defence Distillation (DD) refers to a training method where one (the distilled or defence model) of two AI models(s) trained together, recognises the output probability distributions of another primary (defender) model. Distilled output probability distributions allow for smooth recognition boundaries that allow for making predictions based on inputs.
3. **Feature-Space Hardening:** Feature-Space Hardening (FSH) allows AI to be more effective in differentiating between legitimate users and adversarial (malicious) users by providing the AI system with a wide variety of helpful and important features. The goal of the FSH process is to maximise the amount, quality, and relevance of relevant features that are extracted and represented by the AI and ultimately reduce the ability of malicious inputs to corrupt the model.

Despite the numerous proposals to utilize federated learning, blockchain, homomorphic encryption, and differential privacy for secure autonomous systems, each of these technologies presents significant adoption trade-offs. Federated learning remains susceptible to having the model poisoned and to having significant communication overhead; blockchain solutions can experience limitations due to scalability and latency in near real-time environments; homomorphic encryption can provide very strong privacy guarantees but have high levels of computational cost associated with their use; differential privacy can protect user data, but by adding noise, it can reduce the accuracy of the model. As a result, security architects evaluating these technologies for secure autonomous applications must evaluate these technologies relative to their application needs, rather than relying on one technology or two technologies to fit all situations.

6. REGULATORY AND ETHICAL CHALLENGES IN SECURING AUTONOMOUS SYSTEMS

The ubiquity of the use of autonomous systems in a variety of sectors (such as transportation, healthcare, and smart cities) brings with it a wide array of cybersecurity & regulatory; and ethical; hurdles. Because these technologies are reliant on the use of artificial intelligence (AI), machine learning (ML), as well as a web of interconnected networks, they also present challenges with regard to susceptibility to cyber threats, data privacy, and algorithmic bias.

1. **Lack of Standardized Cybersecurity Regulations:** The lack of standardised Cybersecurity Regulations is one of the major regulatory issues associated with the development and use of autonomous systems. There are many different regulations regarding Cybersecurity for AI, Data Protection for Autonomous Systems and AI Accountability within different jurisdictions and industries; therefore, each organisation and country must attempt to comply with many different regulations (and often cannot do so due to those regulations being inconsistent) (Ighofiomoni et al 2025).
2. **Data Privacy and Compliance with Legal Frameworks:** Collecting and processing copious amounts of personal and sensitive information not only impacts people's ability to maintain their right to privacy but also increases the need for data protection from a legal compliance perspective. The European Union's General Data Protection Regulation (GDPR) and California's Consumer Privacy Protection Act (CCPA), for example, have detailed regulations regarding how data can be obtained, maintained (Holubenko et al., 2025).
3. **Ethical Concerns in AI Decision-Making:** As mentioned previously, an individual's privacy will be compromised; however, in addition to the challenges associated with protecting the individual's privacy, ethical concerns exist as a result of the reliance upon machine learning (ML) models to assist in making decisions. Because of that reliance, the outcome of a decision made based upon a ML model may contain inherent bias or produce unintended consequences.
4. **Security Risks in Autonomous Critical Infrastructure:** Many autonomous systems are integrated into critical infrastructure, such as power grids, traffic management systems, and smart healthcare facilities. A cyberattack on these

infrastructures could lead to catastrophic consequences, including public safety hazards and service disruptions. Regulatory bodies must enforce strict security standards to protect critical autonomous infrastructure from cyber threats. Measures such as intrusion detection systems (IDS), blockchain-based data integrity mechanisms, and AI-driven threat mitigation strategies should be mandated to ensure robust security. Governments and organizations must also conduct regular security audits and risk assessments to proactively address emerging threats (Dhanushkodi and Thejas, 2024).

6.1 Governance, Safety Assurance, and Operational Accountability

Although technical security mechanisms are critical to the successful deployment of autonomous systems, the deployment of autonomous systems also requires governance and operational accountability. Clear policies for the organization must be put in place to govern AI model updates, access control, incident response plans and procedures, and system auditing. The safety assurance framework must outline acceptable risk thresholds, requirements for validation and fallback mechanisms for when systems fail. Continuous monitoring of the systems will be required due to the potential for identifying model drift, performance degradation and new vulnerabilities. Also, there must be an accountability structure that will clarify who is responsible when an autonomous system fails or causes other harm. In these areas, governance considerations will be especially critical in the following areas: healthcare, transportation and critical infrastructure environments; all of which have the potential for security incidents affecting human safety.

6.2 International Regulatory and Governance Frameworks

Autonomous systems function in multiple separate regulatory regimes which directly govern various aspects of security, privacy and governance. The data protection regulations include the General Data Protection Regulation (GDPR) as well as the California Consumer Privacy Act (CCPA), which cover the collection, processing and protecting of personal information. The AI governance initiatives include the European Union Artificial Intelligence Act (EU AI Act), which provide privacy protections, transparency, accountability, a risk classification structure, and the mandate for human oversight of AI systems. The Cybersecurity frameworks include ISO/IEC 27001, the NIST Cybersecurity Framework, and sector-specific standards, which center on the governance of risk, incident response, resilience, and operational security. Although there are commonalities among the frameworks, they are typically implemented in a silo-separation approach, which creates regulatory fragmentation between silos, resulting in compliance issues for organizations deploying and using autonomous technologies in multiple jurisdictions.

7. FUTURE RESEARCH DIRECTIONS AND CHALLENGES

As the technology for Autonomous Systems continues to grow and develop, the focus of future research will also need to be directed to improving security, privacy and resilience against ever-changing cyber threats. Important areas for further review to support the development of robust and reliable autonomous systems have been identified below:

7.1. Future Research Directions in Securing Autonomous Systems

1. **Research on AI and its Defense against Adversarial Attacks:** Future research must improve the resilience of AI-based systems against evolving cybersecurity threats and adversarial attacks. Autonomous systems depend increasingly on the AI-based decision-making process, thereby rendering these systems vulnerable to attacks such as adversarial input, model poisoning, and data manipulation that could potentially compromise performance and safety.
2. **Research on Learning in a Privacy-Preserving Manner:** Continually collecting, processing, and sharing large volumes of sensitive information related to the operation of autonomous systems means that research in the area of learning in a privacy-preserving manner is of great importance. Federated learning, differential privacy, homomorphic encryption, and secure multiparty computation are possible solutions for protecting user privacy while allowing for collaborative model development and platform agnostic secure data analysis.
3. **Decentralized Security Architectures:** The increasing interdependence and complexity of all aspects of the autonomous operating environment necessitates the creation of decentralized security architectures that will facilitate secure communication, trust management capabilities, and collaboration in the area of detecting and reporting threats and significant vulnerabilities to all organizations in the same community. Blockchain-based security mechanisms can provide a mechanism to support integrity, transparency, and tamper-proof record-keeping of data in a distributed system; likewise, distributed intrusion detection systems can increase the available avenues for sharing cooperative threat intelligence among autonomous entities.
4. **Governance/Regulatory Frameworks:** Alongside emerging technology, there is a need for future research to further develop the way that governance,

accountability and regulation are applied to autonomous systems. As these systems continue to be integrated into critical sectors, such as healthcare, transportation, and industrial automation, there will be a need for clear governance mechanisms to establish who is responsible for what; define what constitutes responsibility/accountability; and provide an outline of how risk management will occur. Research efforts will also need to develop safety assurance frameworks, develop standardised compliance mechanisms, and establish effective AI governance models that will facilitate their safe deployment and operation.

7.2 Challenges in Securing Autonomous Systems

Innovation must continue in the creation of AI-based Cybersecurity Frameworks, as well as through cooperation and collaboration between Researchers and Policymakers to develop scalable, resilient, and privacy-preserving solutions to protect the growing threat of Cyber Attacks on Autonomous Systems.

1. **Complexity and Diversity of Autonomous Systems:** Autonomous systems provide solutions across multiple industries and each of these sectors operates with its own unique Cybersecurity criteria; therefore, applying a "one size fits all" Cyber Security Solution to all these sectors is not realistic. Further complicating the security of autonomous systems are the numerous opportunities for a cyber-attack, as a result of the vast number of components that comprise autonomous systems. The use of artificial intelligence (AI), Internet of Things (IOT), Cloud Computing, and Edge Computing creates an extremely large Attack Surface for attackers to exploit, while simultaneously creating barriers to effectively managing vulnerabilities within an autonomous system (Ndibe, 2025).
2. **Vulnerabilities in AI Models and Machine Learning Algorithms:** These ML models are vulnerable to a wide variety of different attacks including: adversarial attacks, model poisoning, and data manipulation, meaning that attackers can leverage weaknesses in AI algorithms to trick autonomous systems to make faulty decisions such as: tricking self-driving cars to read wrong road signs and tricking intelligent healthcare systems into misdiagnosing patients.
3. **Real-Time Threat Detection and Response:** Autonomous systems need real-time threat detection and response capabilities when faced with cyber threats. Existing standard intrusion detection systems (IDS) and cybersecurity solutions usually cannot handle fast, complex autonomous systems since cyber threats are detected and mitigated much sooner than the industry can provide.
4. **Data Privacy and Secure Communication:** Autonomous Vehicles generate and use vast amounts of sensitive information. There are challenges associated

with balancing an individual's right to privacy with security measures taken to secure communications between Autonomous Vehicles that are connected to each other. Recent AI technologies have been developed to help protect an individual's right to privacy (e.g., Federated Learning, Differential Privacy), but they also increase Computational Load and Decrease Performance across the Autonomous Vehicle System.

8. CONCLUSION

As the development of autonomous systems has progressed, the complexity of cybersecurity threats within AI-based environments continues to evolve due to the increase in the number of autonomous systems employing AI-based intrusion detection systems (IDs) and real-time responses (to threats). The need for improved methods for protecting against adversarial attacks on AI-based models being used in autonomous systems indicates a clear opportunity for advancing the methods employed to defend against those adversarial attacks. Adversarial training and explanation-based AI are two methods that can assist in enhancing the security architecture and resilience of AI-based autonomous systems. This chapter compiles all relevant information into an overall descriptive overview, integrating system-level architectural perspectives, domain-specific threat analyses, and critical assessments with regard to the various types of security mechanisms into one complete document. Therefore, through the ongoing provision of context-specific insights, the author seeks to provide readers with informative information that can be effectively incorporated by organizations willing to fill the gap between theoretical research as well as practical implementation in order to build more resistant, scalable, and trustworthy autonomous systems.

REFERENCES

Alqubaysi, T., Asmari, A. F. A., Alanazi, F., Almutairi, A., & Armghan, A. (2025). Federated learning-based predictive traffic management using a contained privacy-preserving scheme for autonomous vehicles. *Sensors (Basel)*, *25*(4), 1116. DOI: 10.3390/s25041116 PMID: 40006346

Andreoni, M., Lunardi, W. T., Lawton, G., & Thakkar, S. (2024). Enhancing autonomous system security and resilience with generative AI: A comprehensive survey. *IEEE Access : Practical Innovations, Open Solutions*, *12*, 109470–109493. DOI: 10.1109/ACCESS.2024.3439363

Cheng, X., Oun, A., & Wince, K. (2025). *The Role of Artificial Intelligence in Boosting Cybersecurity and Trusted Embedded Systems Performance: A Systematic Review on Current and Future Trends*. IEEE.

Dhanushkodi, K., & Thejas, S. (2024). AI enabled threat detection: Leveraging artificial intelligence for advanced security and cyber threat mitigation. *IEEE Access : Practical Innovations, Open Solutions*, *12*, 173127–173136. DOI: 10.1109/ACCESS.2024.3493957

Dhinakaran, D., Sankar, S. M., Selvaraj, D., & Raja, S. E. (2024). Privacy-preserving data in IoT-based cloud systems: A comprehensive survey with AI integration. arXiv preprint arXiv:2401.00794.

Hendaoui, F., Ferchichi, A., Trabelsi, L., Meddeb, R., Ahmed, R., & Khelifi, M. K. (2024). Advances in deep learning intrusion detection over encrypted data with privacy preservation: A systematic review. *Cluster Computing*, *27*(7), 8683–8724. DOI: 10.1007/s10586-024-04424-4

Holubenko, V., Gaspar, D., Leal, R., & Silva, P. (2025). Autonomous intrusion detection for IoT: A decentralized and privacy preserving approach. *International Journal of Information Security*, *24*(1), 7. DOI: 10.1007/s10207-024-00926-9

Ighofiomoni, M. O., Ojerinde, J. S., Olaniyan, I., Issah, P. P., Adepitan, O. S., Oyenuga, O., & Chinonyerem, C. A. (2025). Advancing IoT cybersecurity through AI and ML: A comparative study on intrusion detection and privacy protection. *Asian Journal of Advanced Research and Reports*, *19*(8), 159–174. DOI: 10.9734/ajarr/2025/v19i81122

Laghari, A. A., Khan, A. A., Ksibi, A., Hajjej, F., Kryvinska, N., Almadhor, A., Mohamed, M. A., & Alsubai, S. (2025). A novel and secure artificial intelligence enabled zero trust intrusion detection in industrial internet of things architecture. *Scientific Reports*, *15*(1), 26843. DOI: 10.1038/s41598-025-11738-9 PMID: 40702039

Mollashaik, A. S. (2025). Advancing data security through AI-driven classification: A framework for intelligent threat detection and privacy preservation. [IJCET]. *International Journal of Computer Engineering and Technology*, *15*(6), 467–481. DOI: 10.34218/IJCET_16_01_040

Moulahi, T., Jabbar, R., Alabdulatif, A., Abbas, S., El Khediri, S., Zidi, S., & Rizwan, M. (2023). Privacy-preserving federated learning cyber-threat detection for intelligent transport systems with blockchain-based security. *Expert Systems: International Journal of Knowledge Engineering and Neural Networks*, *40*(5), e13103. DOI: 10.1111/exsy.13103

Moustafa, N., Koroniotis, N., Keshk, M., Zomaya, A. Y., & Tari, Z. (2023). Explainable intrusion detection for cyber defences in the internet of things: Opportunities and solutions. *IEEE Communications Surveys and Tutorials*, *25*(3), 1775–1807. DOI: 10.1109/COMST.2023.3280465

Muneer, S., Farooq, U., Athar, A., Ahsan Raza, M., Ghazal, T. M., & Sakib, S. (2024). A critical review of artificial intelligence-based approaches in intrusion detection: A comprehensive analysis. *Journal of Engineering*, *2024*(1), 3909173. DOI: 10.1155/2024/3909173

Narayan, S. B. (2025). Safeguarding Intelligence: A Comprehensive Analysis of AI Security and Privacy in the Era of Autonomous Systems. Available at *SSRN* 5718122. DOI: 10.2139/ssrn.5718122

Nasir, Z. U. I., Iqbal, A., & Qureshi, H. K. (2024). Securing cyber-physical systems: A decentralized framework for collaborative intrusion detection with privacy preservation. *IEEE Transactions on Industrial Cyber-Physical Systems*, *2*, 303–311. DOI: 10.1109/TICPS.2024.3425794

Ndibe, O. S. (2025). Ai-driven forensic systems for real-time anomaly detection and threat mitigation in cybersecurity infrastructures. *International Journal of Research Publication and Reviews*, *6*(5), 389–411. DOI: 10.55248/gengpi.6.0525.1991

Padmavathi, V., & Saminathan, R. (2025). A federated edge intelligence framework with trust-based access control for secure and privacy preserving IoT systems. *Scientific Reports*, *15*(1), 35832. DOI: 10.1038/s41598-025-19712-1 PMID: 41087484

Sharma, D. P., Habibi Lashkari, A., Firoozjaei, M. D., Mahdavifar, S., & Xiong, P. (2025). Defense Methods for Adversarial Attacks and Privacy Issues in Secure AI. In *Understanding AI in Cybersecurity and Secure AI: Challenges, Strategies and Trends* (pp. 159–195). Springer Nature Switzerland. DOI: 10.1007/978-3-031-91524-6_9

Sharma, S. B., & Bairwa, A. K. (2025). Leveraging AI for Intrusion Detection in IoT Ecosystems: A Comprehensive Study. *IEEE Access : Practical Innovations, Open Solutions*, *13*, 66290–66317. DOI: 10.1109/ACCESS.2025.3550392

Vashishth, T. K., Sharma, V., Chaudhary, S., Sharma, R., Chauhan, P., & Sharma, B. K. (2026). Adoption of Artificial Intelligence Techniques for Enhancing Host-Based Intrusion Detection Systems. In *AI Solutions for Detecting Cyber-Attacks in Information Systems* (pp. 133–164). IGI Global Scientific Publishing.

Vashishth, T. K., Sharma, V., Sharma, K. K., Kumar, B., Chaudhary, S., & Panwar, R. (2024). Intrusion Detection and Prevention Techniques in FL Cloud-Based Healthcare 5.0: A Comprehensive Review. Pioneering Smart Healthcare 5.0 with IoT, Federated Learning, and Cloud Security, 152-174.

Vyas, A., Lin, P. C., Hwang, R. H., & Tripathi, M. (2024). Privacy-preserving federated learning for intrusion detection in IoT environments: A survey. *IEEE Access : Practical Innovations, Open Solutions*, *12*, 127018–127050. DOI: 10.1109/ACCESS.2024.3454211

Zhang, C., Wang, N., Hou, Y. T., & Lou, W. (2025). Machine Learning-Based Intrusion Detection Systems: Capabilities, Methodologies, and Open Research Challenges. *Authorea Preprints*. DOI: 10.1002/9781394293773.ch03

Chapter 9
Healthcare Services Utilizing State-of-the-Art Image Analysis:
A Dilemma Regarding the Right to Privacy

Suchita Arora
http://orcid.org/0000-0003-3191-2144
Poornima University, Jaipur, India

M. V. N. Nagalakshmi
http://orcid.org/0009-0001-4520-6569
Paari School of Business, SRM University AP, India

Yadavalli Venkata Naga Sai Sri Charan Sai Sri Charan
http://orcid.org/0009-0002-6949-227X
DMTS, Department of Sys Architecture, Verizon Data Services, Hyderabad, India

Digvijay Pandey
http://orcid.org/0000-0003-0353-174X
Department of Technical Education, Government of Uttar Pradesh, India

Srijib Shankar Jha
http://orcid.org/0000-0001-7687-7771
SoML, IMS Unison University, India

Pankaj Dadheech
http://orcid.org/0000-0001-5783-1989
Department of Computer Science and Engineering, Swami Keshvanand Institute of Technology, Management, and Gramothan (SKIT), Jaipur, India

ABSTRACT

Many national laws at the federal and state levels protect patients' right to confidentiality in medical records. The A.P. Shah Committee report's privacy principles have been integrated into healthcare organizations' day-to-day operations to the fullest degree practicable. But there are big holes in the policymaking that don't consider what happens to the data once it's been gathered or transferred. To close these gaps, urgent institutional cooperation is required. According to the findings

DOI: 10.4018/979-8-2600-3070-7.ch009

of the research, you should proceed in this manner. If an efficient framework is going to be developed, however, the state will still need to play a part in promoting collaboration between various organizations operating in the public and private sectors across a wide range of industries.

INTRODUCTION

Medical professionals all around the globe are inundated with an overwhelming amount of data, all of which they are required to gather, analyze, and evaluate. Because they are human, they have limitations; specifically, they tire easily, which may have negative effects on both their health and their ability to help their patients. In the healthcare business, 90% of the data collected consists of patient images. Due to an increase in demand for diagnostic imaging services, there is now an ever-increasing volume of data that has to be processed. Because of this, it is now possible to make use of cutting-edge IT systems and software designed specifically for medical picture processing. AI solutions have the potential to shorten the amount of time that patients must wait to obtain their diagnoses, increase the number of individuals who can be evaluated, improve the accuracy of diagnostics, and assist healthcare companies in optimizing their operations.

Image analysis

Image analysis, often known as imagery analysis, is the practice of gleaning useful information from photographs, typically digital ones, by making use of a variety of digital image processing techniques. Image analysis is also sometimes referred to as imagery analysis. Analysis of images is also sometimes referred to as imagery analysis. Projects using image analysis might be as simple as reading barcodes printed on packages, alternatively, they may be as complex as determining someone's identity based purely on external characteristics (Shruthishree, & Tiwari, H., 2017). To conduct tasks that require the analysis of large datasets, the execution of complex computations, or the extraction of quantitative information, computers are indispensable. However, the visual cortex of the human brain is a very effective tool for picture processing, especially for the extraction of more abstract data. And computers still can't replace human analysts in many fields, like medicine, security, and remote sensing. The human visual cortex is also a very efficient structure for visual processing. Because of this, several standard methods for image analysis, such as ED and NN, have been significantly improved, deriving their cues from models of human visual perception. This is the case since these models accurately represent human visual perception (Ker et al., 2017).

Machine Learning in Image Analysis

The technology behind picture analysis relies heavily on machine learning. The software must be appropriately trained to spot certain irregularities regardless of the domain of medicine (or other sectors) under consideration. AI has a very different way of learning than humans do. It uses massive picture datasets that need to be processed and examined by the program. The AI system then learns to identify key trends and applies this information to identify telltale symptoms of various diseases. It's worth noting that Machine Learning-based solutions have the potential to, and have in certain circumstances actually achieved, higher diagnosis accuracy than human physicians (Renukalatha, S., & Suresh, K. V., 2018) of course, there is always going to be a need for some sort of oversight from qualified professionals. The program has certain limitations, particularly when presented with imperfect, partial, or low-quality photos. This is where a human doctor's training and the ability to interpret a picture without first reducing it to binary may be invaluable (Islam & Mondal, 2019).

HEALTHCARE SECTOR

This large group includes not just doctors and hospitals but also drug and device makers, health plans, and other healthcare sector middlemen. In the world of finance, healthcare is one of the 11 S&P sectors or GICS categories that are widely used. It is always one of the top three sectors by weight in the S&P 500. Businesses that develop or sell medical supplies or services are included in this industry's broad definition (Guo Y., 2020).

Machine Learning in Image Analysis

There is a significant amount of reliance on machine learning in the technology that can analyze pictures. Regardless of the field of medicine that is being considered, the software needs to be correctly educated to identify certain anomalies. A significantly different approach to learning is taken by artificial intelligence (AI) in comparison to how humans learn. Large picture collections are utilized, and the application is required to handle and analyze these datasets during the process. The artificial intelligence system then acquires the ability to recognize significant patterns and utilizes this knowledge to recognize telltale indicators of a variety of diseases. It is important to note that solutions based on machine learning have the potential to attain higher diagnosis accuracy than human physicians, and in some cases, they have actually achieved this level of accuracy. With that being said, it is certain that there will always be a requirement for some form of supervision from appropriately trained experts (Zeng N., 2020). A number of restrictions are imposed by the program, particularly when it is supplied with photographs that are imperfect, incomplete, or of poor quality. At this point, the training of a human doctor and the ability to analyse a picture without first reducing it to binary may prove to be quite beneficial.

Medical Image Analysis in Different Areas of Healthcare

Medical imaging, in its various forms, has been crucial to the advancement of medical science for decades. The X-ray was discovered by Wilhelm Röntgen in the 19th century, and its medical applications quickly followed. Patients are typically diagnosed nowadays using pictures generated by a variety of tools and technologies, most of which focus on internal organs. It's hard to conceive of a future in which all medical photos are stored, processed, and manipulated without any digital participation, but IT solutions are currently a popular tool for handling this sort of data. Using technology to examine this data may make it much more helpful (Cai, L., 2020).

Image Analysis Solutions in Medicine

Neurology, cardiology, orthopedics, dentistry, and cancer are just a few of the numerous medical specialties that might benefit from medical image analysis technologies. They can interpret results from X-rays, MRIs, CTs, PET scans, and ultrasounds. Therefore, there is a chance for the automation and acceleration of processes that would otherwise take a long time to do manually. The diagnostic procedure is sped up and accuracy is increased since the software may be trained to spot characteristics in these photos (Wiestler, B., & Menze, B., 2020).

X-ray

The primary use of X-rays in medicine is to create pictures of the patient's interior anatomy. Lung infections and bone fractures are two of the most common medical problems that this technology can diagnose. It's the gold standard of medical imaging and has been around for centuries. More than 22 million X-rays were taken on NHS patients in 2015. Patients had to wait up to a month for their diagnosis since not enough radiologists were available to process the influx of photos (Ziller A., et al.,2020).

CT Scanning

Tumors, vascular abnormalities, abscesses, and many other medical disorders may frequently be detected with the use of CT. It may generate 2D slices or even 3D pictures of the patient's anatomy. The use of this method of examining patients has grown substantially in recent years. Due to the high volume of output, enormous training data sets may be compiled. However, this development opens the door for IT to shoulder more responsibility and speed up the diagnostic process for patients (LungrenM., 2020). Furthermore, as shown by UCF researchers, medical image analysis software is very accurate in its detection of individual disorders. Here, researchers developed a reliable method for spotting lung cancers that are too tiny to be seen by radiologists (Senbekov M.,et al., 2020).

PET scanning

The medical imaging method known as PET may identify cancer, blood flow problems, brain diseases, and abnormal bone development. After injecting this chemical into the patient, a specialized scanner is utilized to capture the resulting pictures. Therefore, doctors can monitor the tracer's progress within the patient's body to get a clearer picture of what's going on. The radioactive tracers used in this procedure provide the largest risk to patients, which is a major downside. In certain ways, this problem may be made less severe with the use of IT solutions. By using appropriate training datasets, image-enhancing and noise-canceling algorithms may be created. As a result, radioactive materials may be used less often. However, there is also the potential for the creation of software that can analyze PET pictures and spot the signs of various illnesses (Asan O., 2020).

MRI

Radio waves and magnetic fields are used in MRI to create a picture of the inside of a patient's body. Common applications include the diagnosis of aneurysms and other circulatory and soft tissue disorders. The patient is not subjected to any radiation during an MRI examination, unlike the previous methods. Nearly 40 million magnetic resonance imaging (MRI) scans were done in the United States in 2016 (Bhattacharya S., 2021). Once again, AI can examine these pictures and identify illnesses. Brain aneurysms may now be accurately detected automatically in MR scans thanks to a deep learning approach developed by researchers at Osaka City University. AI may be used to increase the accuracy of radiologists' diagnoses and decrease their burden in this field.

Ultrasound

Multiple sectors make use of ultrasound imaging technologies. Medical professionals may use it to capture high-definition video and still photographs of their patients' skeletal muscles, tendons, and blood vessels. It's also used to monitor a fetus's growth in the womb. In the medical field, ultrasounds are widely used because of their noninvasive nature (Puttagunta, M., & Ravi, S., 2021). Medical image analysis software finds this field particularly fruitful due to the massive amounts of data being generated. Radiologists spend a lot of time reading and analyzing these pictures. Artificial intelligence (AI) systems that use Machine Learning can handle a significant chunk of this job. According to a study published in 2018 by the National Centre for Biotechnology Information (NCBI), deep learning software can utilize ultrasound scans to detect breast cancer with an accuracy that is on par with radiologists. This is of paramount importance in places where medical professionals are in low supply, like many developing nations (Raman R., et al., 2021).

LITERATURE REVIEW

Shruthishree, & Tiwari, H., 2017 focused on the processing of medical images. When it comes to therapeutic evaluation and treatment, as well as medical education and study, etc., the medical picture was invaluable. However, its utility lies more in the realm of physiology than morphology. The discipline of medicine has been profoundly impacted by the advancements in computer and imaging technology that have led to medical imaging. The importance of high-quality medical pictures in making accurate diagnoses has led to a surge of interest in the field of medical IP, and clinical apps that wish to archive and recover images for later use require a straightforward system for doing so.

J. Ker, et al.(2017) reviewed deep learning in diagnostic imaging technology. Recent years have seen a rapid rise in the use of computerized medical data and diagnostic imagery, coinciding with the great success of machine learning algorithms at picture identification tasks. This article serves as an introduction to the therapeutic applications of machine learning methods in the area of medical picture analysis, with an emphasis on CNN. Machine learning is useful in the age of medical big data because it can find important hierarchical connections within the data automatically, without the need for time-consuming feature engineering. Classification, localization, recognition, segmentation, and alignment of medical images were among the topics they explore. They address some of the challenges, new developments, and potential future paths in this area of study.

Renukalatha, S., & Suresh, K. V., (2018) presented work on images used in medicine; a survey. Biology, science, medicine, and engineering are just some of the fields that contribute to bio-medical image analysis' multidisciplinary nature. The focus is on using picture processing methods to solve health and medicinal issues. Medical pictures contain a wealth of detail about the physical structure under study, which can be used to make an accurate diagnostic and guide treatment decisions. The majority of the time, doctors physically analyze these medical pictures by looking at them. However, human viewers' ability to visually analyze these pictures was constrained by factors such as inter-observer perception variance, fatigue-induced mistakes, environmental disruptions, and subjectivity. On the other hand, using machines equipped with the right methods for analyzing these pictures supports objective analysis by an expert, which in turn increases diagnosis confidence and precision. The vast amounts of information available on biological picture analysis have been compiled in this study.

Islam & Montal (2019) did research on medical image analysis based on image enhancement. This article describes a method for improving photos, with a focus on medical pictures. Picture improvement allows you to see previously concealed features and adjust the brightness of a picture. The border of a picture was the starting point for any analysis involving that image. Edge recognition and improvement are crucial to achieving accurate findings in picture analysis. The effectiveness of this created technique for improving medical pictures was evaluated by applying it to low-contrast medical images.

Y. Guo, et al. (2020) focused on AI in medical treatment. The purpose of this research was to do a complete bibliometric assessment of healthcare articles relating to AI across time. As a result of this study, academics, policymakers, and practitioners will have a better grasp of the evolution of AI research in the field of healthcare and its potential practice consequences. The disparities between AI health care studies and practical uses should be the focus of future AI research.

N. Zeng, et al.(2020) provided work on medical neuroimaging data analysis using artificial intelligence. Researchers in the field of artificial intelligence for brain picture analysis were encouraged to share their work and insights into this Research Topic, which aimed to solicit novel additions to the field. They were grateful to the many writers who have submitted their most recent findings on the use of AI in medical picture analysis. After extensive evaluations, only 19 of 29 applications were approved. China, the UK, the USA, and many other nations and areas added to it.

L. Cai, et al.(2020)reviewed the classification and segmentation of medical images using deep learning: a literature survey. Big data analysis and illness detection are only two of the applications of DL and intelligent imaging that are discussed in this article, drawing from the most recent findings in the field of big data analysis of medical images as well as our team's own efforts in this area.

Wiestler, B., & Menze, B., 2020 did research on DL for the study of medical images. In this summary, they will provide a short introduction to neural networks, focusing on CNN in particular. They will describe how these networks autonomously divide structures of interest in the image volume, how they learn to correlate imaging findings with relevant (clinical) traits like genetics, and why they can be so effective at finding pertinent features. They will also talk about some of the obstacles that prevent these methods from being used more widely.

S. Bhattacharya, et al.(2021) introduced medical picture analysis and DL for the COVID-19 coronavirus outbreak. they begin by providing a concise overview of the most recent findings from the field of deep learning as it pertains to COVID-19 medical IP. Then, they summarize the deep learning field and its recent healthcare uses. At last talk about a few problems and difficulties with DL implementations for COVID-19 medical IP that are likely to spur more research into stopping the spread of the virus and ending the crisis, ultimately leading to wise, healthy communities.

M. Puttagunta, et al.(2021) presented work on deep learning-based medical picture analysis. This article details the progress made in ANN, including a thorough examination of DLA that has exciting potential in medical imaging. X-ray, CT, mammogram, and digital histology pictures are typically the focus of DLA deployments. It offers a comprehensive analysis of the literature on the use of DLA in medical picture categorization, recognition, and segmentation. This summary will help academics conceive of effective ways to apply DLA to medical picture analysis.

B. M. Rashed, et al. (2022) focused on the state of the art in automated illness diagnosis using medical images. They efficiently sorted through publications using the PRISMA approach, and towards the end, we had forty studies over the last five years (2017-2021) that were relevant to our study concerns. Medical IP and analysis methods, including those utilized for preprocessing, segmentation, FE, and diagnosis, were identified, explored, and reviewed. Machine learning and deep learning are also extensively explained in this article. Also, the best medical IP techniques used in these articles and the best methodologies for future approaches were discussed, and the collection was proposed as a comprehensive reference source for their use in future medical diagnosis systems.

Suganyadevi, S., et al. (2022) reviewed DL for medical picture analysis. The medical field was one of the many that have recently benefited from deep learning's widespread application. Research conducted in the following domains was briefly summarized: the nervous system; eye; lungs; computerized disease; breasts; bones; digestive system; muscles; and skeleton. Successful applications of deep learning networks to big data include information exploration, knowledge deployment, and knowledge-based prediction. This article provides introductory material and cutting-edge applications of deep learning to the study of medical image processing and analysis. The fundamental goals of this work were to identify and execute the most essential principles that have arisen from medical image processing research and to present an overview of this field.

Problem Statement

It is important to note that this research has several limitations. To begin, our study is qualitative research; so, rather than attempting to quantify the predominance of opinions, we would like to highlight the range of problems that need to be investigated in relation to the confidentiality of digital health information. We are unable to guarantee that our experts accurately reflect the entire community of specialists in the disciplines from which they were selected because the sample size for the qualitative method is quite small. Despite the fact that efforts were made to create a broad sample, it is possible that certain points of view are not well represented. The second factor is the consistently shifting landscape of online privacy and the attention that the general public is paying to it. The results are representative of the time period in which the research was conducted, which is presently in the year 2018. In the third place, our interview guide did not make any attempt to arrive at policy answers, and we did not collect sufficient data from our experts in order to identify the full spectrum of viewpoints on privacy legislation and possible policy responses. In conclusion, it is impossible to completely eliminate the impact of social standards.

Proposed Methodology

Regarding the interpretation of the right to privacy, there is not yet a general agreement. It's a fluid idea whose definition and scope change depending on the circumstances. A number of characteristics are associated with the right to privacy, each of which is contingent upon the particular circumstances in which it is exercised. However, when it comes to this broad right, physical anonymity has been the most strictly protected. The right to privacy over one's own body, which includes the organs, genetic material, and biological processes that comprise one's health, is an inherent right that does not begin with the state. This is in contrast to other types of privacy, such as communication or transactional privacy, which are derived from the state. Because this right is based on the concept of the right to life as defined in natural law, the state can only revoke it under extraordinary circumstances that affect the right to life of a larger number of people.

Following the preprocessing of the data for equal shaping, which is shown in figure 1, that data pertaining to the healthcare sector is then compressed. The image is encrypted once it has been compressed. Following that, the photograph is sent to its final destination. The image is decompressed and decrypted once it reaches the receiving end. Next, the accuracy and performance of the model are taken into consideration.

To this point, however, the discussion that has led to the creation of a right to privacy that applies everywhere has been limited to how it can be read as an extension of Article 21's fundamental right to life and liberty and Articles 19(1)(a) and (b)'s freedom of expression and movement. This is because the discussion has been limited to how it can be read as an extension of these rights. Despite the fact that this viewpoint might be accurate, it restricts the scope of the right to just encompass activities that are conducted against the official state. It is important to note, however, that the scope of the right to privacy extends far beyond the bounds of the state. As can be seen in Figure 1, there is an immediate need for a robust legal and regulatory framework that safeguards the personal information of persons from companies that are not necessarily a part of the state.

Figure 1. Process flow of Visual encryption for healthcare sector

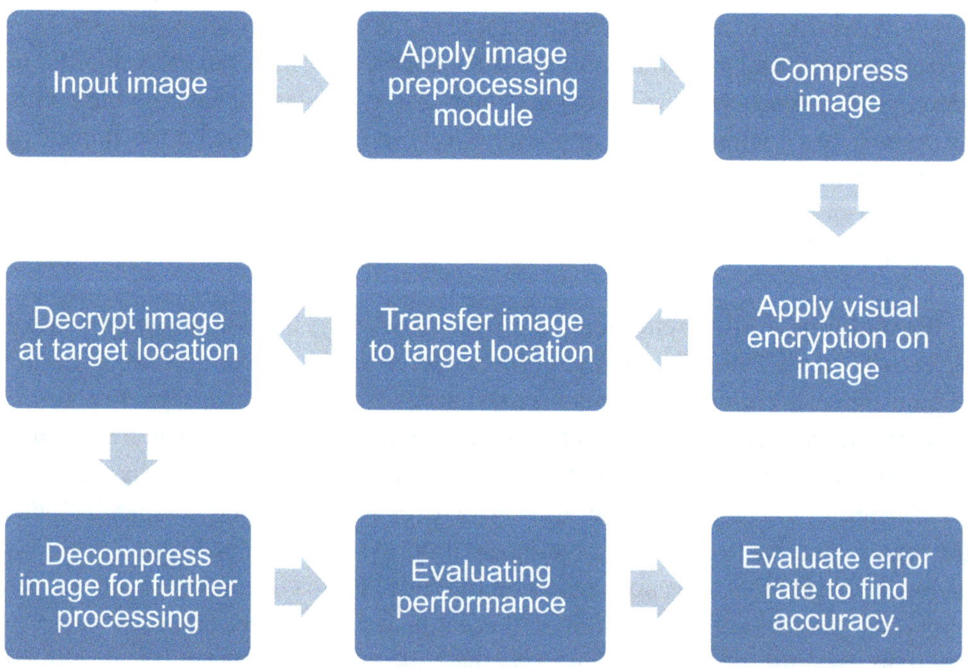

This investigation looks at how privacy is currently understood in the healthcare industry, what measures are in place to safeguard personal information, and how those safeguards are really put to use in the field. In addition, it identifies concrete policy gaps in the current framework and makes concerted efforts to offer efficient recommendations for repairing these gaps and developing a system that effectively achieves the overarching goal of making the Right to Privacy a reality on the individual, state, and institutional levels.

Purpose

A chapter that offers an overview of the synergy, structure and execution of privacy legislation in the healthcare industry in India is the primary purpose of the study. This chapter will be produced as a result of the study. The study investigates the evolution of domestic legislation across various sectors of the healthcare industry with a specific emphasis on privacy regulations that protect patients medical data and DNA samples from prying eyes, aiming to aid therapeutic and scientific growth. This focuses on the regulations that protect patients' medical data and DNA samples. The implementation of appropriate safeguards that are incorporated into the routines of data collection, administration, and storage is required for businesses operating in the healthcare industry that have the intention of restricting the sorts of data they gather as well as the quantity of data they obtain. Because of this, the objective of this study is to compile a list of the many privacy protection systems that are now in place. These systems come in the form of laws, regulations, and guidelines. This research will examine the similarities and differences between these systems and the real procedures that are carried out in diagnostic laboratories, public and private hospitals and other medical facilities. The goal of this comparison is to assess the effectiveness of these laws in satisfying the necessary standards for privacy protection. The findings of this study offer suggestions for enhancing the efficiency of the methods that are now in place to avoid unjustified intrusions into the privacy of patients. Such as implementing stricter regulations and improving training for healthcare professionals on privacy standards. This scholarly inquiry not only offers a comprehensive review of privacy protection processes carried out in different parts of the world, but it also offers recommendations.

Importance

Though it is on pace with worldwide standards in terms of diagnosis and the use of cutting-edge technology, India healthcare industry is still in its infancy in terms of the nature and scope of its engagement with the law. The several aspects of medical care balance between the public interest and the patient's right to make their own decisions. The right to privacy is one such factor that is progressively developing. Many individual case laws reflecting a changing social structure have brought to light the many dimensions of this right, which aims to balance the socioeconomic rights that formerly ruled society with the individual interests that the public is just now beginning to recognize. There are some controversial issues in healthcare include a person's right to reveal the nature of his illness, a woman's right not to be forced to undergo a blood test, a couple's right to decide whether or not to have children, a woman's right to choose whether or not to have an abortion, and a man and a woman's right to joint custody of a child. By analyzing the framework of current domestic legislation and regulations and their subsequent application, this study aims to identify crucial gaps in the development of law and policy. The study's overarching goal is to provide a foundation for future policy considerations and legal modifications by drawing appropriate findings to remedy these gaps and making suggestions based on worldwide best practices.

METHODOLOGY

This inquiry was conducted in two distinct parts. The first part of this paper analyses the current condition of domestic legislation and assesses its efficacy. Several broad privacy principles are laid forth in the A.P. Shah Committee report on Privacy Protection, which may be used to evaluate whether or not the provisions of the Act comply with these principles. Only secondary sources, both print and electronic, are used in this portion of the research report. The second part of the research focuses on the actual methods of patient data integration, organization, use, and storage employed by public and commercial hospitals and diagnostic facilities. Data from a diagnostic center, three independent hospitals, and one large public hospital were included in this study. Medical record keepers at these facilities freely participated in an anonymous online survey. The information was gathered and processed to reveal how effectively these businesses follow the privacy guidelines detailed by the Group of Experts' Report as shown i**n Table 1.**

The Domestic Legal Formalization of Privacy Regulation

This study analyses the effectiveness of domestic legislation in curtailing practices related to the privacy of persons' healthcare, drawing judgments about the strategy's viability. By using this technique, healthcare providers can create a culture of good privacy regulation by following best practices, self-regulating, and putting policy ideas into action, all while following the law. To do this, we looked into national laws that protect patients' privacy. There has been more investigation in the prospect that the rule will be added to the standard operating procedures, norms, and standards that both public and private healthcare facilities follow. We have studied how effective this strategy is for achieving the perambulatory goals of providing safe and unobtrusive procedures while allowing the patient to rest and seek therapy, as well as how widely it has been used.

Regulations use the concept of "privacy" in many countries. It is most often used when talking about the trust that exists between a doctor and a patient. Section 20(A) of the Indian Medical Council Act of 1952 recognizes the fiduciary relationship between a doctor and his or her patient because both parties reasonably expect to trust each other. There are several kinds of privacy that are important in healthcare, such as decisional privacy, associational privacy, proprietary privacy, and physiological privacy.

Privacy Violations stem from policy and information gaps: Healthcare policy violations can happen when policies are made or put into action, or when data is collected that isn't useful or accurate. One example is when data is collected for no cause at all, as when a customer can't get their medical information or when a patient isn't told about a data breach in a timely manner. It could be embarrassing, stigmatizing, or even discriminatory to have your medical history made public. Also, unlimited access to medical information could put a lot of things at risk, like jobs, life insurance, and health insurance.

It is not a violation of a patient's right to privacy to share his or her health information during a referral, in response to a court or police order, in accordance with the Insurance Act when a patient has waived his or her rights in taking out insurance, or by the requirements of workers' compensation, consumer protection, or other similar laws. Patients have the right to keep things private.

Table 1. Evaluation of accuracy and performance in various researches

	Deep learning	Health care	Image processing	Security	Performance
Asan, O.(2020)	No	Yes	No	No	No
Bhattacharya, S.(2021)	Yes	Yes	Yes	No	No
Cai, L. (2020)	Yes	Yes	Yes	No	No
Puttagunta, M. (2021)	Yes	Yes	Yes	No	No
Raman, R., et al., (2021)	Yes	Yes	Yes	No	Yes
Ziller, A., et al., (2020)	No	Yes	Yes	Yes	No

CONCLUSION

There are several domestic laws that were enacted to address concerns relating to healthcare, and one of these laws protects the right to keep medical records confidential. It is an additional point of interest that healthcare organizations have incorporated, to the maximum extent practically possible, the privacy principles outlined in the report compiled by the A.P. Shah Committee into their standard operating procedures. The data that are shown in Table 1 indicate that conventional research did not take into account all of the relevant elements, which include deep learning, healthcare, image processing, security, and performance. On the other hand, the language of the policy has several fundamental flaws, the most significant of which is that it does not take into account what happens to the data after it has been obtained or how it will be transferred in the future. This is the most significant of the policies flaws. Because of this, there is an immediate requirement for institutional collaboration to quickly fill in the gaps in coverage of the gaps. The findings of the research contain recommendations that are similar to these in a manner that is analogous, specifically suggesting that institutional collaboration is essential to address the identified flaws in policy coverage. In order to develop an effective framework, the state must actively promote collaboration among a diverse range of institutions operating in both the public and private sectors, representing a wide range of industries. This is necessary to achieve the goal of establishing an efficient framework. Insurance corporations, internet servers that host patient information databases, and advocacy organizations that fight for patients' rights to privacy when demanding access to medical records under the Freedom of Information Act are all examples of enterprises that fall under this category. In addition, this category includes organizations that protect patients' rights to privacy. It is possible to establish a solid foundation that will enable the right to privacy to be constructed in a timely and effective manner if everyone works together. This foundation may be laid when everyone works together.

REFERENCES

Asan, O., Bayrak, A. E., & Choudhury, A. (2020). Artificial Intelligence and Human Trust in Healthcare: Focus on Clinicians. *Journal of Medical Internet Research*, *22*(6), 1–7. DOI: 10.2196/15154 PMID: 32558657

Bhattacharya, S., Reddy Maddikunta, P. K., Pham, Q. V., Gadekallu, T. R., & Krishnan, S. (2021). Deep learning and medical image processing for coronavirus (COVID-19) pandemic: A survey. *Sustainable Cities and Society*, *65*(November), 102589. DOI: 10.1016/j.scs.2020.102589 PMID: 33169099

Cai, L., Gao, J., & Zhao, D. (2020). A review of the application of deep learning in medical image classification and segmentation. *Annals of Translational Medicine*, *8*(11), 713–713. DOI: 10.21037/atm.2020.02.44 PMID: 32617333

Guo, Y., Hao, Z., Zhao, S., Gong, J., & Yang, F. (2020). Artificial intelligence in health care: Bibliometric analysis. *Journal of Medical Internet Research*, *22*(7), 1–12. DOI: 10.2196/18228 PMID: 32723713

Islam, S. M., & Mondal, H. S. (2019). Image Enhancement Based Medical Image Analysis. 2019 10th International Conference on Computing, Communication and Networking Technologies, ICCCNT 2019, 1–5. DOI: 10.1109/ICCCNT45670.2019.8944910

Ker, J., Wang, L., Rao, J., & Lim, T. (2017). Deep Learning Applications in Medical Image Analysis. *IEEE Access : Practical Innovations, Open Solutions*, *6*, 9375–9379. DOI: 10.1109/ACCESS.2017.2788044

Puttagunta, M., & Ravi, S. (2021). Medical image analysis based on deep learning approach. *Multimedia Tools and Applications*, *80*(16), 24365–24398. DOI: 10.1007/s11042-021-10707-4 PMID: 33841033

Raman, R., Rajalakshmi, R., Surya, J., Ramakrishnan, R., Sivaprasad, S., Conroy, D., Thethi, J. P., Mohan, V., & Netuveli, G. (2021). Impact on health and provision of healthcare services during the COVID-19 lockdown in India: A multicentre cross-sectional study. *BMJ Open*, *11*(1), 1–11. DOI: 10.1136/bmjopen-2020-043590 PMID: 33468529

Renukalatha, S., & Suresh, K. V. (2018). A review on biomedical image analysis. *Biomedical Engineering : Applications, Basis, and Communications*, *30*(4), 1830001. Advance online publication. DOI: 10.4015/S1016237218300018

Senbekov, M., Saliev, T., Bukeyeva, Z., Almabayeva, A., Zhanaliyeva, M., Aitenova, N., Toishibekov, Y., & Fakhradiyev, I. (2020). The recent progress and applications of digital technologies in healthcare: A review. *International Journal of Telemedicine and Applications*, *2020*, 1–18. Advance online publication. DOI: 10.1155/2020/8830200 PMID: 33343657

Shruthishree, & Tiwari, H. (2017). a Review Paper on Medical Image Processing. International Journal of Research -GRANTHAALAYAH, 5(4RACSIT), 21–29. DOI: 10.29121/granthaalayah.v5.i4RACSIT.2017.3344

Suganyadevi, S., Seethalakshmi, V., & Balasamy, K. (2022). A review on deep learning in medical image analysis. *International Journal of Multimedia Information Retrieval*, *11*(1), 19–38. DOI: 10.1007/s13735-021-00218-1 PMID: 34513553

Wiestler, B., & Menze, B. (2020). Deep learning for medical image analysis: A brief introduction. *Neuro-Oncology Advances*, *2*(Supplement_4), IV35–IV41. DOI: 10.1093/noajnl/vdaa092 PMID: 33521639

Zeng, N., Zuo, S., Zheng, G., Ou, Y., & Tong, T. (2020). Editorial: Artificial Intelligence for Medical Image Analysis of Neuroimaging Data. *Frontiers in Neuroscience*, *14*(May), 1–2. DOI: 10.3389/fnins.2020.00480 PMID: 32508575

Ziller, A., Passerat-Palmbach, J., Ryffel, T., Usynin, D., Trask, A., Junior, I. D. L. C., Mancuso, J., Makowski, M., Rueckert, D., Braren, R., & Kaissis, G. (2020).Privacy-preserving medical image analysis.https://arxiv.org/abs/2012.06354

Compilation of References

Abdel-Wahab, A., Pulipati, V., Joshi, S., Srikanteswara, R., Menon, S., & Dutta, P. (2025). Deep Learning Framework for Breast Cancer Detection and Segmentation Using EfficientNet and U-Net with Hyperparameter Optimization. *SN Computer Science*, *6*(5), 528. DOI: 10.1007/s42979-025-03900-x

Adepoju, D. A., & Adepoju, A. G. (2025). Establishing ethical frameworks for scalable data engineering and governance in AI-driven healthcare systems. *International Journal of Research Publication and Reviews*, *6*(4), 8710–8726. DOI: 10.55248/gengpi.6.0425.1547

Ahmad, R. (2025). *Developing trustworthy and ethically-based healthcare systems*. Applied Computing and Informatics., DOI: 10.1108/ACI-05-2025-0203

Akhmetov, A., Latif, Z., Tyler, B., & Yazici, A. (2025). Enhancing healthcare data privacy and interoperability with federated learning. *PeerJ. Computer Science*, *11*, e2870. DOI: 10.7717/peerj-cs.2870 PMID: 40567682

Akila, K., Gopinathan, R., Arunkumar, J., & Malar, B. S. B. (2025). The Role of Artificial Intelligence in Modern Healthcare: Advances, Challenges, and Future Prospects. *The European Journal of Cardiovascular Medicine*, *15*, 615–624.

Akter, M., Moustafa, N., & Turnbull, B. (2024). SPEI-FL: Serverless privacy edge intelligence-enabled federated learning in smart healthcare systems. *Cognitive Computation*, *16*(5), 2626–2641. DOI: 10.1007/s12559-024-10310-3

Alaka, E., Abiodun, K., Jinadu, S. O., Igba, E., & Ezeh, V. N. (2025). Data integrity in decentralized financial systems: A model for auditable, automated reconciliation using blockchain and AI. *International Journal of Management and Commerce Innovations*, *13*(1), 136–158.

Al-Amiery, A. (2025). The ethical implications of emerging artificial intelligence technologies in healthcare. *MedMat*, *2*(2), 85–100. DOI: 10.1097/mm9.0000000000000015

Alasmary, H. (2024). Scalable Digital Health (SDH): An IoT-Based scalable framework for remote patient monitoring. *Sensors (Basel), 24*(4), 1346. DOI: 10.3390/s24041346 PMID: 38400504

Albshaier, L., Almarri, S., & Albuali, A. (2025). Federated Learning for Cloud and Edge Security: A Systematic Review of Challenges and AI opportunities. *Electronics (Basel), 14*(5), 1019. DOI: 10.3390/electronics14051019

Alenoghena, C. O., Onumanyi, A. J., Ohize, H. O., Adejo, A. O., Oligbi, M., Ali, S. I., & Okoh, S. A. (2022). eHealth: A survey of architectures, developments in mHealth, security concerns and solutions. *International Journal of Environmental Research and Public Health, 19*(20), 13071. DOI: 10.3390/ijerph192013071 PMID: 36293656

Alghamdi, A., Zhu, J., Yin, G., Shorfuzzaman, M., Alsufyani, N., Alyami, S., & Biswas, S. (2022). Blockchain Empowered Federated Learning Ecosystem for Securing Consumer IoT Features. *Analysis & Sensing, 22*(18), 6786. Advance online publication. DOI: 10.3390/s22186786 PMID: 36146134

Almogadwy, B., & Alqarafi, A. (2025). Fused federated learning framework for secure and decentralized patient monitoring in healthcare 5.0 using IoMT. *Scientific Reports, 15*(1), 24263. DOI: 10.1038/s41598-025-06574-w PMID: 40624105

Alotaibi, B., Khan, F. A., & Mahmood, S. (2024). Communication Efficiency and Non-Independent and Identically Distributed Data Challenge in Federated Learning: A Systematic Mapping study. *Applied Sciences (Basel, Switzerland), 14*(7), 2720. DOI: 10.3390/app14072720

Alowais, S. A., Alghamdi, S. S., Alsuhebany, N., Alqahtani, T., Alshaya, A. I., Almohareb, S. N., Aldairem, A., Alrashed, M., Saleh, K. B., Badreldin, H. A., Yami, M. S. A., Harbi, S. A., & Albekairy, A. M. (2023). Revolutionizing healthcare: The role of artificial intelligence in clinical practice. *BMC Medical Education, 23*(1), 689. DOI: 10.1186/s12909-023-04698-z PMID: 37740191

Alqubaysi, T., Asmari, A. F. A., Alanazi, F., Almutairi, A., & Armghan, A. (2025). Federated learning-based predictive traffic management using a contained privacy-preserving scheme for autonomous vehicles. *Sensors (Basel), 25*(4), 1116. DOI: 10.3390/s25041116 PMID: 40006346

Anandavally, B. B. (2024). Improving Clinical Support Through Retrieval-Augmented Generation Powered Virtual Health Assistants. *Journal of Computer and Communications, 12*(11), 86–94. DOI: 10.4236/jcc.2024.1211006

Andreoni, M., Lunardi, W. T., Lawton, G., & Thakkar, S. (2024). Enhancing autonomous system security and resilience with generative AI: A comprehensive survey. *IEEE Access : Practical Innovations, Open Solutions*, *12*, 109470–109493. DOI: 10.1109/ACCESS.2024.3439363

Ansari, R. A., Senapati, S. G., Ahluwalia, V., Panjwani, G. A. R., Kaur, A., Yerrapragada, G., & Asadimanesh, N. (2025). Artificial intelligence-guided neuromodulation in heart failure with preserved and reduced ejection fraction: Mechanisms, evidence, and future directions. *Journal of Cardiovascular Development and Disease*, *12*(8), 314. DOI: 10.3390/jcdd12080314 PMID: 40863380

Arikumar, K. S., Prathiba, S. B., Alazab, M., Gadekallu, T. R., Pandya, S., Khan, J. M., & Moorthy, R. S. (2022). FL-PMI: Federated learning-based person movement identification through wearable devices in smart healthcare systems. *Sensors (Basel)*, *22*(4), 1377. DOI: 10.3390/s22041377 PMID: 35214282

Arunprasath, S., & Annamalai, S. (2024). Improving patient centric data retrieval and cyber security in healthcare: Privacy preserving solutions for a secure future. *Multimedia Tools and Applications*, *83*(27), 70289–70319. DOI: 10.1007/s11042-024-18253-5

Asan, O., Bayrak, A. E., & Choudhury, A. (2020). Artificial Intelligence and Human Trust in Healthcare: Focus on Clinicians. *Journal of Medical Internet Research*, *22*(6), 1–7. DOI: 10.2196/15154 PMID: 32558657

Ashraf, M., & Haile, A. (2023). Data protection and AI: Navigating regulatory compliance in AI-driven systems. In: ed.

Babar, M., Qureshi, B., & Koubaa, A. (2024). Investigating the impact of data heterogeneity on the performance of federated learning algorithm using medical imaging. *PLoS One*, *19*(5), e0302539. DOI: 10.1371/journal.pone.0302539 PMID: 38748657

Bacha, A., & Shah, H. H. (2025). AI-Powered Virtual Health Assistants: Transforming Patient Care and Engagement. *Global Insights in Artificial Intelligence and Computing*, *1*(1), 15–30.

Bagdasaryan, E., Veit, A., Hua, Y., Estrin, D., & Shmatikov, V. (2020). How to backdoor federated learning. *Proceedings of the 23rd International Conference on Artificial Intelligence and Statistics (AISTATS)*, 2938–2948.

Bajwa, J., Munir, U., Nori, A., & Williams, B. (2021). Artificial intelligence in healthcare: Transforming the practice of medicine. *Future Healthcare Journal*, *8*(2), e188–e194. DOI: 10.7861/fhj.2021-0095 PMID: 34286183

Bala, I., Pindoo, I. A., Mijwil, M. M., Abotaleb, M., & Yundong, W. (2024). Ensuring Security and Privacy in Healthcare Systems: A Review Exploring Challenges, Solutions, Future Trends, and the Practical Applications of Artificial Intelligence. *Jordan Medical Journal*, *58*(2), 250–270. DOI: 10.35516/jmj.v58i2.2527

Barkas, G. I., Dimeas, I. E., & Kotsiou, O. S. (2025). Bug Wars: Artificial Intelligence Strikes Back in Sepsis Management. *Diagnostics (Basel)*, *15*(15), 1890. DOI: 10.3390/diagnostics15151890 PMID: 40804855

Basharat, I., & Shahid, S. (2024). AI-enabled chatbots healthcare systems: An ethical perspective on trust and reliability. *Journal of Health Organization and Management*. Advance online publication. DOI: 10.1108/JHOM-10-2023-0302

Batista, A. S. (2025). The Transforming Clinical Practice: The Role of AI-Powered Medical Assistants in Enhancing Healthcare Efficiency and Decision-Making. Journal of Next-Generation Research 5.0.

Bebortta, S., Tripathy, S. S., Basheer, S., & Chowdhary, C. L. (2023). FedEHR: A Federated Learning Approach towards the Prediction of Heart Diseases in IoT-Based Electronic Health Records. *Diagnostics (Basel)*, *13*(20), 3166. DOI: 10.3390/diagnostics13203166 PMID: 37891987

Bembinov, M., & Soenardi, N. (2023). An assessment of client and clinician satisfaction in veterinary teleconsultation compared to in-person consultations. *Vet. Evid*, *7*, 1–17. PMID: 42006178

Bhattacharya, S., Reddy Maddikunta, P. K., Pham, Q. V., Gadekallu, T. R., & Krishnan, S. (2021). Deep learning and medical image processing for coronavirus (COVID-19) pandemic: A survey. *Sustainable Cities and Society*, *65*(November), 102589. DOI: 10.1016/j.scs.2020.102589 PMID: 33169099

Bhosale, Y. (2025). Real-Time Monitoring of Fetal Arrhythmias Using AI-Driven Cardiotocography Systems. *Vascular and Endovascular Review (ISSN: 2516-3302)*.

Blanchard, P., El Mhamdi, E. M., Guerraoui, R., & Stainer, J. (2017). Machine learning with adversaries: Byzantine tolerant gradient descent. *Advances in Neural Information Processing Systems (NeurIPS)*, 30.

Bonawitz, K., Ivanov, V., Kreuter, B., Marcedone, A., McMahan, B., Patel, S., Ramage, D., Segal, A., & Seth, K. (2017). Practical secure aggregation for privacy-preserving machine learning. *Proceedings of the 2017 ACM SIGSAC Conference on Computer and Communications Security (CCS)*, 1175–1191. https://doi.org/DOI: 10.1145/3133956.3133982

Boukaf, M., Fadli, F., & Meskin, N. (2024). A comprehensive review of digital twin technology in building energy consumption forecasting. *IEEE Access : Practical Innovations, Open Solutions, 12*, 187778–187799. DOI: 10.1109/ACCESS.2024.3498107

Branda, F., Stella, M., Ceccarelli, C., Cabitza, F., Ceccarelli, G., Maruotti, A., Ciccozzi, M., & Scarpa, F. (2025). The Role of AI-Based Chatbots in Public Health Emergencies: A Narrative Review. *Future Internet, 17*(4), 145. DOI: 10.3390/fi17040145

Brian Brenner, M. D., Scott Brancolini, M. D., Yashar Eshraghi, M. D., Maged Guirguis, M. D., Shravani Durbhakula, M. D., David Provenzano, M. D., & Kevin Vorenkamp, M. D. (2022). Telemedicine implementation in pain medicine: A survey evaluation of pain medicine practices in spring 2020. *Pain Physician, 25*, 387–390. PMID: 35901479

Cai, L., Gao, J., & Zhao, D. (2020). A review of the application of deep learning in medical image classification and segmentation. *Annals of Translational Medicine, 8*(11), 713–713. DOI: 10.21037/atm.2020.02.44 PMID: 32617333

Chakraborty, C., Gupta, B., & Ghosh, S. K. (2013). A review on telemedicine-based WBAN framework for patient monitoring. *Telemedicine Journal and e-Health, 19*(8), 619–626. DOI: 10.1089/tmj.2012.0215 PMID: 23841489

Chauhan, S., Paliwal, M., Manchanda, N., & Gupta, M. (2024). AI and Machine Learning in Modern Healthcare. In Transforming Gender-Based Healthcare with AI and Machine Learning (pp. 1-13). CRC Press. DOI: 10.1201/9781003473435-1

Chavali, D., Dhiman, V. K., & Katari, S. C. (2024). AI-Powered Virtual Health Assistants: Transforming Patient Engagement through Virtual Nursing. *International Journal of Pharma Sciences, 2*, 613–624.

Cheng, X., Oun, A., & Wince, K. (2025). *The Role of Artificial Intelligence in Boosting Cybersecurity and Trusted Embedded Systems Performance: A Systematic Review on Current and Future Trends*. IEEE.

Chen, Y., Qin, X., Wang, J., Yu, C., & Gao, W. (2020). FedHealth: A federated transfer learning framework for wearable healthcare. *IEEE Intelligent Systems, 35*(4), 83–93. DOI: 10.1109/MIS.2020.2988604

Chiruvella, V., & Guddati, A. K. (2021). Ethical issues in patient data ownership. *Interactive Journal of Medical Research, 10*(2), e22269. DOI: 10.2196/22269 PMID: 34018968

Dara, S., Kanapala, A., Babu, A. R., Dhamercherala, S., Vidyarthi, A., & Agarwal, R. (2022). Scalable Federated-Learning and Internet-of-Things enabled architecture for Chest Computer Tomography image classification. *Computers & Electrical Engineering*, *102*, 108266. DOI: 10.1016/j.compeleceng.2022.108266

Datta, S., & Namasudra, S. (2024). Blockchain-based smart contract model for securing healthcare transactions by using consumer electronics and mobile-edge computing. *IEEE Transactions on Consumer Electronics*, *70*(1), 4026–4036. DOI: 10.1109/TCE.2024.3357115

Devaraj, S. J., & Ezra, K. (2011, April). Current trends and future challenges in wireless telemedicine system. In 2011 3rd International Conference on Electronics Computer Technology (Vol. 4, pp. 417-421). IEEE. DOI: 10.1109/ICECTECH.2011.5941933

Dhanka, S., Kumar, A., Sharma, A., Vundavilli, H., Maini, S., & Rajasekar, E. (2025). Advances in machine learning and deep learning for hormonal disorder diagnosis: An exhaustive review on PCOS, thyroid, and optimization techniques. *Archives of Computational Methods in Engineering*, •••, 1–45.

Dhanushkodi, K., & Thejas, S. (2024). AI enabled threat detection: Leveraging artificial intelligence for advanced security and cyber threat mitigation. *IEEE Access : Practical Innovations, Open Solutions*, *12*, 173127–173136. DOI: 10.1109/ACCESS.2024.3493957

Dhinakaran, D., Sankar, S. M., Selvaraj, D., & Raja, S. E. (2024). Privacy-preserving data in IoT-based cloud systems: A comprehensive survey with AI integration. arXiv preprint arXiv:2401.00794.

Dhinakaran, D., Selvaraj, D., Dharini, N., Raja, S. E., & Priya, C. S. L. (2023). Towards a Novel Privacy-Preserving Distributed Multiparty Data Outsourcing Scheme for Cloud Computing with Quantum Key Distribution. *International Journal of Intelligent Systems and Applications in Engineering*, *12*(2), 286–300.

Dinh-Le, C., Chuang, R., Chokshi, S., & Mann, D. (2019). Wearable Health Technology and Electronic Health Record Integration: Scoping review and Future Directions. *JMIR mHealth and uHealth*, *7*(9), e12861. DOI: 10.2196/12861 PMID: 31512582

Doshi-Velez, F., & Kim, B. (2017). Towards a rigorous science of interpretable machine learning. *arXiv preprint arXiv:1702.08608.*

Dwork, C., & Roth, A. (2014). The algorithmic foundations of differential privacy. *Foundations and Trends in Theoretical Computer Science*, *9*(3–4), 211–407. DOI: 10.1561/0400000042

Edwin Raja, S., Ramathilagam, A., Jeno Jasmine, J., & Suganya, S. (2025). Ensuring privacy and security of EHR with secure collaborative transfer learning (SCTL). In *Generative AI techniques for sustainability in healthcare security* (p. 30). DOI: 10.4018/979-8-3693-6577-9.ch012

Edwin Raja, S., Ramesh, T., Thevahi, B., & Prabaharan, G. (2025). SI-CL-SDEO algorithm for improving HDFS performance and data reliability. *Results in Engineering*, *26*, 104773. DOI: 10.1016/j.rineng.2025.104773

Elkhateeb, S., & Anwar, R. (2025). Parametric Optimization of Urban Street Tree Placement: Computational Workflow for Dynamic Shade Provision in Hot Climates. *Urban Science (Basel, Switzerland)*, *9*(12), 504. DOI: 10.3390/urbansci9120504

Esmaeilzadeh, P. (2023). Evolution of health information sharing between health care organizations: Potential of nonfungible tokens. *Interactive Journal of Medical Research*, *12*, e42685. DOI: 10.2196/42685 PMID: 37043269

European Commission. (2021). *Proposal for a regulation laying down harmonised rules on artificial intelligence*. Artificial Intelligence Act.

European Parliament and Council of the European Union. (2016). *Regulation (EU) 2016/679 (General Data Protection Regulation)*. Official Journal of the European Union.

Everard, K. M., Schiel, K. A., Xu, E., & Kulshreshtha, A. (2022). Use of telemedicine in the family medicine clerkship: A CERA study. *PRiMER: Peer-Reviewed Reports in Medical Education Research*, *6*, 25. DOI: 10.22454/PRiMER.2022.105712 PMID: 36119909

Ezz, M., Alaerjan, A. S., & Mostafa, A. M. (2025). Ethical AI in Healthcare: Integrating Zero-Knowledge Proofs and Smart Contracts for Transparent Data Governance. *Bioengineering (Basel, Switzerland)*, *12*(11), 1–30. DOI: 10.3390/bioengineering12111236 PMID: 41301192

Fahad, M., Abbasi, N., Qayyum, M. U., Fnu, N., & Zeb, S. (2024). Ethical and Legal Challenges in AI-Driven Healthcare: Patient Privacy, Data Security, Legal Framework, and Compliance. *Article in International Journal of Innovative Research in Science Engineering and Technology*, *13*(8). Advance online publication. DOI: 10.15680/IJIRSET.2024.1308136

Fang, C., Dziedzic, A., Zhang, L., Oliva, L., Verma, A., Razak, F., Papernot, N., & Wang, B. (2024). Decentralised, collaborative, and privacy-preserving machine learning for multi-hospital data. *EBioMedicine*, *101*, 105006. DOI: 10.1016/j.ebiom.2024.105006 PMID: 38377795

Ferraiolo, D. F., & Kuhn, D. R. (1992). Role-based access controls. *15th National Computer Security Conference*, 554–563.

Fredrikson, M., Jha, S., & Ristenpart, T. (2015). Model inversion attacks that exploit confidence information and basic countermeasures. *Proceedings of the 22nd ACM SIGSAC Conference on Computer and Communications Security (CCS)*, 1322–1333. https://doi.org/DOI: 10.1145/2810103.2813677

Galiana, L. I., Gudino, L. C., & González, P. M. (2024)... *Revista Clínica Española, 224*, 178–186. DOI: 10.1016/j.rceng.2024.02.003 PMID: 38355097

Gerke, S., Minssen, T., & Cohen, G. (2020). Ethical and legal challenges of artificial intelligence-driven healthcare. In *Artificial Intelligence in Healthcare*. INC., DOI: 10.1016/B978-0-12-818438-7.00012-5

Goktas, P., & Grzybowski, A. (2025). Shaping the Future of Healthcare: Ethical Clinical Challenges and Pathways to Trustworthy AI. *Journal of Clinical Medicine, 14*(5), 1–28. DOI: 10.3390/jcm14051605 PMID: 40095575

Goodfellow, I. J., Shlens, J., & Szegedy, C. (2015). Explaining and harnessing adversarial examples. *International Conference on Learning Representations (ICLR)*.

Gopalakrishnan, S., Selvaraj, D., Girija, M. S., & Prabaharan, G. (2025). Mining privacy-preserving association rules using transaction hewer allocator and facile hash algorithm in multi-cloud environments. *MethodsX, 14*, 103317. DOI: 10.1016/j.mex.2025.103317 PMID: 40331027

Grataloup, A., Jonas, S., & Meyer, A. (2024). A review of federated learning in renewable energy applications: Potential, challenges, and future directions. *Energy and AI, 17*, 100375. DOI: 10.1016/j.egyai.2024.100375

Guo, Y., Hao, Z., Zhao, S., Gong, J., & Yang, F. (2020). Artificial intelligence in health care: Bibliometric analysis. *Journal of Medical Internet Research, 22*(7), 1–12. DOI: 10.2196/18228 PMID: 32723713

Gu, X., Sabrina, F., Fan, Z., & Sohail, S. (2023). A review of privacy enhancement methods for federated learning in healthcare systems. *International Journal of Environmental Research and Public Health, 20*(15), 6539. DOI: 10.3390/ijerph20156539 PMID: 37569079

Habehh, H., & Gohel, S. (2021). Machine learning in healthcare. *Current Genomics, 22*(4), 291–300. DOI: 10.2174/1389202922666210705124359 PMID: 35273459

Harrath, Y., Adohinzin, O., Kaabi, J., & Saathoff, M. (2025). Bridging Domains: Advances in Explainable, Automated, and Privacy-Preserving AI for Computer Science and Cybersecurity. *Computers, 14*(9), 374. DOI: 10.3390/computers14090374

Hasan, M. M. (2025). Federated Learning Models for Privacy-Preserving AI In Enterprise Decision Systems. *International Journal of Business and Economics Insights, 5*(3), 238–269. DOI: 10.63125/ry033286

Hassan, S. U., Abdulkadir, S. J., Zahid, M. S. M., & Al-Selwi, S. M. (2024). Local interpretable model-agnostic explanation approach for medical imaging analysis: A systematic literature review. *Computers in Biology and Medicine, 185*, 109569. DOI: 10.1016/j.compbiomed.2024.109569 PMID: 39705792

Hendaoui, F., Ferchichi, A., Trabelsi, L., Meddeb, R., Ahmed, R., & Khelifi, M. K. (2024). Advances in deep learning intrusion detection over encrypted data with privacy preservation: A systematic review. *Cluster Computing, 27*(7), 8683–8724. DOI: 10.1007/s10586-024-04424-4

Hindelang, M., Sitaru, S., & Zink, A. (2024). Transforming Health Care through Chatbots for Medical History-Taking and Future Directions: Comprehensive Systematic Review. *JMIR Medical Informatics, 12*(1), e56628. DOI: 10.2196/56628

Holubenko, V., Gaspar, D., Leal, R., & Silva, P. (2025). Autonomous intrusion detection for IoT: A decentralized and privacy preserving approach. *International Journal of Information Security, 24*(1), 7. DOI: 10.1007/s10207-024-00926-9

Hosen, M. S., Fakir, M., Hawlader, S. C., Rahman, F., Karim, T., & Uddin, M. H. (2025). Generative AI-Driven Decision-Making for Disease Control and Pandemic Preparedness Model 4.0 in Rural Communities of Bangladesh: Management Informatics Approach. *arXiv preprint arXiv:2508.01142.*

Hou, J., Cheng, X., Liao, J., & Zhang, Z. (2026). *Ethical concerns of AI in healthcare : A systematic review of qualitative studies. 33*(371), 428–449. DOI: 10.1177/09697330251385024

Husnain, A. (2025). Smarter Healthcare: Harnessing AI for Faster, More Accurate, and Accessible Medicine. *Global Trends in Science and Technology, 1*(2), 1–22. DOI: 10.70445/gtst.1.2.2025.1-22

Ighofiomoni, M. O., Ojerinde, J. S., Olaniyan, I., Issah, P. P., Adepitan, O. S., Oyenuga, O., & Chinonyerem, C. A. (2025). Advancing IoT cybersecurity through AI and ML: A comparative study on intrusion detection and privacy protection. *Asian Journal of Advanced Research and Reports, 19*(8), 159–174. DOI: 10.9734/ajarr/2025/v19i81122

Ikegwu, A. C., Alo, U. R., Nweke, H. F., & Ebem, D. U. (2026). Advancing federated learning frameworks for privacy-preserving cyber threat detection in healthcare systems. *International Journal of Computational Intelligence Systems*, *19*(1), 169. DOI: 10.1007/s44196-026-01274-3

Islam, S. M., & Mondal, H. S. (2019). Image Enhancement Based Medical Image Analysis. 2019 10th International Conference on Computing, Communication and Networking Technologies, ICCCNT 2019, 1–5. DOI: 10.1109/ICCCNT45670.2019.8944910

Islam, M. J., Rahman, A., Kabir, S., Karim, M. R., Acharjee, U. K., Nasir, M. K., Band, S. S., Sookhak, M., & Wu, S. (2021). Blockchain-SDN-Based Energy-Aware and distributed secure architecture for IoT in smart cities. *IEEE Internet of Things Journal*, *9*(5), 3850–3864. DOI: 10.1109/JIOT.2021.3100797

Islam, M., & Khan, F. (2024). *Adaptive Software Engineering: Integrating AI-driven Techniques for Software Development.* IUB, CSE, Jayanthi, S., Suhasini, S., Sharmili, N., Laxmi Lydia, E., Shwetha, V., Dash, B. B., & Bachute, M. (2025). A deep dive into artificial intelligence with enhanced optimization-based security breach detection in internet of health things enabled smart city environment. *Scientific Reports*, *15*(1), 22909. PMID: 39358471

Jagadish Kumar, N., Ponnuviji, N. P., & Praveen Kumar, B. (2025). Safeguarding confidentiality and privacy in cloud-enabled healthcare systems with spectrasafe encryption and dynamic k-anonymity algorithm. *Expert Systems with Applications*, *279*, 127584. DOI: 10.1016/j.eswa.2025.127584

Javed, H., Muqeet, H. A., Danesh, A., Rehman, A. U., Javed, T., & Bermak, A. (2024). Impact of AI and Dynamic Ensemble Techniques in Enhancing Healthcare Services: Opportunities and Ethical Challenges. *IEEE Access : Practical Innovations, Open Solutions*, *12*(July), 141064–141087. DOI: 10.1109/ACCESS.2024.3443812

Johannssen, A., & Chukhrova, N. (2025). The crucial role of explainable artificial intelligence (XAI) in improving health care management. *Health Care Management Science*, *28*(3), 565–570. DOI: 10.1007/s10729-025-09720-y PMID: 41026402

Kairouz, P., McMahan, H. B., Avent, B., Bellet, A., Bennis, M., Bhagoji, A. N., Bonawitz, K., Charles, Z., Cormode, G., Cummings, R., D'Oliveira, R., Eichner, H., El Rouayheb, S., Evans, D., Gardner, J., Garrett, Z., Gascón, A., Ghazi, B., Gibbons, P. B., & Zhao, S. (2021). Advances and open problems in federated learning. *Foundations and Trends in Machine Learning*, *14*(1–2), 1–210. DOI: 10.1561/2200000083

Kasralikar, P., Polu, O. R., Chamarthi, B., Veer Samara Sihman Bharattej Rupavath, R., Patel, S., & Tumati, R. (2025). Blockchain for Securing AI-Driven Healthcare Systems: A Systematic Review and Future Research Perspectives. *Cureus*, *17*(4). Advance online publication. DOI: 10.7759/cureus.83136 PMID: 40438823

Ker, J., Wang, L., Rao, J., & Lim, T. (2017). Deep Learning Applications in Medical Image Analysis. *IEEE Access : Practical Innovations, Open Solutions*, *6*, 9375–9379. DOI: 10.1109/ACCESS.2017.2788044

khan, A. A., Ghodhbani, R., Alsufyani, A., Alsufyani, N., & Mohamed, M. A. (2025). Leveraging blockchain-integrated explainable artificial intelligence (XAI) for ethical and personalized healthcare decision-making: a framework for secure data sharing and enhanced patient trust. The Journal of Supercomputing, 81(15), 1353.

Khan, L. U., Saad, W., Han, Z., Hossain, E., & Hong, C. S. (2021). *Federated learning for Internet of Things: Recent advances, taxonomy, and open challenges*. arXiv. https://doi.org//arXiv.2009.13012DOI: 10.48550

Khan, A. (2025). DEVELOPMENT OF PERSONALIZED, NON-HORMONAL, AI-DRIVEN TREATMENT PATHWAYS FOR HEAVY MENSTRUAL BLEEDING BASED ON MENSTRUAL BLOOD BIOMARKERS AND UTERINE MICROBIOME PROFILING. *Pakistan Journal of Medical & Cardiological Review*, *4*(2), 332–361.

Kim, J., Kim, J., Hur, K., & Choi, E. (2026). Federated learning for heterogeneous electronic health record systems with cost effective participant selection. *Scientific Reports*, *16*(1), 6876. DOI: 10.1038/s41598-026-38299-9 PMID: 41622329

Kindervag, J. (2010). *No more chewy centers: Introducing the zero trust model of information security*. Forrester Research.

Kjwan, A. H., & Mohammad, O. H. (2024). Enhancing Medical Data Analysis with Federated Learning in the Internet of Medical Things. *International Journal of Research in Science & Engineering*, *43*(43), 38–52. DOI: 10.55529/ijrise.43.38.52

Kodete, C. S., Thuraka, B., & Pasupuleti, V. (2024). A systematic review of AI-driven and quantum-resistant security solutions for cyber-physical systems: Blockchain, federated learning, and emerging technologies. In *Proceedings of the 2024 International Conference on Computer and Applications (ICCA)* (pp. 1–6). DOI: 10.1109/ICCA62237.2024.10927942

Kolhar, A. & Sridevi. (2026). Secure and Ethically Aligned AI Solutions for Cybersecurity and Threat Detection. In *Ethical AI Applications for Software Engineering and Development*., DOI: 10.4018/979-8-3373-6038-6.ch011

Kolhar, A., & Gundoor, T. K. (2026). API Security Testing and Exploitation Techniques. *Advanced Cybersecurity for Threats Exploitation and Digital Risk*, 87–116. DOI: 10.4018/979-8-2600-0747-1.ch004

Kolhar, A., & Sridevi. (2025). Principles and Emerging Trends of Healthcare Robotics. *Robotics and IoT Synergy in Next-Generation Healthcare*, 401–428. DOI: 10.4018/979-8-3373-5447-7.ch012

Kolhar, A. (2025). *Sridevi, Soni, H., & Kant, K.* Blockchain and AI Secure Wireless Transactions., DOI: 10.4018/979-8-3373-3576-6.ch007

Koshechkin, K., & Khokholov, A. (2024). Ethical issues in implementing artificial intelligence in healthcare. *Медицинская Этика*, *2024*(1), 11–17. DOI: 10.24075/medet.2024.006

Kumar, K. S., Nelson, L., & Jibinsingh, B. R. (2025). Systematic review of privacy-preserving Federated Learning in decentralized healthcare systems. *Franklin Open*, *13*, 100440. DOI: 10.1016/j.fraope.2025.100440

Laghari, A. A., Khan, A. A., Ksibi, A., Hajjej, F., Kryvinska, N., Almadhor, A., Mohamed, M. A., & Alsubai, S. (2025). A novel and secure artificial intelligence enabled zero trust intrusion detection in industrial internet of things architecture. *Scientific Reports*, *15*(1), 26843. DOI: 10.1038/s41598-025-11738-9 PMID: 40702039

Laxminarayan, S., & Istepanian, R. S. (2000). UNWIRED E-MED: The next generation of wireless and internet telemedicine systems. *IEEE Transactions on Information Technology in Biomedicine*, *4*(3), 189–193. DOI: 10.1109/TITB.2000.5956074 PMID: 11026588

Laymouna, M., Ma, Y., Lessard, D., Schuster, T., Engler, K., & Lebouché, B. (2024). Roles, users, benefits, and limitations of chatbots in health care: Rapid review. *Journal of Medical Internet Research*, *26*, e56930. DOI: 10.2196/56930

Lazaros, K., Koumadorakis, D. E., Vrahatis, A. G., & Kotsiantis, S. (2024). Federated Learning: Navigating the Landscape of Collaborative Intelligence. *Electronics (Basel)*, *13*(23), 4744. Advance online publication. DOI: 10.3390/electronics13234744

Li, F., Ruijs, N., & Lu, Y. (2023). Ethics & AI: A Systematic Review on Ethical Concerns and Related Strategies for Designing with AI in Healthcare. *AI*, *4*(1), 28–53. DOI: 10.3390/ai4010003

Lim, W. Y. B., Luong, N. C., Hoang, D. T., Jiao, Y., Liang, Y.-C., Yang, Q., Niyato, D., & Miao, C. (2020). Federated learning in mobile edge networks: A comprehensive survey. *IEEE Communications Surveys and Tutorials*, *22*(3), 2031–2063. DOI: 10.1109/COMST.2020.2986024

Liu, M., Wang, L., Jia, R., Ji, S., Wu, Y., Wu, Y., Xie, L., & Dong, M. (2025). Cross-Modal and Contrastive Optimization for Explainable Multimodal Recognition of Predatory and Parasitic Insects. *Insects, 16*(12), 1187. DOI: 10.3390/insects16121187 PMID: 41465627

Li, X., Gu, Y., Dvornek, N., Staib, L. H., Ventola, P., & Duncan, J. S. (2020). Multi-site fMRI analysis using privacy-preserving federated learning and domain adaptation: ABIDE results. *Medical Image Analysis, 65*, 101765. DOI: 10.1016/j.media.2020.101765 PMID: 32679533

Ma, B., Feng, Y., Chen, G., Li, C., & Xia, Y. (2023). Federated adaptive reweighting for medical image classification. *Pattern Recognition, 144*, 109880. DOI: 10.1016/j.patcog.2023.109880

Maher, C., Singh, B., Wylde, A., & Chastin, S. (2024). Virtual health assistants: A grand challenge in health communications and behavior change. *Frontiers in Digital Health, 6*, 1418695. DOI: 10.3389/fdgth.2024.1418695

Manesh, M. T., Hoonejani, M. R., Gousheh, S. G., Abdolmaleki, A., Dehnavi, A. N., & Shahrashoob, A. (2025). AI-driven control algorithm using machine learning and genetic optimization for enhancing visual comfort in adaptive façades. *Automation in Construction, 179*, 106474. DOI: 10.1016/j.autcon.2025.106474

Martínez, A. L., Pérez, M. G., & Ruiz-Martínez, A. (2023). A comprehensive model for securing sensitive patient data in a clinical scenario. *IEEE Access : Practical Innovations, Open Solutions, 11*, 137083–137098. DOI: 10.1109/ACCESS.2023.3338170

Masood, I., Daud, A., Wang, Y., Banjar, A., & Alharbey, R. (2024). A blockchain-based system for patient data privacy and security. *Multimedia Tools and Applications, 83*(21), 60443–60467. DOI: 10.1007/s11042-023-17941-y

Mathew, J., & Krishnan, A. (2025). Artificial Intelligence in Computer Science and Information Technology: A Synergy for Intelligent Systems and Software Engineering. *GRJESTM, 1*(3), 135–141.

Matta, S. S., & Bolli, M. (2025). Federated Learning for Privacy-Preserving Healthcare Data Sharing: Enabling Global AI Collaboration. *American Journal of Scholarly Research and Innovation, 4*(01), 320–351. DOI: 10.63125/jga18304

McGraw, G. (2006). *Software security: Building security in.* Addison-Wesley.

McMahan, B., Moore, E., Ramage, D., & Hampson, S. Arcas, B.A.y. (2017). Communication-Efficient Learning of Deep Networks from Decentralized Data. Proceedings of the 20th International Conference on Artificial Intelligence and Statistics, in Proceedings of Machine Learning Research 54:1273-1282 Available from https://proceedings.mlr.press/v54/mcmahan17a.html.

McMahan, H. B., Moore, E., Ramage, D., Hampson, S., & Arcas, B. A. Y. (2017). Communication-efficient learning of deep networks from decentralized data. *Proceedings of the 20th International Conference on Artificial Intelligence and Statistics (AISTATS)*, 1273–1282.

Mennella, C., Maniscalco, U., De Pietro, G., & Esposito, M. (2024). Ethical and regulatory challenges of AI technologies in healthcare: A narrative review. *Heliyon, 10*(4), e26297. DOI: 10.1016/j.heliyon.2024.e26297 PMID: 38384518

Mishra, A., Saha, S., Mishra, S., & Bagade, P. (2023). A federated learning approach for smart healthcare systems. *CSI Transactions on ICT, 11*(1), 39–44. DOI: 10.1007/s40012-023-00382-1

Mishra, S., Chaudhury, P., Tripathy, H. K., Sahoo, K. S., Jhanjhi, N. Z., Hassan Elnour, A. A., & Abdelmaboud, A. (2024). Enhancing health care through medical cognitive virtual agents. *Digital Health, 10*, 20552076241256732. DOI: 10.1177/20552076241256732

Mohsin Khan, M., Shah, N., Shaikh, N., Thabet, A., alrabayah, T., & Belkhair, S. (2024, December). alrabayah, T., & Belkhair, S. (2025). Towards secure and trusted AI in healthcare: A systematic review of emerging innovations and ethical challenges. *International Journal of Medical Informatics, 195*, 105780. DOI: 10.1016/j.ijmedinf.2024.105780 PMID: 39753062

Mollashaik, A. S. (2025). Advancing data security through AI-driven classification: A framework for intelligent threat detection and privacy preservation. [IJCET]. *International Journal of Computer Engineering and Technology, 15*(6), 467–481. DOI: 10.34218/IJCET_16_01_040

Moore, M. (1999). The evolution of telemedicine. *Future Generation Computer Systems, 15*(2), 245–254. DOI: 10.1016/S0167-739X(98)00067-3

Moshawrab, M., Adda, M., Bouzouane, A., Ibrahim, H., & Raad, A. (2023). Reviewing federated machine learning and its use in diseases prediction. *Sensors (Basel), 23*(4), 2112. DOI: 10.3390/s23042112 PMID: 36850717

Moulahi, T., Jabbar, R., Alabdulatif, A., Abbas, S., El Khediri, S., Zidi, S., & Rizwan, M. (2023). Privacy-preserving federated learning cyber-threat detection for intelligent transport systems with blockchain-based security. *Expert Systems: International Journal of Knowledge Engineering and Neural Networks*, *40*(5), e13103. DOI: 10.1111/exsy.13103

Moustafa, N., Koroniotis, N., Keshk, M., Zomaya, A. Y., & Tari, Z. (2023). Explainable intrusion detection for cyber defences in the internet of things: Opportunities and solutions. *IEEE Communications Surveys and Tutorials*, *25*(3), 1775–1807. DOI: 10.1109/COMST.2023.3280465

Muneer, S., Farooq, U., Athar, A., Ahsan Raza, M., Ghazal, T. M., & Sakib, S. (2024). A critical review of artificial intelligence-based approaches in intrusion detection: A comprehensive analysis. *Journal of Engineering*, *2024*(1), 3909173. DOI: 10.1155/2024/3909173

Muschol, J., Heinrich, M., Heiss, C., Knapp, G., Repp, H., Schneider, H., Thormann, U., Uhlar, J., Unzeitig, K., & Gissel, C. (2022). Assessing telemedicine efficiency in follow-up care with video consultations for patients in orthopedic and trauma surgery in Germany: Randomized controlled trial. *Journal of Medical Internet Research*, *24*(7), e36996. DOI: 10.2196/36996 PMID: 35896015

N, P. S., Shelke, N., Saini, D. K. J. B., Pimpalkar, A., Pal, M., & Chirchi, V. (2025). Explainable federated learning for secure and transparent medical diagnosis in IoT-based smart hospitals. In *2025 5th International Conference on Soft Computing for Security Applications (ICSCSA)* (pp. 883–889). IEEE. https://doi.org/DOI: 10.1109/ICSCSA66339.2025.11171173

Naib, P., Park, J., Abedin, P., & King, C. (2026). *Defining an Ethical Explainability Metric for Measuring AI Trustworthiness in Connected Healthcare Systems*. 1–19.

Nankya, M., Mugisa, A., Usman, Y., Upadhyay, A., & Chataut, R. (2024). Security and privacy in e-health systems: A review of AI and machine learning techniques. *IEEE Access : Practical Innovations, Open Solutions*, *12*(October), 148796–148816. DOI: 10.1109/ACCESS.2024.3469215

Narayan, S. B. (2025). Safeguarding Intelligence: A Comprehensive Analysis of AI Security and Privacy in the Era of Autonomous Systems. Available at *SSRN* 5718122. DOI: 10.2139/ssrn.5718122

Nasir, Z. U. I., Iqbal, A., & Qureshi, H. K. (2024). Securing cyber-physical systems: A decentralized framework for collaborative intrusion detection with privacy preservation. *IEEE Transactions on Industrial Cyber-Physical Systems*, *2*, 303–311. DOI: 10.1109/TICPS.2024.3425794

National Institute of Standards and Technology (NIST). (2020). *Security and privacy controls for information systems and organizations (SP 800-53 Rev. 5)*. U.S. Department of Commerce.

National Institute of Standards and Technology (NIST). (2021). *Software bill of materials (SBOM) considerations*. U.S. Department of Commerce.

Nazari, A., Jazaeri, S. S., Omidi, A., & Mansoorizadeh, M. (2025). An AI-driven multi-stage routing protocol for energy-efficient IoT networks. *Telecommunication Systems*, *88*(3), 113. DOI: 10.1007/s11235-025-01344-5

Ndibe, O. S. (2025). Ai-driven forensic systems for real-time anomaly detection and threat mitigation in cybersecurity infrastructures. *International Journal of Research Publication and Reviews*, *6*(5), 389–411. DOI: 10.55248/gengpi.6.0525.1991

Nivedhitha, D. P., Madhumitha, G., Sri, J. J., Jayashree, S., Surya, J., & Divya, D. M. (2024, April). Conversational AI for healthcare to improve member efficiency. In *2024 International Conference on Science Technology Engineering and Management (ICSTEM)* (pp. 1-6). IEEE. DOI: 10.1109/ICSTEM61137.2024.10561046

Noor, A., Chaman, U. M., & Kabir, M. S. (2026). Federated learning in healthcare: A comprehensive survey on privacy, scalability and clinical applications. *ICT Express*. Advance online publication. DOI: 10.1016/j.icte.2026.05.011

Noorzai, E., Bakmohammadi, P., & Garmaroudi, M. A. (2023). Optimizing daylight, energy and occupant comfort performance of classrooms with photovoltaic integrated vertical shading devices. *Architectural Engineering and Design Management*, *19*(4), 394–418. DOI: 10.1080/17452007.2022.2080173

Oh, W., & Nadkarni, G. N. (2023). Federated Learning in Health care Using Structured Medical Data. *Advances in Kidney Disease and Health*, *30*(1), 4–16. DOI: 10.1053/j.akdh.2022.11.007 PMID: 36723280

Padmavathi, V., & Saminathan, R. (2025). A federated edge intelligence framework with trust-based access control for secure and privacy preserving IoT systems. *Scientific Reports*, *15*(1), 35832. DOI: 10.1038/s41598-025-19712-1 PMID: 41087484

Pandian, P. S., Safeer, K. P., Shakunthala, D. T. I., Gopal, P., & Padaki, V. C. (2007). Store and Forward Applications in Telemedicine for Wireless IP Based Networks. *J. Networks*, *2*(6), 58–65. DOI: 10.4304/jnw.2.6.58-65

Pattichis, C. S., Kyriacou, E., Voskarides, S., Pattichis, M. S., Istepanian, R., & Schizas, C. N. (2002). Wireless telemedicine systems: An overview. *IEEE Antennas & Propagation Magazine*, *44*(2), 143–153. DOI: 10.1109/MAP.2002.1003651

Paul, D., Sanap, G., Shenoy, S., Kalyane, D., Kalia, K., & Tekade, R. K. (2020). Artificial intelligence in drug discovery and development. *Drug Discovery Today*, *26*(1), 80–93. DOI: 10.1016/j.drudis.2020.10.010 PMID: 33099022

Paul, M., Maglaras, L., Ferrag, M. A., & Almomani, I. (2023). Digitization of healthcare sector: A study on privacy and security concerns. *ICT Express*, *9*(4), 571–588. DOI: 10.1016/j.icte.2023.02.007

Periáñez, Á., Fernández Del Río, A., Nazarov, I., Jané, E., Hassan, M., Rastogi, A., & Tang, D. (2024). The digital transformation in health: How AI can improve the performance of health systems. *Health Systems and Reform*, *10*(2), 2387138. DOI: 10.1080/23288604.2024.2387138 PMID: 39437247

Pham, Q. V., Dev, K., Maddikunta, P. K. R., Gadekallu, T. R., & Huynh-The, T. (2021). *Fusion of federated learning and industrial Internet of Things: A survey* (arXiv:2101.00798). arXiv. https://arxiv.org/abs/2101.00798

Ponnusamy, S., Assaf, M., Antari, J., Singh, S., & Kalyanaraman, S. (2024). *Digital twin technology and AI implementations in future-focused businesses*. IGI Global. DOI: 10.4018/979-8-3693-1818-8

Prabaharan, G., Valarmathi, K., Sankar, S. U., & Sugumar, R. (2025). Safeguarding privacy by utilizing SC-DℓDA algorithm in cloud-enabled multi-party computation. *KSII Transactions on Internet and Information Systems*, *19*(2), 635–656. DOI: 10.3837/tiis.2025.02.014

Pustokhina, I. V., Pustokhin, D. A., Gupta, D., Khanna, A., Shankar, K., & Nguyen, G. N. (2020). An effective training scheme for deep neural network in edge computing enabled Internet of Medical Things (IOMT) systems. *IEEE Access : Practical Innovations, Open Solutions*, *8*, 107112–107123. DOI: 10.1109/ACCESS.2020.3000322

Puttagunta, M., & Ravi, S. (2021). Medical image analysis based on deep learning approach. *Multimedia Tools and Applications*, *80*(16), 24365–24398. DOI: 10.1007/s11042-021-10707-4 PMID: 33841033

Qayyum, A., Ahmad, K., Ahsan, M. A., Al-Fuqaha, A., & Qadir, J. (2021). Collaborative Federated Learning for Healthcare: Multi-Modal COVID-19 Diagnosis at the Edge. ArXiv. https://arxiv.org/abs/2101.07511

Qin, Z., Liang, L., Wang, Z., Jin, S., Tao, X., Tong, W., & Li, G. Y. (2024). AI empowered wireless communications: From bits to semantics. *Proceedings of the IEEE*. DOI: 10.1109/JPROC.2024.3437730

Qi, P., Chiaro, D., Guzzo, A., Ianni, M., Fortino, G., & Piccialli, F. (2023). Model aggregation techniques in federated learning: A comprehensive survey. *Future Generation Computer Systems*, *150*, 272–293. DOI: 10.1016/j.future.2023.09.008

Rahman, A., Hossain, M. S., Muhammad, G., Kundu, D., Debnath, T., Rahman, M., Khan, M. S. I., Tiwari, P., & Band, S. S. (2022b). Federated learning-based AI approaches in smart healthcare: Concepts, taxonomies, challenges and open issues. *Cluster Computing*, *26*(4), 2271–2311. DOI: 10.1007/s10586-022-03658-4 PMID: 35996680

Rajagopal, S. M., M, S., & Buyya, R. (2023). FedSDM: Federated learning based smart decision making module for ECG data in IoT integrated Edge–Fog–Cloud computing environments. *Internet of Things : Engineering Cyber Physical Human Systems*, *22*, 100784. DOI: 10.1016/j.iot.2023.100784

Ramani, R., Edwin Raja, S., & Selvaraj, D. (2026). Enhancing clinical data security with the contextual polynomial-based data protection model (CPDPM). *Biomedical Signal Processing and Control*, *111*, 108329. DOI: 10.1016/j.bspc.2025.108329

Raman, R., Rajalakshmi, R., Surya, J., Ramakrishnan, R., Sivaprasad, S., Conroy, D., Thethi, J. P., Mohan, V., & Netuveli, G. (2021). Impact on health and provision of healthcare services during the COVID-19 lockdown in India: A multicentre cross-sectional study. *BMJ Open*, *11*(1), 1–11. DOI: 10.1136/bmjopen-2020-043590 PMID: 33468529

Rani, S., Kataria, A., Kumar, S., & Tiwari, P. (2023). Federated learning for secure IoMT-applications in smart healthcare systems: A comprehensive review. *Knowledge-Based Systems*, *274*, 110658. DOI: 10.1016/j.knosys.2023.110658

Rao, D., & Sharma, S. (2024). Secure and Ethical Innovations: Patenting AI Models for Precision Medicine, Personalized Treatment and Drug Discovery in Healthcare. *International Journal of Business, Management and Visuals*, *6*(September 2023), 1–8.

Rao, S., & Seema, M. VijayaDurga, D., Nallametti, N., Manasa, S., & Keerthana, N. (2025). *Enhancing Big Data Forecasting with Gradient Boosting Machine Learning Framework*. Paper presented at the 2025 9th International Conference on Electronics, Communication and Aerospace Technology (ICECA).

Reddy, K. V., Saketh, G., Priyanshu, S. S., Nitesh, M., Hussain, S. K., & Sharma, K. V. (2025). AI-Driven Healthcare Management Platform: Enhancing Accessibility, Efficiency, and Security in Digital Health Systems. Synthesis: A Multidisciplinary Research Journal, 3(1), 1-14.

Reddy, K. D., & Gadekallu, T. R. (2023). A comprehensive survey on federated learning techniques for healthcare informatics. *Computational Intelligence and Neuroscience, 2023*(1), 8393990. DOI: 10.1155/2023/8393990 PMID: 36909974

Renukalatha, S., & Suresh, K. V. (2018). A review on biomedical image analysis. *Biomedical Engineering : Applications, Basis, and Communications, 30*(4), 1830001. Advance online publication. DOI: 10.4015/S1016237218300018

Rieke, N., Hancox, J., Li, W., Milletarì, F., Roth, H. R., Albarqouni, S., Bakas, S., Galtier, M. N., Landman, B. A., Maier-Hein, K., Ourselin, S., Sheller, M., Summers, R. M., Trask, A., Xu, D., Baust, M., & Cardoso, M. J. (2020). The future of digital health with federated learning. *NPJ Digital Medicine, 3*(1), 119. DOI: 10.1038/s41746-020-00323-1 PMID: 33015372

Saeidnia, H. R., Hashemi Fotami, S. G., Lund, B., & Ghiasi, N. (2024). Ethical considerations in artificial intelligence interventions for mental health and well-being: Ensuring responsible implementation and impact. *Social Sciences (Basel, Switzerland), 13*(7), 381. DOI: 10.3390/socsci13070381

Saltzer, J. H., & Schroeder, M. D. (1975). The protection of information in computer systems. *Proceedings of the IEEE, 63*(9), 1278–1308. DOI: 10.1109/PROC.1975.9939

Samala, A. D., & Rawas, S. (2024). Generative AI as Virtual Healthcare Assistant for Enhancing Patient Care Quality. *International Journal of Online & Biomedical Engineering, 20*(5), 174–187. DOI: 10.3991/ijoe.v20i05.45937

Sandhu, S. S., Gorji, H. T., Tavakolian, P., Tavakolian, K., & Akhbardeh, A. (2023). Medical imaging applications of federated learning. *Diagnostics (Basel), 13*(19), 3140. DOI: 10.3390/diagnostics13193140 PMID: 37835883

Santos, M. R., Guedes, A., & Sanchez-Gendriz, I. (2024). SHapley Additive ExPlanations (SHAP) for efficient feature selection in rolling bearing fault diagnosis. *Machine Learning and Knowledge Extraction, 6*(1), 316–341. DOI: 10.3390/make6010016

Seh, A. H., Zarour, M., Alenezi, M., Sarkar, A. K., Agrawal, A., Kumar, R., & Khan, R. A. (2020). Healthcare data breaches: Insights and implications. *Health Care, 8*(2), 133. DOI: 10.3390/healthcare8020133 PMID: 32414183

Selvaraj, D., Jeno, J., Ramani, R., Dhinakaran, D., & Prabaharan, G. (2025). AFCP data security model for EHR data using blockchain. *Journal of Cybersecurity and Information Management, 15*(1), 22–33. DOI: 10.54216/JCIM.150103

Senbekov, M., Saliev, T., Bukeyeva, Z., Almabayeva, A., Zhanaliyeva, M., Aitenova, N., Toishibekov, Y., & Fakhradiyev, I. (2020). The recent progress and applications of digital technologies in healthcare: A review. *International Journal of Telemedicine and Applications*, *2020*, 1–18. Advance online publication. DOI: 10.1155/2020/8830200 PMID: 33343657

Shaheen, M., Farooq, M. S., Umer, T., & Kim, B. S. (2022). Applications of Federated Learning; Taxonomy, Challenges, and Research Trends. *Electronics (Basel)*, *11*(4), 670. Advance online publication. DOI: 10.3390/electronics11040670

Shaik, T., Tao, X., Higgins, N., Li, L., Gururajan, R., Zhou, X., & Acharya, U. R. (2023). Remote patient monitoring using artificial intelligence: Current state, applications, and challenges. *Wiley Interdisciplinary Reviews. Data Mining and Knowledge Discovery*, *13*(2), e1485. Advance online publication. DOI: 10.1002/widm.1485

Shanmugam, S., & Arumugam, C. (2025). Hybrid ladybug Hawk optimization-enabled deep learning for multimodal Parkinson's disease classification using voice signals and hand-drawn images. *Network (Bristol, England)*, •••, 1–43. DOI: 10.1080/0954898X.2025.2457955 PMID: 40035544

Sharma, D. P., Habibi Lashkari, A., Firoozjaei, M. D., Mahdavifar, S., & Xiong, P. (2025). Defense Methods for Adversarial Attacks and Privacy Issues in Secure AI. In *Understanding AI in Cybersecurity and Secure AI: Challenges, Strategies and Trends* (pp. 159–195). Springer Nature Switzerland. DOI: 10.1007/978-3-031-91524-6_9

Sharma, S. B., & Bairwa, A. K. (2025). Leveraging AI for Intrusion Detection in IoT Ecosystems: A Comprehensive Study. *IEEE Access : Practical Innovations, Open Solutions*, *13*, 66290–66317. DOI: 10.1109/ACCESS.2025.3550392

Sharma, V., Vashishth, T. K., Kumar, B., Sharma, K. K., Vidyant, S., & Chaudhary, S. (2023, December). Health Interpretation of Covid-19 Patients using Artificial Intelligence. In *2023 International Conference on Artificial Intelligence for Innovations in Healthcare Industries (ICAIIHI)* (Vol. 1, pp. 1-5). IEEE Computer Society. DOI: 10.1109/ICAIIHI57871.2023.10488924

Sheller, M. J., Edwards, B., Reina, G. A., Martin, J., Pati, S., Kotrotsou, A., Milchenko, M., Xu, W., Marcus, D., Colen, R. R., & Bakas, S. (2020). Federated learning in medicine: Facilitating multi-institutional collaborations without sharing patient data. *Scientific Reports*, *10*(1), 12598. DOI: 10.1038/s41598-020-69250-1 PMID: 32724046

Sheller, M. J., Reina, G. A., Edwards, B., Martin, J., & Bakas, S. (2019). Multi-institutional deep learning modeling without sharing patient data: A feasibility study on brain tumor segmentation. *Lecture Notes in Computer Science*, *11383*, 92–104. DOI: 10.1007/978-3-030-11723-8_9 PMID: 31231720

Shoghli, A., Darvish, M., & Sadeghian, Y. (2024). Balancing Innovation and Privacy: Ethical Challenges in AI-Driven Healthcare. *Journal of Research in Medical Sciences : the Official Journal of Isfahan University of Medical Sciences*, *4*(1), 31. DOI: 10.22034/jrms.2024.494112.1034

Shojaei, P., Vlahu-Gjorgievska, E., & Chow, Y. (2024). Security and Privacy of Technologies in Health Information Systems: A Systematic Literature review. *Computers*, *13*(2), 41. DOI: 10.3390/computers13020041

Shokri, R., Stronati, M., Song, C., & Shmatikov, V. (2017). Membership inference attacks against machine learning models. *2017 IEEE Symposium on Security and Privacy*, 3–18. https://doi.org/DOI: 10.1109/SP.2017.41

Shostack, A. (2014). *Threat modeling: Designing for security*. Wiley.

Shruthishree, & Tiwari, H. (2017). a Review Paper on Medical Image Processing. International Journal of Research -GRANTHAALAYAH, 5(4RACSIT), 21–29. DOI: 10.29121/granthaalayah.v5.i4RACSIT.2017.3344

Singh, M., Mittal, M., Dewan, P., Kaur, A., Kaur, G., & Gupta, A. (2024, February). From Text to Treatment: An Overview of Artificial Intelligence Chatbots in Healthcare. In 2024 11th International Conference on Computing for Sustainable Global Development (INDIACom) (pp. 690-696). IEEE.

Singh, S., Rathee, T., & Singhal, N. (2025). AI-Enabled Medical Chatbots: Advancements in Patient Query Handling and Automated Healthcare Delivery. *International Journal of Environmental Sciences*, *11*(4s), 796–810. DOI: 10.64252/1n1waz11

Sofiyan, U. (2021). Machine Learning-Based Supervised Classifiers for Phishing Detection and DoS Mitigation in Large-Scale Big Data Environments.

Sridevi, & Kolhar, A. (2025a). Energy-Efficiency Strategies for Wireless Sensor Networks in IoT. *Energy-Efficient Deep Learning Approaches in IoT, Fog, and Green Blockchain Revolution*, 167–191. DOI: 10.4018/979-8-3373-0300-0.ch006

Sridevi, & Kolhar, A. (2025b). Machine learning algorithms and IoT sensors for securing the networks. *Exploiting Machine Learning for Robust Security*, 183–209. DOI: 10.4018/979-8-3693-7758-1.ch009

Sridhar, N., Peeriga, R., Thouti, S., Sravanthi, G., Sangeetha, V., Ghatasheh, M., & Flah, A. (2025). Sustainable Plant Disease Management with Real-Time Crop Optimization. *Engineering, Technology &. Applied Scientific Research, 15*(6), 30580–30585.

Srinivasan, L., Selvaraj, D., & Anish, T. P. (2025). A novel privacy preservation of healthcare data with information entropy-based multi-scheme fully homomorphic encryption and Rivest–Shamir–Adleman techniques. *Biomedical Engineering : Applications, Basis, and Communications, 37*(4), 2450060. Advance online publication. DOI: 10.4015/S1016237224500601

Sthankiya, K., Saeed, N., McSorley, G., Jaber, M., & Clegg, R. G. (2024). A Survey on AI-driven Energy Optimisation in Terrestrial Next Generation Radio Access Networks. *IEEE Access : Practical Innovations, Open Solutions, 12*, 157540–157555. DOI: 10.1109/ACCESS.2024.3482561

Stroud, A. M., Anzabi, M. D., Wise, J. L., Barry, B. A., Malik, M. M., McGowan, M. L., & Sharp, R. R. (2025). Toward Safe and Ethical Implementation of Health Care Artificial Intelligence: Insights From an Academic Medical Center. *Mayo Clinic Proceedings. Digital Health, 3*(1), 100189. DOI: 10.1016/j.mcpdig.2024.100189 PMID: 40206995

Suganyadevi, S., Seethalakshmi, V., & Balasamy, K. (2022). A review on deep learning in medical image analysis. *International Journal of Multimedia Information Retrieval, 11*(1), 19–38. DOI: 10.1007/s13735-021-00218-1 PMID: 34513553

Sulaiman, K. Al, Alharthi, A. F., Alqahtani, R., Aljouie, A., Khan, A., Al-jedai, A., Almoeen, A., Alshennawi, M., Badreldin, H. A., Alnasser, L. A., Alshehri, A. M., Alzahrani, M., Alhaidal, H. A., Alhajaji, R., Alotaibi, S., Redhwan, E. Z., Alharthi, F., Alghamdi, B. G., Alquayt, A., & Aljuhani, O. (2026). Ethical, data security, and resource allocation considerations in AI integration for healthcare during Hajj: task force insights and future directions. *International Journal of Medical Informatics, 205*(August 2025), 106123. DOI: 10.1016/j.ijmedinf.2025.106123

Suvarnamukhi, B., Praveena, A., Prakash, C. R. C., & Babu, K. N. (2025). Automated Chatbot for Healthcare Using NLP and ML. *International Journal of Information Technology and Computer Engineering, 13*(1), 1–10.

Teo, Z. L., Jin, L., Liu, N., Li, S., Miao, D., Zhang, X., Ng, W. Y., Tan, T. F., Lee, D. M., Chua, K. J., Heng, J., Liu, Y., Goh, R. S. M., & Ting, D. S. W. (2024). Federated machine learning in healthcare: A systematic review on clinical applications and technical architecture. *Cell Reports Medicine, 5*(2), 101419. DOI: 10.1016/j.xcrm.2024.101419 PMID: 38340728

Tharini, V. J., & Vijayarani, S. (2019). IoT in healthcare. In *Advances in medical technologies and clinical practice book series* (pp. 1–22). https://doi.org/DOI: 10.4018/978-1-7998-1090-2.ch001

Tian, S., Yang, W., Grange, J. M. L., Wang, P., Huang, W., & Ye, Z. (2019). Smart healthcare: Making medical care more intelligent. *Global Health Journal (Amsterdam, Netherlands)*, *3*(3), 62–65. DOI: 10.1016/j.glohj.2019.07.001

Timofte, E. M., Dimian, M., Graur, A., Potorac, A. D., Balan, D., Croitoru, I., Hri can, D. F., & Pu ca u, M. (2024). Federated Learning for Cybersecurity: A Privacy-Preserving Approach. *Applied Sciences (Basel, Switzerland)*, *15*(12), 6878. DOI: 10.3390/app15126878

U.S. Department of Health & Human Services. (1996). Health Insurance Portability and Accountability Act of 1996 (HIPAA). *Public Law*, •••, 104–191.

Umer, N., Deng, M., Zhang, Y., Zhang, M., & Khan, S. (2025). Quantum resilient security framework for privacy preserving AI in Apple MM1 on device architecture. *Scientific Reports*, *15*(1), 38297. DOI: 10.1038/s41598-025-22056-5 PMID: 41184318

Vashishth, T. K., Sharma, V., Kumar, B., Panwar, R., Sharma, K. K., & Chaudhary, S. (2024). AI-Integrated IoT in Healthcare Ecosystem: Opportunities, Challenges, and Future Directions. AI and IoT Technology and Applications for Smart Healthcare Systems, 37-54.

Vashishth, T. K., Sharma, V., Sharma, K. K., Kumar, B., Chaudhary, S., & Panwar, R. (2024). Intrusion Detection and Prevention Techniques in FL Cloud-Based Healthcare 5.0: A Comprehensive Review. Pioneering Smart Healthcare 5.0 with IoT, Federated Learning, and Cloud Security, 152-174.

Vashishth, T. K., Sharma, V., Sharma, K. K., Kumar, B., Kumar, A., & Panwar, R. (2024). Artificial Intelligence (AI)–Powered Chatbots: Providing Instant Support and Personalized Recommendations to Guests 24/7. In Technology and Luxury Hospitality (pp. 211-236). Routledge.

Vashishth, T. K., Sharma, V., Chaudhary, S., Sharma, R., Chauhan, P., & Sharma, B. K. (2026). Adoption of Artificial Intelligence Techniques for Enhancing Host-Based Intrusion Detection Systems. In *AI Solutions for Detecting Cyber-Attacks in Information Systems* (pp. 133–164). IGI Global Scientific Publishing.

Vashishth, T. K., Sharma, V., Sharma, K. K., Kumar, B., Chaudhary, S., & Agarwal, S. (2025). IoT-Enabled Multimedia Applications in Healthcare, Telemedicine, and Imaging. *Multimedia Technologies in the Internet of Things Environment*, *4*(173), 135–160. DOI: 10.1007/978-981-96-4356-1_7

Vinoth Kumar, V., Jagadish Kumar, N., & Selvaraj, D. (2025). Secured and privacy-preserved aggregation of data in edge computing using blockchain-based secured aggregation (BSA). In Convergence of cybersecurity and cloud computing (p. 34). DOI: 10.4018/979-8-3693-6859-6.ch007

Vyas, A., Lin, P. C., Hwang, R. H., & Tripathi, M. (2024). Privacy-preserving federated learning for intrusion detection in IoT environments: A survey. *IEEE Access : Practical Innovations, Open Solutions*, *12*, 127018–127050. DOI: 10.1109/ACCESS.2024.3454211

Wah, J. N. K. (2025). Revolutionizing e-health: The transformative role of AI-powered hybrid chatbots in healthcare solutions. *Frontiers in Public Health*, *13*, 1530799. DOI: 10.3389/fpubh.2025.1530799

Wiestler, B., & Menze, B. (2020). Deep learning for medical image analysis: A brief introduction. *Neuro-Oncology Advances*, *2*(Supplement_4), IV35–IV41. DOI: 10.1093/noajnl/vdaa092 PMID: 33521639

Williamson, S. M., & Prybutok, V. (2024). Balancing Privacy and Progress: A Review of Privacy Challenges, Systemic Oversight, and Patient Perceptions in AI-Driven Healthcare. *Applied Sciences (Basel, Switzerland)*, *14*(2), 675. Advance online publication. DOI: 10.3390/app14020675

Xie, Z., Wang, H., Dai, L., Wang, Z., Song, H., & Qian, J. (2026). *Ethical issues in multi-agent AI systems for healthcare : a narrative review. April*, 1–15. DOI: 10.3389/fpubh.2026.1792627

Xu, J., Glicksberg, B. S., Su, C., Walker, P., Bian, J., & Wang, F. (2020). Federated Learning for Healthcare Informatics. *Journal of Healthcare Informatics Research*, *5*(1), 1–19. DOI: 10.1007/s41666-020-00082-4 PMID: 33204939

Yamin, M. A. Y., & Alyoubi, B. A. (2020). Adoption of telemedicine applications among Saudi citizens during COVID-19 pandemic: An alternative health delivery system. *Journal of Infection and Public Health*, *13*(12), 1845–1855. DOI: 10.1016/j.jiph.2020.10.017 PMID: 33172819

Yang, D., Xu, Z., Li, W., Myronenko, A., Roth, H. R., Harmon, S., Xu, S., Turkbey, B., Turkbey, E., Wang, X., Zhu, W., Carrafiello, G., Patella, F., Cariati, M., Obinata, H., Mori, H., Tamura, K., An, P., Wood, B. J., & Xu, D. (2021). Federated semi-supervised learning for COVID region segmentation in chest CT using multi-national data from China, Italy, Japan. *Medical Image Analysis*, *70*, 101992. DOI: 10.1016/j.media.2021.101992 PMID: 33601166

Yang, Q., Liu, Y., Chen, T., & Tong, Y. (2019). Federated Machine Learning. *ACM Transactions on Intelligent Systems and Technology*, *10*(2), 1–19. DOI: 10.1145/3298981

Yao, A. C. (1982). Protocols for secure computations. *23rd Annual Symposium on Foundations of Computer Science (FOCS)*, 160–164. DOI: 10.1109/SFCS.1982.38

Yousefi, Z., Alesheikh, A. A., Rezaie, F., & Lee, S. (2025). An Explainable Geospatial Artificial Intelligence Approach for Spatiotemporal Assessment of Climate Change Effects on Landslide Susceptibility. *Earth Systems and Environment*, •••, 1–29.

Zaman Wani, R. U., & Can, O. (2025). FED-EHR: A Privacy-Preserving Federated Learning Framework for Decentralized Healthcare Analytics. *Electronics (Basel)*, *14*(16), 3261. Advance online publication. DOI: 10.3390/electronics14163261

Zendehbad, S. A. (2025). *Trustworthy AI in Telehealth : Navigating Challenges, Ethical Considerations, and Future Opportunities for Equitable Healthcare Delivery*. 1–26. DOI: 10.1049/htl2.70020

Zeng, N., Zuo, S., Zheng, G., Ou, Y., & Tong, T. (2020). Editorial: Artificial Intelligence for Medical Image Analysis of Neuroimaging Data. *Frontiers in Neuroscience*, *14*(May), 1–2. DOI: 10.3389/fnins.2020.00480 PMID: 32508575

Zhang, C., Wang, N., Hou, Y. T., & Lou, W. (2025). Machine Learning-Based Intrusion Detection Systems: Capabilities, Methodologies, and Open Research Challenges. *Authorea Preprints*. DOI: 10.1002/9781394293773.ch03

Zhang, F., Shuai, Z., Kuang, K., Wu, F., Zhuang, Y., & Xiao, J. (2023). Unified fair federated learning for digital healthcare. *Patterns (New York, N.Y.)*, *5*(1), 100907. DOI: 10.1016/j.patter.2023.100907 PMID: 38264718

Zhang, P., & Kamel Boulos, M. N. (2022). Privacy-by-Design Environments for Large-Scale Health Research and Federated Learning from Data. *International Journal of Environmental Research and Public Health*, *19*(19), 11876. Advance online publication. DOI: 10.3390/ijerph191911876 PMID: 36231175

Zhang, Q., Wong, A. K. C., & Bayuo, J. (2024). The role of Chatbots in enhancing health Care for Older Adults: A scoping review. *Journal of the American Medical Directors Association*, *25*(9), 105108. DOI: 10.1016/j.jamda.2024.105108

Zhou, Q., & Xue, F. (2025). *L-SCOPE: An LLM-Assisted Interactive Platform for Efficient Building Design Optimization.* Paper presented at the Proceedings of Smart and Sustainable Built Environment Conference Series. DOI: 10.66408/sasbe.2025.2554

Zhu, L., Liu, Z., & Han, S. (2019). Deep leakage from gradients. *Advances in Neural Information Processing Systems (NeurIPS)*, 32.

Ziller, A., Passerat-Palmbach, J., Ryffel, T., Usynin, D., Trask, A., Junior, I. D. L. C., Mancuso, J., Makowski, M., Rueckert, D., Braren, R., & Kaissis, G. (2020). Privacy-preserving medical image analysis.https://arxiv.org/abs/2012.06354

Zulzilah, S., & Isa, J. R. (2024). Decoding Patient Interactions with AI-Based Virtual Health Assistants. *CARAKA: Indonesia Journal of Communication*, *5*(2), 180–190. DOI: 10.25008/caraka.v5i2.173

About the Contributors

Hanh Le is a dedicated researcher, Full Stack Software Developer, and manager of a software development team. She holds a Ph.D. in Information Technology and a Master's degree in Computer Science. Her research interests include artificial intelligence (AI), software development, data analytics, data science, and cloud computing. Dr. Le's work focuses on leveraging AI and data-driven technologies to enhance decision-making and optimize software systems across industries such as healthcare, law enforcement, and retail. With expertise in both front-end and back-end development, she designs object-oriented, database-driven applications and values interdisciplinary collaboration to drive innovation and discovery.

***

Sachin Chaudhary is involved in academic development and scholarly activities. He is member of International Association of Engineers, The Society of Digital Information and Wireless Communications, Global Professors Welfare Association, International Association of Academic plus Corporate (IAAC), Computer Science Teachers Association and Internet Society .

Pankaj Dadheech is currently working as a Professor in the Department of Computer Science & Engineering (NBA Accredited), Swami Keshvanand Institute of Technology, Management & Gramothan (SKIT), Jaipur, Rajasthan, India (Accredited by NAAC A++ Grade, An Autonomous Institute Affiliated to Rajasthan Technical University, Kota). He is declared as World Top 2% Scientist by Stanford/Elsevier's in year 2025. He is Convener R&D Cell & DRC Chairman (CSE Department) at SKIT, Jaipur. He has more than 20 years of experience in teaching. He has published 125+ papers in many reputed journals in high indexed outlets, 8 international patents from Australia, Germany, South Africa and USA, 28 patents & 2 copyrights from India, 5 authored books, 4 edited books & several book chapters.

He has been awarded with best paper awards, and several other recognitions. He is a Sr. Member of IEEE (#99561311) and Member of Professional Organizations like the IEEE Computer Society, ACM, CSI, IAENG & ISTE. He is Ph.D. Research Supervisor in the Department of Computer Science & Engineering at SKIT, Jaipur recognized Research Centre of Rajasthan Technical University (RTU), Kota. He has Chaired Technical Sessions in various International Conferences & Contributed as Resource Person in various FDP's, Workshops, STTP's, and Conferences. He is also acting as a Guest Editor of the various reputed Journals, Conference Proceedings and Bentham Ambassador of Bentham Science Publisher. His area of interest includes High Performance Computing, Cloud Computing, Information Security, Big Data Analytics, Artificial Intelligence, Intellectual Property Right and Internet of Things.

D. Dhinakaran, is an Associate Professor in the Department of Computer Science and Engineering at Vel Tech Rangarajan Dr. Sagunthala R&D Institute of Science and Technology, Chennai. He holds a B.E., M.E., and Ph.D. in Computer Science from Anna University. His research expertise includes Privacy-Preserving Data Mining, Artificial Intelligence, Internet of Things (IoT), MANETs, Cloud Computing, and Image Processing. A prolific researcher, he has presented over 30 papers at international conferences, published more than 60 articles in reputed international journals, and filed three patents. He has been honoured as one of the Top 2% Scientists globally by Elsevier and Stanford University. He is actively supervising Ph.D. scholars and serves as a reviewer for reputed international journals and conferences, reflecting his strong commitment to academic excellence and research advancement. His innovative contributions and dedication to academia have made a significant impact on the evolving fields of Computer Science and Engineering.

Selvaraj Damodaran is working as a professor in the Department of Electronics and Communication Engineering at Panimalar Engineering College. He obtained his B.E Degree from Madras University, ME degree from Anna University and Ph.D. from Sathyabama University. He has a vast teaching experience of 21 years. He has published more than 75 papers at various refereed journals and conferences. His area of interest is in the field of signal processing, image processing, Biomedical Instrumentation, wireless communication, Artificial Intelligence, Machine learning, Data Mining and Antenna Design. He is a member of IEEE and life member of IETE.

Papri Das is presently working as an Associate Professor, School of Information Technology, Auro University, Surat. She has to her credit a Ph.D. in cloud data security and Masters in IT Apart from being an Academician, Dr. Das is also a keen researcher. Her research papers are presented in various Conferences and Seminars.

She also has to her credit publication of papers in various journals of National and International repute. Her areas of interest are security, computer networks, wireless communication and Cloud computing.

A. Shaji George is a highly respected and accomplished figure in the fields of education and the ICT industry. With over 30 years of experience in designing and deploying large-scale projects, Dr. George has made significant contributions to industry. He has a passion for working with clients to help them overcome complex business challenges, drive innovation, and deliver results. Dr. George is recognized as an expert in the field of ICT and has published over 250 research papers in national and international journals and conferences. He is also the author of 30 books that have been published by reputed international publishers. His extensive contributions to the field have earned him 20 awards, recognizing his outstanding achievements and contributions to the industry. Dr. George is the founder of PU Publications, PUIRJ, PUIIJ and PUIRP International Journal. He has a keen interest in wireless networking, cloud computing, big data analytics, the Internet of Things, and industrial automation systems. He works with clients from a wide range of industries to develop strategies and implement next-generation solutions that transform their businesses. Dr. George's wealth of knowledg

T. K Gundoor Dedicated researcher and academic professional with experience in both research and teaching at the postgraduate level, specializing in the critical intersection of Cybersecurity and Artificial Intelligence (AI). He currently serves as an Assistant Professor at the National Forensic Science University (NFSU), Goa. Ph.D. in Computer Science (Cybersecurity) from Karnatak University, Dharwad, focusing his doctoral research on the vital domain of Design an effective algorithm to detect Non-Portable Executable (Non-PE) Malicious Files. He is a Qualified NET and SET candidate in Computer Science and Application and holds a Certified Artificial Intelligence Professional certification from the Defense Institute of Advanced Technology (DIAT, DRDO). His academic foundation includes a Master of Computer Application (MCA) from Visvesvaraya Technological University, Belagavi, and a Bachelor of Computer Application (BCA) from Karnatak University, Dharwad. His research work is highly focused on emerging technology and security, with a track record of significant academic contributions: He has published 6 journal papers including Scopus, Elsevier, springer, two conference papers, and has contributed 10 book chapters, 1 Edited book to publications by renowned international publishers like IGI Global, CRC Apple Press, Bentham science and Wiley, with several being Scopus-indexed. Demonstrating a commitment to continuous learning, he has attended a total of 60+ Faculty Development Programs (FDPs), courses, and training programs, with recent attendance in advanced topics such as Cyber Security, Blockchain, AI, Machine Learning, and Data Science, including multiple programs. Actively contributes to maintaining the quality of scholarly work, receiving a Certificate of Recognition from Bentham Science Publishers for his peer-review contributions. Is a lifetime member of the IAENG International Association of Engineering and holds memberships with the IEEE Student Member, IFERP (Institute for Educational Research and Publication), and the CSTA (Computer Science Teachers Association). His dedication is defined by a passion for helping organizations reach their full potential and a consistent drive to excel in the academic and research fields.

Anitha K is a dynamic and research-oriented Associate Professor and Head (Management Studies & Visual Communication) at Meenakshi Academy of Higher Education and Research (MAHER), Chennai, with additional roles as Assistant Director of Online Education and Placement Officer at MAHER. She holds a PhD in Management, an M.Phil. in Management (University First, Distinction), and dual UGC-NET qualifications in HRM (2014) and Management (2022). Her academic specialization blends Human Resource Management and Marketing, strengthened by industry experience with Microsoft and Velan Info Services in sales and customer relations. Dr. Anitha has demonstrated excellence in teaching, research, and administration—evidenced by her leadership in IQAC, placement coordination, entrepreneurship development, and online program management. Her approach emphasizes experiential learning, student engagement, and digital pedagogy. She has Authored 20+ research papers in reputed UGC CARE and Scopus-indexed journals.Contributed 24 book chapters with top international publishers such as Springer, Taylor & Francis, Wiley, Emerald, and IGI Global (USA). Published one book: "Harmony Within: Mastering Self-Management for a Balanced Life."Her research Focus areas include Artificial Intelligence in HR, Employee Engagement, Organizational Sustainability, and Digital Transformation. Published five patents (2024–2025) on automation, AI-driven toll systems, appointment kiosks, and sanitary innovations. Her accolades include • Best Women Outstanding Researcher (2025) – PARA Awards. • Best Placement Officer Award (2023–24) – Bharat Education Excellence Awards. • Multiple Research Excellence Awards (2020–2024) from MAHER. • International Women's Day Achievement Award (2025) – Brain O Vision. Delivered numerous guest lectures and workshops on AI, HR innovation, gamification, online education, and digital marketing. Presented papers at over 20 national and international conferences (including Springer and IEEE-affiliated events). Completed professional certifications from IIT Madras, IIT Kharagpur, IIT Roorkee, Annamalai University, and Coursera (University of Minnesota, UC Irvine).

Shivani Kharra Experienced Risk Management Data Scientist in the Gas Transmission Management division with a strong background in Big Data Analytics with M Tech in Geomatics and MS in Information Systems. With over 7 years of experience in the Renewable Energy and Mapping industry, I excel in creating and deploying AI algorithms, constructing robust data science infrastructure, and proficiently engaging in data analytics and modeling. Currently focused on creating and updating threat models to assess and mitigate risks, and actively developing a location-based consequence model to enhance decision-making processes. Specializing in Geographic Information Systems (GIS) and Remote Sensing, I have contributed to the development of GIS-based enterprise web applications using Arcpy and ArcGIS API for Python. Proficient in GIS databases, Spatial Analysis Techniques, and Esri ArcGIS, I actively participate in architecting logical and physical models for GIS-based enterprise web applications.

Keerthana N V is an Assistant Professor with 8 Years of experience in teaching and 1-year experience in research (IUCAA LIGO Data Centre, Pune). Her area of interest is Network Security, Blockchain Security, and Machine Learning Algorithms. She is pursuing PhD at Anna University in Security in Blockchain. She has a working experience in High-Performance Computing (HTCondor) in LIGO INDIA Project. She has written many research articles in Network Security and assisted Scientists in analyzing Datasets in HTCondor.

Swathi Pothala is an academician and researcher in Computer Science with expertise in Artificial Intelligence, Machine Learning, Big Data Analytics, Internet of Things (IoT), and computational bioinformatics. She earned her Ph.D. from Sri Padmavathi Mahila Viswa Vidyalayam (SPMVV), Tirupati, in 2023, focusing on diabetic retinopathy detection using big data analytics and RNA-based computational techniques. She holds an M.Tech in Computer Science and Engineering from RVR & JC College of Engineering and an MCA from Bharath University, both with distinction. She currently serves as an Academic Consultant at Sri Venkateswara University, Tirupati. Dr. Swathi has published research papers in IEEE, Springer, and Scopus-indexed journals and conferences. She has also contributed to textbooks and academic book chapters in the areas of AI, IoT, and big data analytics. Her research interests include AI-driven healthcare applications, cloud computing, IoT, and RNA data analysis. She is an innovator with multiple patents in AI-based systems.

S. Edwin Raja, Associate Professor, Department of Computer Science and Engineering in Vel Tech Rangarajan Dr.Sagunthala R&D Institute of Science and Technology, Chennai. He has completed his Ph.D. in Information and Communication Engineering from Anna University-chennai in the year 2021. He obtained his M.Tech. (Network Engineering) in the year 2010 from Kalasalingam University, Krishnan kovil and B.E. (Computer Science and Engineering) in the year 2006 from C.S.I Institute of Technology, Thovalai. He has more than thirteen plus years of teaching experience and his area of interests are Cyber Security, Big Data Analytics, Machine Learning & Computer Networks. He has published more than 4 research articles in various journals and conferences. Also, he has published 3 patents, acted as reviewer in reputed journals.

Vikas Sharma is an active academician and researcher in the field of computer science with 7 years of experience. He earned M. Tech degree specialized in Computer Science. He is involved in academic development and scholarly activities. He is member of International Association of Engineers, The Society of Digital Information and Wireless Communications, Global Professors Welfare Association, International Association of Academic plus Corporate (IAAC), Computer Science Teachers Association and Internet Society. His research interest includes Cloud Computing, Artificial Intelligence, Machine Learning; published more than 55 research articles with 4 books and 75 book chapters in edited books. He is contributing as member of editorial and reviewers' boards in conferences and various computer journals and edited books published by Elsevier, CRC Press, Taylor and Francis, Springer, IGI global, Wiley Publication, IET Publication, De Gruyter, River Publication etc.

Shashiraj Teotia is member of International Association of Engineers, The Society of Digital Information and Wireless Communications, Global Professors Welfare Association, International Association of Academic plus Corporate (IAAC), Computer Science Teachers Association and Internet Society .

Blessy Thankachan is currently working as Associate Professor and Dy. HoD in School of Computer Applications, JECRC University, Jaipur. She has more than a decade of teaching experience. She also have an illustrious experience of research and administrative work too. She has one patent to her credit, and multiple research publications in national and international journals. Dr. Blessy has endued her time in authoring books for University students in Computer Science. She adheres to equal participation in presenting papers in Conferences too. Currently she is guiding around half a dozen research scholars on the topics Software Engineering and Reliability, Big Data, Internet of Things and Machine Learning.

Tarun Kumar Vashishth is an active academician and researcher in the field of Computer Science with 22 years of experience. He earned Ph.D. Mathematics degree specialized in Operations Research; served several academic positions such as Dy. Director, HoD, NAAC Coordinator, Academic Coordinator, Member Secretary of Department Research Committee, Assistant Center Superintendent and Head Examiner in University Examinations. He is involved in academic development and scholarly activities. He is member of International Association of Engineers, The Society of Digital Information and Wireless Communications, Global Professors Welfare Association, International Association of Academic plus Corporate (IAAC), Computer Science Teachers Association and Internet Society . His research interest includes Cloud Computing, Artificial Intelligence, Machine Learning and Operations Research; published more than 50 research articles & conference papers with 2 book and 90+ book chapters. He is contributing as member of editorial and reviewers boards in conferences and various computer journals and edited books published by Elsevier, CRC Press, Taylor and Francis, Springer, IGI global, Wiley Publication, IET Publication, De Gruyter, River Publication etc.

Pushpendra Verma Academic Coordinator, Member Secretary of Department Research Committee, Assistant Center Superintendent and Head Examiner in University Examinations. He is involved in academic development and scholarly activities. He is member of International Association of Engineers, The Society of Digital Information and Wireless Communications, Global Professors Welfare Association, International Association of Academic plus Corporate (IAAC), Computer Science Teachers Association and Internet Society . His research interest includes Cloud Computing, Artificial Intelligence, Machine Learning and Operations Research; published more than 50 research articles & conference papers with 2 book and 90+ book chapters.

Index

R

S

T

V

www.ingramcontent.com/pod-product-compliance
Lightning Source LLC
LaVergne TN
LVHW081524300926
849161LV00006B/1286